Arts
Therapies

For Elsevier:
Commissioning Editor: Susan Young
Development Editor: Catherine Jackson
Project Manager: Morven Dean
Senior Designer: Stewart Larking
Illustration Manager: Bruce Hogarth

Arts
Therapies
A RESEARCH-BASED MAP OF THE FIELD

Vassiliki (Vicky) Karkou PhD MEd PgDip(DMT) BEd Sc(Hons)
Lecturer in Art Therapy,
Queen Margaret University College,
Edinburgh;
Postdoctoral Research Fellow,
University of Hertfordshire,
Hatfield, UK

Patricia Sanderson PhD MA AdvDipEd(Dist)
Lecturer in Arts Education,
The University of Manchester,
Manchester, UK

4/08

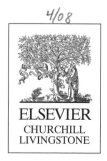

ELSEVIER
CHURCHILL
LIVINGSTONE

Edinburgh   London   New York   Oxford   Philadelphia   St Louis   Sydney   Toronto   2006

ELSEVIER
CHURCHILL
LIVINGSTONE

An imprint of Elsevier Limited

First published 2006

ISBN 0 443 07256 6

British Library Cataloguing in Publication Data
A catalogue record for this book is available from the British Library

Library of Congress Cataloguing in Publication Data
A catalog record for this book is available from the Library of Congress

Notice
Medical knowledge is constantly changing. Standard safety precautions must be followed, but as new research and clinical experience broaden our knowledge, changes in treatment and drug therapy may become necessary or appropriate. Readers are advised to check the most current product information provided by the manufacturer of each drug to be administered to verify the recommended dose, the method and duration of administration, and contraindications. It is the responsibility of the practitioner, relying on experience and knowledge of the patient, to determine dosages and the best treatment for each individual patient. Neither the Publisher nor the author assumes any liability for any injury and/or damage to persons or property arising from this publication.

The Publisher

Printed in Great Britain by MPG Books Ltd, Bodmin, Cornwall

Elsevier are grateful to Dr Raymond MacDonald for kindly allowing us to use a selection of his art for the book cover. The front cover image is 'Station Map' and the back cover images are (top to bottom) 'Thelonious', 'Bird on Verve' and 'Scottish Sky No. 1'.

Contents

Preface

When we first thought about looking at the field of arts therapies as a whole we were aware that our task was ambitious. We knew that the field is complex, as any field involving social interaction is likely to be, but it is even more so because arts therapies involve multilayered therapeutic endeavours. The use of the arts and associated creativity and imagination also suggest limitless applications. Moreover, there are different traditions within the field deriving from subdivisions into music, art, drama and dance therapy fields, each with its own huge variety of practices. Therefore, attempting to describe such a complex and diverse field was not always easy. Attempting to do so while both of us were in full-time employment was an additional challenge.

However, a major aid to this task has been the fact that a substantial part of this book was based on our empirical research work completed over a number of years at the School of Education at The University of Manchester. This study was supported financially by the Economic and Social Research Council (ESRC) as part of the PhD work completed by one of the authors and supervised by the other. A large number of arts therapists offered their time and expertise as participants in the study through interviews and/or through responding to the survey questionnaire. Key participants in the first interview stage were, amongst others: Laurence Higgens, Steve Mitchell, Dr Helen Payne and Susan Scarth. The 580 arts therapists practising in the UK who responded to the survey also need to be acknowledged.

In a follow-up research project, financial support and time was offered by the Department of Art and Arts Therapies at the University of Hertfordshire. During this second research period, leading figures in the field made additional contributions in the form of case vignette material and explanations about their own practice; many of these contributions have been included in the book. For their input, we need to thank: Madeline Andersen-Warren, Dr Gary Ansdell, Professor Leslie Bunt, Sue Curtis, Dr Alida Gersie, Dr Sue Jennings, Dr Alison Levinge, Helen Odell-Miller, Nina Papadopoulos, Kay Sobey and Derryn Thomas.

We are also thankful to: Alex Chew, Katrina Hyvonen, Dr Raymond MacDonald, Pauline McGee and Patti Parfitt who, during the revision process of the manuscript, commented on certain specialised chapters (especially those in Section 2) from a discipline-specific perspective. Given our consistent attempts to include the voices of practitioners from within the field during all the stages of our research work, it has been vital to check whether practitioners' voices were indeed recognised by their colleagues from the same discipline in the final delivery of this work, i.e. this book. Ultimately, we hope that the arts therapists reading this book will offer additional comments, perspectives and ideas and will engage in fruitful discussions about its content.

Finally, we need to thank: Mark Elliott, Dr Colin Lees, Themis Kokolakakis, Professor Frank Sanderson and Dr Dimitris Sirakos who read substantial sections of the book, identified areas of ambiguity, asked questions about the content and commented on the overall style of our writing. We found that their input contributed towards making this book accessible to a much wider audience than the arts therapies field. We will be glad if this will indeed prove to be the case.

Vicky Karkou and Patricia Sanderson, 2005

Preface

Introduction

Both authors have experienced the blank looks on the faces of people when they first hear about arts therapies:

'Arts what?'

'Therapy for whom . . .?'

Or on a more positive note:

'Oh, yes, I understand. When I listen to my favourite music, I find it so relaxing.'

'It's about self-expression.'

'It's when you use people's drawings to find out what sort of problems they have.'

Nevertheless, the message is clear: the field is new and largely unknown to the general public. Thus, we often find ourselves in the position of having to introduce, explain or correct:

'It's not about relaxation only.'

'It's not just about self-expression . . .'

'It's not just a diagnostic tool (although it may be used as one).'

Undoubtedly, such misconceptions suggest that arts therapies are not sufficiently known and understood by the public. Although arts therapies (otherwise known as creative arts therapies) are becoming increasingly recognised within health services, schools and social or voluntary organisations, we believe that even amongst colleagues in these settings there is limited understanding of what the field stands for. Similarly, although there is a growth in availability of postgraduate training courses within established higher education structures and an increasing number of publications and research studies in the area, we are aware that these developments have not been as extensive or as rapid, as we, along with many members of the profession, would wish.

A major aim of this book is therefore to offer explicit descriptions and explanations of arts therapies practices that make the field accessible to lay readers and other professionals. Indeed, not to do this will perpetuate misconceptions, will inevitably limit the progress of the profession, and will lead to questioning of the quality of the service provided to the public.

Another important aim of this book is to inform arts therapists themselves about the field as a whole and/or other practices that exist alongside their own. The arts therapies field consists of four professions: art therapy (AT), music therapy (MT), dramatherapy (DT) and dance movement therapy (DMT). Despite the common threads amongst these four professions, each of them has a separate history and training, separate professional organisations and indeed different theoretical and methodological preferences. Although these days there are a number of arts therapies teams consisting of DT, MT, AT and/or DMT, the majority of arts therapists still find themselves working in isolation with limited connections with professionals from other arts therapies disciplines. This book aims to bring these isolated practices together, outline similarities and differences and offer a broad picture within which practitioners can make connections between their own work and the work of their colleagues.

In order to achieve the above aims, this book is based extensively on our research work in the field. Our research perspective is different from those frequently adopted in the relevant published literature. For example, this book does not limit itself to case study material from one practitioner with one client, one client group and/or in one setting. It does not limit itself to one arts therapies discipline either. Instead, it offers general demographic information, overall trends and a collection of case vignettes that are found across a variety of arts therapies practices. The voices of as many practising arts therapists in the UK as possible are incorporated in the book, either as analysed findings from contributions from a large number of research participants, or as direct quotes and summaries from a selected few. Grounded theory has offered philosophical justification for our research design (the study was 'grounded' in the field – Glaser & Strauss 1967), while creativity, an important aspect for arts therapies practice and research (Meekums 1993), has been a characteristic of our methodological choices (see Appendix 1 for further details on research methodology).

With empirical research work to back up our writing, this book claims to offer a first broad picture of the field in the UK. Although references to arts therapies in the USA are also made (there is substantial literature originating from there), our emphasis remains on arts therapies in the UK. With few exceptions, British arts therapies literature is primarily used to discuss relevant concepts and findings from our study. We are aware that locating arts therapies in the context of the whole of the UK is an ambitious undertaking, especially as the individualistic nature of practice is characteristic of the work in the UK; Woddis (1986) for example, acknowledges this culture within British *art* therapy; we find this to be true for the field as a whole. At the same time, we believe that, despite this diversity, there are a number of commonalities across arts therapies practices. As the American dramatherapist Landy (1995) claims: 'The . . . differences among our modalities of treatment are ultimately insignificant for, as professionals, we are more alike than different' (p. 84). A number of voices from within the field (the majority of them are American) call for developing closer links between different arts therapies (e.g. Johnson 1994, 1999, Levine 1997, McNiff 1986). In Europe, the ECArTE (European Consortium for Arts Therapies Education) plays an important role in promoting such links across arts therapies and across nations. In the UK, all four modalities fall under one group for professional registration with the Health Professions Council (HPC), while work across disciplines is currently undertaken in a number of areas (e.g. standards of practice, benchmarking, research and education). Waller, leading the way for arts therapies towards HPC registration, has argued that the four arts therapies share enough in common to be regarded 'as a single professional body for regulatory purposes' (cited in ADMT UK 1997, p. 15). However, there have been no substantial attempts, as yet, to delineate common ground between disciplines in terms of theory and practice in a manner that goes beyond anecdotal testimonies or short scale projects.

In an attempt to foster close links amongst arts therapies in the UK, this book offers an overall description of professional groupings and identifies common areas of clinical practice. At the same time it refers to arts therapies as separate disciplines. We can see these different arts therapies as different 'cultures' or better 'subcultures'. With such associations, our work can be seen as holding a cross-cultural perspective. One of the major discussions within cross-cultural studies is the preference for either an absolute or relative position, otherwise known as the etic-emic debate (Shiraev & Levy 2001). With the first perspective, commonalities are highlighted. With the second, differences are valued. Both of these approaches have their limitations as well as their strengths. Strict absolutism bears the danger of making comparisons between things that are different, e.g. comparing an apple to an orange. Strict relativism has the disadvantage of prohibiting any comparisons between fields assuming that everything is context-specific. Our position is that arts therapies share between them a number of common features that can be studied and presented through the search for common beliefs and practices (absolutism). We also see each of the arts therapies disciplines as having their own idiosyncrasies and unique character that make sense within a specific context (relativism). In this book we will be shifting from one position to the other. According to Shiraev & Levy (2001, p 5) 'there are not two cultures that are either entirely similar or entirely different'. This statement is even truer for arts therapies within which separate disciplines are perceived as subcultures of a greater whole. Looking at arts therapies as one whole and arts therapies as separate disciplines is reflected in Sections 1 and 2 of the book, respectively.

In particular, in Section 1, we place the field in the wider western context from which it mainly originates and make a brief review of the development of arts therapies in the UK. We present and discuss common issues surrounding arts therapies professional associations, training courses, professional developments and important working environments. We also refer briefly to the range of client groups currently working with arts therapies. We argue that arts therapies is a field that is different from therapeutic arts, arts education or 'talking therapies' (i.e. psychotherapy and counselling), areas incidentally, which often overlap with arts therapies.

By examining a number of definitions associated with each of the arts therapies subfields, which are discussed in the literature, we endeavour to redefine the field and highlight common aspects across all arts therapies. Some of the common topics we discuss are: principles and assumptions about the use of the arts, the emphasis on creativity, the role of imagery and imagination, symbolism and metaphors, non-verbal communication, the significance of the client–therapist relationship and the type of therapeutic aims relevant to arts therapies. There are a number of other aspects that are not covered in our list of essential common features of arts therapies. For example, all arts therapists are engaged in routine assessment/evaluation practices. This aspect of arts therapies work deserves specialised attention and research. Readers interested in this topic can consult sections/chapters within discipline-specific books or arts therapies publications such as Feder & Feder (1998) and Wigram (2000).

Section 1 also deals with the need to locate arts therapies work within therapeutic frameworks that support, explain and guide practice. The role of theory and those therapeutic frameworks most frequently drawn upon by arts therapists are given close attention. We discuss the humanistic, psycho-analytic/psychodynamic, developmental, artistic/creative, active/directive and eclectic/integrative trends in relation to major principles, models and/or methodological relevance to arts therapies practice. Throughout Section 1 we consider the field as a whole.

In Section 2, we address arts therapies as separate modalities and focus on the uniqueness of each discipline in terms of both their separate profession-al developments and current practices. Some important approaches to MT, AT, DT and DMT are presented, compared and contrasted. Case examples illustrate these different approaches and present opportunities for some understanding of practices in each modality.

Although it is not our intention to offer in-depth accounts of each of the different disciplines (key texts in each separate discipline are more appropri-ate readings for this), the interplay between closeness (distinctive practices – Section 2) and distance from the subject (field as one whole – Section 1) will offer the lay reader of this book the possibility of a first, comprehensive understanding of the field. Comparisons between practices and between dis-ciplines will give an opportunity to the more informed reader to think about what is common and what is unique in the field and, if the reader is an arts therapies practitioner, to locate his or her own practices within the wider pic-ture. We believe that mapping the field in this way will provide a sound basis from which information can be acquired, discussion can be triggered and fur-ther development can proceed.

References

- Association for Dance Movement Therapy (ADMT UK), 1997 UK news: Council for Professions Supplementary to Medicine (CPSM): about the setting up of the Arts Therapists Board, E-motion. ADMT UK Quarterly IX(2):15
- Feder B, Feder E 1998 The art and science of evaluation in the arts therapies: how do we know what's working? Charles C Thomas, Springfield, IL.
- Glaser B G, Strauss A L 1967 The discovery of grounded theory: strategies for qualitative research. Aldine, Chicago
- Johnson D R 1994 Shame dynamics among creative arts therapies. The Arts in Psychotherapy 21(3):1999 173–178
- Johnson D R 1999 Essays on the creative arts therapies. Charles C Thomas, Springfield, IL
- Landy R J 1997 Isolation and collaboration in the creative arts therapies – the implications of crossing borders. The Arts in Psychotherapy 22(2):83–86
- Levine S 1997 Expressive arts therapy: a call for dialogue. The Arts in Psychotherapy 23(5):431–434
- McNiff S 1986 Educating the creative arts therapist. Charles C Thomas, Springfield, IL
- Meekums B 1993 Research as an act of creation. In: Payne H (ed) Handbook of inquiry in the arts therapies: one river, many currents. Jessica Kingsley, London, p130–137
- Peter M 1998 'Good for them, or what?' The arts and pupils with SEN. British Journal of Special Education 25(4):168–172.
- Shirae, E, Levy D 2001 Introduction to cross-cultural psychology: critical thinking and con-temporary application. Allyn and Bacon, London
- Wigram T 2000 Assessment and evaluation in the arts therapies: art therapy, music therapy and dramatherapy. Harper House Publications, Radlett
- Woddis J 1986 Reflections: judging from appearances. The Arts in Psychotherapy 13:147–149.

Section 1
Arts Therapies as One Field

For this section of the book we will discuss arts therapies as one field in order to identify patterns of practice that are shared amongst different disciplines of art therapy (AT), music therapy (MT), dramatherapy (DT) and dance movement therapy (DMT). The main reason for our 'global' approach to the field is our belief that arts therapies have a lot of things in common that are hardly ever discussed in any depth within existing arts therapies literature. The silence on the topic is even more curious given the fact that arts therapies disciplines currently come under the same umbrella insofar as professional registration with the Health Professions Council (HPC) is concerned. Although they retain separate professional identities, they manage to represent the field with one voice when faced with governmental negotiations. We find that the fact that arts therapies are collaborating closely in relation to professional issues is not just the result of a strategic decision for professional recognition, although, as McNiff (1986) argues, this can also play an important role. Over the years, members of the different arts therapies disciplines have felt strong affiliations with each other. We think that this tendency reflects the common ground shared across arts therapies, for example in terms of theoretical principles and ethos of practice. Section 1 looks at exactly this, i.e. the areas of overlap across the four disciplines.

What Section 1 does not attempt to do is to make a case for all four disciplines to become one. Initiatives to bring arts therapies together in one professional body that emerged during the early days of professional development were finally abandoned as theoretically unsound and professionally dangerous. It was believed that the depth of knowledge and understanding of the art form would be jeopardized, and consequently clinical practice would become superficial and thus questionable. Such initiatives were also seen as putting already limited resources into further danger. Policy makers could easily settle for cheap solutions in relation to anything to do with the arts, and as a consequence, also anything to do with arts therapies. Similar debates had already taken place in arts education. Movements that supported an arts education system in which all arts were taught as one subject were subsequently dropped with a similar rationale.

Instead, Section 1 attempts to look at similarities amongst arts therapies in order to foster closer links between practices, contribute to further development of collaborative work amongst practitioners and strengthen the theoretical and practical positions of each of the four disciplines. While differences may offer richness and depth in the field, common features may create a clearer and thus stronger basis for further developments.

From a cross-cultural perspective, Section 1 is closely aligned with absolutism (an etic view) in that it steps back from each of the separate disciplines and attempts to describe the bigger picture of the field as a whole. While it throws light on what is common amongst the disciplines, with few exceptions, it leaves in the shadow what is different and unique about each of them separately. Section 2 will focus more on the 'different' and 'unique' in each discipline.

References

• McNiff S 1986 Educating the creative arts therapist. Charles C Thomas, Springfield, IL

Chapter 1

Professional Development of Arts Therapies

Key issues:

- The idea of the arts for healing has been in and out of favour throughout western history. This view was highly regarded in classical Greece, but lost favour during the Middle Ages. During the Renaissance and the Age of Enlightenment the healing purpose was reinstated, but again was suppressed during the Victorian era.

- Modern psychology/psychotherapy, artistic movements at the beginning of the 20th century, and movements within social psychiatry and education during and after the Second World War, opened the way for the development of arts therapies.

- Official recognition of the professional status of arts therapies began in the second half of the 20th century as a result of political action initiated by artists, teachers and other health professionals.

- Arts therapies are organised according to each art form into separate professional associations. The aims of all these associations are similar: to represent members' interests, to negotiate conditions of work, and jointly with the Health Professions Council to assure quality of practice.

- Training for qualified arts therapist status takes place at postgraduate level. Currently there are more than 15 universities offering or validating arts therapies training courses at a Master's level.

- Arts therapists work mainly in hospitals, in education or in community-based settings with a range of client groups; the most important areas of work are in mental health and learning disabilities.

Introduction

Arts therapies is a field that, in the west, has developed significantly during the 20th century. However, the use of the arts for healing purposes is much older. A brief overview is presented in order to locate some of the historical roots of arts therapies and provide a perspective on the use of the arts for healing and/or well-being. A background to the re-emergence and growth in popularity of arts therapies since the end of the 19th century will assist us in describing the immediate roots of the field, in the UK in particular. Current professional developments are described particularly in relation to British professional associations, training courses and main areas of work. With the exception of the broad sources of information utilised in the first sections of this chapter and some references to government documents later on, findings from our study are discussed in relation to relevant arts therapies literature.

The healing role of the arts: an historical perspective

The arts have been used as therapy and/or healing for centuries (see Fig. 1.1). For example, evidence from prehistoric times and anthropological studies of contemporary indigenous cultures suggests that the arts had functional purposes of a magico-religious nature (Fleshman & Fryrear 1981). The connection of the arts in rituals with the supernatural has served, and in some places continues to serve, as the predominant means of preventing or curing physical and mental illness, of not only the individual but also the community as a whole. In the west, and classical Greece in particular, there was a strong belief in the integrated nature of mind and body, and a strong connection between music and medicine. Apollo, the god of music, was also a physician to the other gods, with sons such as Aesculapius, the god of medicine, and Orpheus, the god of soothing and curative music. Similar emphasis was placed on the power of music by Pythagorean thinkers, who perceived specific types of music as contributing towards the promotion of individual and universal harmony. The belief in harmony and balance was extended to all the other arts and theatre enactment in particular. Aristotle (trans. 1961), for example, regarded drama as promoting catharsis through identification of the audience with the ordeals of the actors, emotional crescendo and eventual return to a more normal balance of emotions. Similarly dance, as part of ancient Greek theatre, ceremonies and rituals, was regarded as contributing to emotional balance and therefore mental health.

However, such confidence in the power of the arts for mental health was not retained during subsequent periods in Greek history, starting with Plato. The arts were banned from his ideal city (Plato, trans. 1957) because artistic engagement was regarded as enabling people to get in touch with feelings that would make them 'emotional and softer than they ought to be' (Plato, trans. 1957 p. 84). Furthermore, the 'world of ideas' attained a superior position and the mind–body division was introduced for the first time in the western world.

During the Middle Ages, Christianity, which spread rapidly throughout Europe, was a major influence, and it embraced this premise (Feder & Feder 1981). However, the Christian Church held an ambivalent attitude towards

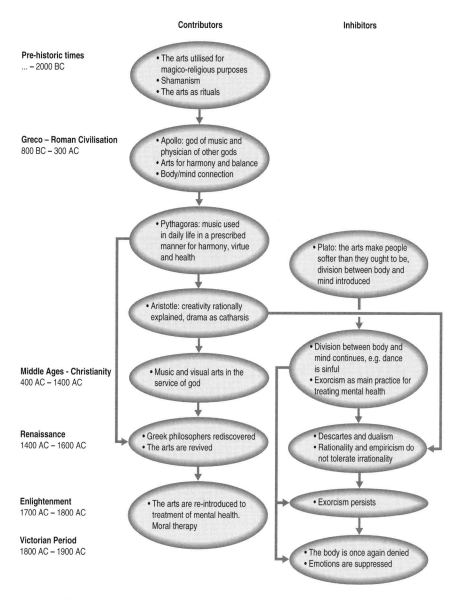

Contributors   **Inhibitors**

Pre-historic times
... – 2000 BC

- The arts utilised for magico-religious purposes
- Shamanism
- The arts as rituals

Greco – Roman Civilisation
800 BC – 300 AC

- Apollo: god of music and physician of other gods
- Arts for harmony and balance
- Body/mind connection

- Pythagoras: music used in daily life in a prescribed manner for harmony, virtue and health

- Plato: the arts make people softer than they ought to be, division between body and mind introduced

- Aristotle: creativity rationally explained, drama as catharsis

- Division between body and mind continues, e.g. dance is sinful
- Exorcism as main practice for treating mental health

Middle Ages - Christianity
400 AC – 1400 AC

- Music and visual arts in the service of god

Renaissance
1400 AC – 1600 AC

- Greek philosophers rediscovered
- The arts are revived

- Descartes and dualism
- Rationality and empiricism do not tolerate irrationality

Enlightenment
1700 AC – 1800 AC

- The arts are re-introduced to treatment of mental health. Moral therapy

- Exorcism persists

Victorian Period
1800 AC – 1900 AC

- The body is once again denied
- Emotions are suppressed

Figure 1.1: *The arts as healing in western Europe.*

the arts as a form of expression that involved both the body and the mind. On the one hand it regarded dance as sensual and therefore sinful, yet on the other, enlisted music and the visual arts in the service of God (Clark 1966). It is also likely that the Church, despite officially holding some anti-arts doctrines, integrated preChristian rituals and arts practices into its religious services. This ambiguous relationship between the Church and the arts continued for a long time.

Major shifts of thought occurred during periods such as the Renaissance and Enlightenment. The former for example, signified a shift towards rationality and empiricism through the revival of Greek philosophers and Aristotle in particular. With this revival, the status of the arts increased compared to that in the Middle Ages. However, this period also signified the re-establishment of dualism initially introduced by Plato in classical Greece. Descartes (1947 [trans.]), the philosopher with whom dualism is most often connected, was searching for truth. According to him the truth could only be achieved through rational thought and the mind, a process that was distinct and superior to sensory experience and the body. Consequently, the arts that involved the senses and the body had nothing to do with the truth and were perceived as more closely aligned with mere amusement. Similarly, the treatment of mental illness did not improve. On the contrary, the belief in rationality led to a decreased tolerance towards irrationality and consequently towards mental illness. Exorcism remained the means of dealing with mental illness, often employing harsh methods of 'separating the devil from abnormally behaving victims' (Fleshman & Fryrear 1981, pp. 12–13). It was not until the Age of Enlightenment that the arts were re-introduced in the treatment of people with mental health problems, mainly through the moral reform movement, and as a form of occupational therapy (Fleshman & Fryrear 1981). The Victorian period of the 19th century signified yet another backlash: emotions were suppressed and there was only limited acceptance of the interdependence of body and mind.

The emergence of arts therapies in the 20th century

Arts therapies emerged as a result of changes in a number of related areas (see Fig. 1.2). For example, between the end of the 19th and beginning of the 20th centuries, a number of revolutionary changes occurred in the arts and their relationship to mental health. The 'Art of the Insane' and Cizek's 'Child Art' movements in visual arts (Waller 1991), the contribution of Isadora Duncan, Mary Wigman and most importantly, Laban to dance (Levy 1992), and Stanislavski's, Evreinov's and Artaud's approaches to the theatre (Jones 1996), are some examples of the roots of arts therapies found in the arts world during this period. Although most of these artists and movements were very different from each other in terms of emphasis, content and direction of their work, they shared common themes: they emphasised self-expression, placed value on emotions, attempted to connect the artists' artistic work with psychological states, made sociological and political references and interventions, and stressed new ways to relate to the audience or the spectators.

Simultaneous with revolutionary developments in the arts world, psychotherapy emerged with the writings of Freud and the founding of psychoanalysis. After centuries of Aristotelian thinking, Freud's writings signified a

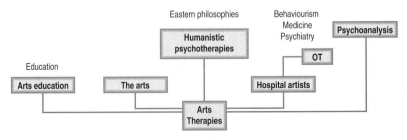

Figure.1.2: *Contributors to the emergence of arts therapies in the 20th century in the UK.*

challenge to rational materialism. The concept of the unconscious was introduced and intrapsychic forces were acknowledged. The belief in the presence of the unconscious opened up the way to make connections with the arts and provided starting points for the development of arts therapies. For example, the surrealist movement was particularly inspired by Freudian writings. Open expression, spontaneous play and acknowledgement of the irrational characterised this artistic movement and was closely connected with Freud's free association technique which had been introduced as a means of accessing the unconscious material of the individual (Chilvers et al 1988, Hogan 2001).

Other thinkers linked with the psychoanalytic tradition offered even further support for the development of arts therapies. For example, Jung (1990) regarded imagination and creativity as healing forces within his analytical psychology approach. Similarly to dreams, they were regarded as having potential to throw light onto the 'shadow' self (i.e. the primitive side of the self that is generally unacceptable to the individual concerned and hence is experienced as either inferior or uncontrollable). According to Jung (1990), the shadow self consists of the personal and the 'collective unconscious' (the collective unconscious refers to aspects of the psyche that are common to all humankind, transmitted genetically and that consist of universal images called 'archetypes'). The arts were therefore seen as allowing the individual to access personal as well as deeply located archetypal images and to contribute towards accepting and coming to terms with or integrating the shadow self. Having given such a valuable role to the arts, Jung inspired the work of many pioneers in the arts therapies, who not only incorporated his theoretical principles into their own practice but also adopted and adapted some of his techniques. For example, 'active imagination', a technique introduced and developed by Jung as a means of freeing personal and collective unconscious associations, has been in extensive use within the arts therapies field up until the present day.

Finally, deriving from the same psychoanalytic tradition there has been another important development in psychotherapy that has had an impact upon the emergence of arts therapies: object relations theory, with Melanie Klein and Winnicott as the main representatives. Object relations theory introduced a major shift from the primacy of instinctual drives within classical psychoanalysis to relational bonds between the self and the 'object' (i.e. inner representations of a real or phantasised person or aspects of a person that either satisfies or frustrates individual needs). It highlighted symbolic play as a means of understanding the inner world of children (Klein 1975) and the creative process as an important indicator of healthy psychological development (Winnicott 1971).

As a result of development in psychoanalytic thinking, psychoanalytically-trained psychiatrists began to pay attention to the value of visual art, drama and music as adjunctive tools to their work (Hogan 2001, Jones 1996, Waller 1991) and boosted therapeutic activity that involved the arts. For example, Hogan (2001) describes how drawings and paintings created outside the therapy sessions were analysed by a number of psychoanalytically trained psychiatrists such as Pickford, Kris and Pailthorpe.

Humanistic psychology, another major school of thought that evolved in parallel and as a reaction to psychoanalysis, offered even stronger support for the emergence of arts therapies. Moreno, the person often regarded as the founder of humanistic psychotherapy, was a contemporary of Freud in Vienna at the beginning of the 20th century. His work diverged from Freudian thinking in that he introduced group psychotherapeutic work, in the form of psychodrama (an early precursor of dramatherapy [DT]) and gave theoretical 'permission' for the development of action therapies. During the 1960s and 1970s, humanistic psychotherapies became increasingly popular in various ways and with a number of different names, for example client-centred therapy (Rogers 1951), Gestalt therapy (Perls et al 1969) and transactional therapy (Berne 1961). Common elements of all of them are: (i) a rejection of psychoanalytic determinism over the development of human potential, (ii) an emphasis on the here-and-now of the therapy rather an exploration of the past, and (iii) a belief in a close relationship between the client and therapist, a relationship in which both client and therapist are regarded as equal partners in their therapeutic journey. Humanistic psychotherapists have also regarded self-expression and creativity as important aspects of their therapeutic work. The active nature of these therapies, taken in conjunction with their emphases on self-expression and creativity, has had a direct impact on the development of arts therapies.

In contrast to psychoanalytic thinking and the numerous humanistic traditions, behaviourism, the third important school of thought within modern psychology, has had much less contribution to the emergence of arts therapies. Behaviourism, rooted in the physiological tradition of the 19th century, focuses on observable behaviour that may be explained as a response to a stimulus. Underlying causes for such responses are not explored, the idea of the unconscious is rejected, while laws of learning theory are utilised to explain, predict and control behaviour. The more esoteric and holistic claims made by arts therapists have neither found very fertile ground within this tradition nor within the numerous types of therapies that derived from this major school of thought (e.g. behaviour modification, rational-emotive, cognitive, cognitive behaviour therapy).

Nevertheless, there have been many physicians who have shown an interest in the effects of the arts upon human physiology and/or on psychology. For example, there have been a number of experimental studies that have attempted to establish direct links between certain types of movement, music or art with either physiological or psychological health and its opposite, pathology. Systematic reviews of such studies made by people like Biley (2000), Cambrera & Lee (2000), Hacking & Foreman (2001), Kneafsey (1997) and Thomas & Jolly (1998) offer, in some cases, strong evidence that some such links are present (e.g. regarding movement and physiological changes, music and alleviation of chronic pain). In other cases, despite extensive research literature completed on such topics, the results remain inconclusive. Overall, arts therapists in the UK have been particularly sceptical towards such work. Edwards (2004) for example, argues that in most cases, the value of these findings for either the arts therapists or their clients has been questionable. This can be due to the fact that such studies often presented a limited understanding of the nature of the arts. There have also been some inherent difficulties in the translation of results from the controlled environment of a laboratory into the complexity of daily practice. Despite these criticisms, the interest shown by the medical profession towards the arts meant that some physicians have been particularly open towards encouraging the use of the arts with their patients. For example, as early as the 1920s and 1930s they invited musicians to play 'sedative' music for large numbers of patients (Bunt 1994) or artists to draw pictures for hospital walls (Waller 1991).

In the UK however, it was primarily during and particularly after the Second World War that active use of the arts by patients was encouraged. It was also during this period that such usage was considered for purposes other than mere entertainment and/or aesthetic cultivation. This shift of perspectives was closely linked with a growing awareness of the psychological needs of war veterans, the development of therapeutic communities and the growth of the social psychiatry movement. During this climate of change, the profession of occupational therapy emerged; it was the first health profession that openly acknowledged the potential contribution of the arts towards well-being. Bunt (1994) records that initial state recognition of arts therapies in the UK was achieved in 1982 under the remit of occupational therapy. Distinctions between occupational therapy and arts therapies are still not clearly understood by people outside the two professions; a discussion of some of these differences is included in Chapter 2.

Movements such as 'the arts for all' and 'the arts for health' also grew at that time and artists became regularly employed in hospitals, therapeutic communities and community settings. Although the early work of artists was very exploratory and their theoretical frameworks often ill-defined, their work constituted the first serious attempt, in modern times and in the western world, to involve the arts directly in improving health within the wider community (Bunt 1994, Waller 1991). 'Community' and 'hospital' artists contributed to the development of arts therapies but then continued as distinctive practices from arts therapies. Clear differences between 'therapeutic arts' (a generic term referring to all the practices that use the arts therapeutically) and arts therapies were outlined for the first time in 1985 with the Attenborough Report; this will be further discussed in Chapter 2.

In the post-war era, changes in attitudes also took place within education. The contribution of the American educator Dewey had a significant effect upon existing practices (Waller 1991). Child-centred education, with its emphasis on personal, emotional and social development, became the preferred theoretical framework for many arts teachers (Bunt 1994, Waller 1991) and contributed to the development of arts therapies in the UK. Jennings (1987), Payne (1992) and Waller (1991), for example, testify to the educational background of many of the pioneers of arts therapies. Moreover, Waller (1992) claims that, during the early days of the profession, arts therapies were often regarded as sensitive forms of arts teaching. This trend persisted until the end of the 1980s. The introduction of the National Curriculum of England and Wales in 1988 signified the end of child-centred education and created obvious differences between arts education and arts therapies. Within the current arts education climate, increasing emphasis is placed upon specific artistic/aesthetic learning outcomes, which are different from the emotional and social objectives of the previous period and different from the therapeutic aims of current arts therapies practice (see Ch. 2 for further discussion of differences between the two fields).

Professional associations

Formal organisation of practitioners working with the arts in a therapeutic way began during the 1950s and 1960s. In 1958 the pioneer Julliette Alvin founded the first organisation for practitioners working with the arts and special needs populations; it was called the Society for Music Therapy and Remedial Music. Jones (1996) and Waller (1991) describe how individuals, with a special interest in the therapeutic use of visual arts and drama/theatre, also formed their own groups in order to exchange experiences and promote existing work to potential employers.

Developing a common body of knowledge amongst the members of these first groups was particularly difficult. Individuals involved in these groupings were used to working on their own in a variety of different settings and with various factors supporting or inhibiting their work; this was particularly apparent for example, in the development of the dramatherapy profession. The diverse and often disconnected approaches adopted by practitioners created a number of inter-professional battles (Waller 1991), but gradually a less individual character began to emerge, common characteristics were agreed and a number of common practices developed. However, the choice of the artistic medium (visual art, music, drama/theatre or dance and movement) remained an important distinguishing factor for subgroupings. A vigorous debate started between the supporters of the maintenance of separate identities for each of the arts therapies, and those believing in the existence of substantial common ground shared by all the arts therapies types. The supporters of a common ground for arts therapies initiated the movement of the study of arts therapies as a whole in 1977; the latter was connected with the Sesame Institute and was chaired by Antony Storr (Jones 1996). A parallel debate was taking place in the USA, with arguments that arts therapies share a clear, definite and common identity. McNiff (1986) for example, considered the existence of separate professional identities as a characteristic of the 1980s and 1990s based on an unjustifiable and unsound 'media-related' division of creativity. He explained this division as being the result of political rather than philosophical or theoretical choices. Those supporting separate identities argued that merging the arts therapies together into one professional association bore the danger of developing practices with questionable depth in the understanding of the art form, and thus questionable therapeutic value (Waller 1991). They also warned of the danger of minimising opportunities for funding within a context where there were already limited budgets for anything relating to the arts.

As a result of such arguments, separate developments in the arts therapies remained the rule. Some exceptions to this rule have been: the 'expressive arts therapies' movement in the USA and the Institute for the Arts in Therapy and Education in the UK. The latter has pursued an integrative arts route and is currently affiliated with the UKCP (UK Chartered Psychotherapists: the regulatory organisation for psychotherapists that holds a voluntary register for practitioners as opposed to the obligatory registration required for arts therapies practitioners). For most arts therapists in the UK however, the main forums for political action were separate professional associations, namely the BAAT (British Association of Art Therapists), APMT

(Association of Professional Music Therapists), BADth (British Association of Dramatherapists) and ADMT UK (Association for Dance Movement Therapy UK) (see Appendix 3 for contact details). BAAT, one of the first associations to be formed (1964), is currently the professional body with the longest list of registered practitioners (more than 1000 members; BAAT 2004). ADMT UK is the most recent professional body to be established. It was founded in 1982 by Crane, Garvie and Payne (Payne 1992), and since then it has expanded to currently more than 140 qualified members (ADMT UK 2004/2005). Current sizes of each of these associations are reflected in Figure 1.3.

Despite their separate developments, all arts therapies associations have similar aims and responsibilities and often cooperate in representing the professional interests of their members, such as negotiating conditions of work. For example, they have pursued, and in 1982, partly succeeded in gaining recognition as professionals working within the National Health Service (NHS), with initial state recognition under the remit of OT (DHSS 1982). Since then, arts therapists have become recognised allied health professionals within the NHS with a similar status to occupational therapists, physiotherapists and speech and language therapists, and have continued expanding and establishing practices in a number of other areas as we will see later in this chapter. Arts therapies professional associations have been instrumental to these changes. Current alliance with AMICUS, a very active trade union, is expected to strengthen associations' ongoing attempts to improve conditions of work and payment and contribute towards further professional recognition and status.

In return, arts therapies associations have realised the need to ensure high quality of practice for all their members. For example, all arts therapists are obliged to follow explicit codes of ethics, attend ongoing clinical supervision and show commitment to continuing professional development (CPD). Evidence of CPD work is currently becoming increasingly formalised for all arts therapists and it is expected that it will eventually become mandatory especially insofar as re-registration is concerned. Arts therapies professional

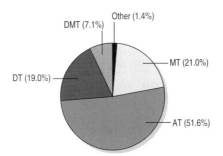

Figure 1.3: *Indicative sizes of arts therapies professional associations. The questionnaire for our study was fully completed by 580 arts therapists, around 40% of all arts therapists registered with arts therapies professional associations at the time of the study. The make-up of the final sample of the study in terms of representation of different arts therapies is shown. More than half of the respondents were registered art therapists, with the music therapists and dramatherapists making up around 20% each. Dance movement therapists constituted only 7% of the total sample.*

associations have also pursued and achieved independent regulation for their members through the Health Professions Council (HPC). The HPC is an independent regulatory body that assures high quality of training and high standards of service provision for most health professions in the country (HPC 2003). Arts therapists are now, and have been since 1999, represented in the HPC as a separate health profession through an umbrella arts therapies board that represents the different arts therapies disciplines. Title protection is an additional assurance of quality, since only HPC-registered, and consequently sufficiently-monitored practitioners, are allowed to practice as arts therapists.

During the recent history of the profession there have been a number of interdisciplinary arts therapies groups that work on areas of common interest. Committees for arts therapies in education and in prisons, the Joint Quality Assurance Committee, National Arts Therapies Research Committee, and the Research Forum for Allied Health Professions and the National (Scottish) Network for Clinical Effectiveness and Practice Development are some examples. Representatives from each of the different arts therapies associations are members of these groups.

Training courses

The first training course in the arts therapies was set up by Alvin in 1968 at the Guildhall School of Music and Drama in London, followed soon after by two courses in art therapy (AT) in at the Birmingham School of Art (as part of the Diploma and later the MA in Art Education) and at the St Albans School of Art (a Certificate in Remedial Art course). According to Waller (1991), between 1965 and 1972, discussions were taking place about the possibility of offering an Advanced Diploma incorporating art, music and movement at the Institute of Education, University of London; however, Waller (1991) claims that the plan for such training was possibly overly ambitious at the time.

During the following period a number of training courses were developed in various forms. For example, much of the initial training schemes for dramatherapy (DT) comprised short courses or weekend and summer schools. Training of a similar short duration and format was also developed for the first dance movement therapy (DMT) courses established in the UK. Very soon however, these courses adopted a more formal structure and, following the example of the courses in music therapy (MT) and AT, entry requirements, curricula and recognition were established. Today, programmes that lead to a licence to practise are at a Master's level and are approved by higher education (HE) institutions, their respective arts therapies associations and the HPC. Information about the length of these courses, the degrees awarded and the specific university they are validated by is included in Appendix 2.

Arts therapies training courses are currently validated by more than 15 HE institutions. Some of these courses are based within arts, health, social sciences, humanities or education faculties, while others are run independently (e.g. as charities) and receive academic validation without using university premises. In some cases there is more than one arts therapies programme; the same institution may be offering training for professionals in more than one discipline. When this is the case, often although separate programmes are followed, some common aspects of these programmes are shared (e.g. modules on psychotherapy or research methods). For instance, Goldsmiths College has recently developed a new DMT course alongside its much older AT training programmes. At the University of Roehampton, programmes incorporating all four arts therapies are available. Derby University has developed postgraduate training courses (Diploma/Master) alongside an undergraduate course. (Note: A licence to practise is granted only to graduates from Diploma/Master courses. This is a characteristic of British training; in the Netherlands, for example, arts therapies training is primarily offered at an undergraduate level.) Also available in the UK are foundation courses that prepare applicants to reach appropriate entry requirements for professional qualification training, as well as opportunities for post-qualification studies at an MPhil/PhD level. Such programmes can be followed in most universities that offer arts therapies postgraduate training (see Appendix 2).

After lengthy debates within and between professional associations, there is currently consensus across disciplines and courses on some of the important 'ingredients' of arts therapies training programmes. In most cases, both Diploma and the more recent Master courses attempt to combine experiential knowledge and academic studies. According to the handbook of the Joint Quality Assurance Committee (JQAC 2002), the practical/experiential part often comprises:

- a number of supervised placements
- training in relevant skills and the art form central to the specific arts therapies
- experience in individual and group work as participants and facilitators
- some experience in other arts and arts therapies
- experience of writing clinical reports and keeping records.

Recent studies of experiential groups within training and placement learning (Karkou et al 2002, Payne 2001) highlight the value of this type of work for personal and professional development. The academic/theoretical part of the work usually covers areas such as:

- the theory of the modality and the art form central to it
- relevant psychological, psychiatric, sociological, psychotherapeutic and medical aspects
- theories of group and individual work
- a deep understanding of the therapeutic relationship and the management of the process
- issues related to equal opportunities, culture, age, gender, disability and ethics
- assessment and evaluation.

Introduction to the code of ethics, regulations and relevant legislations is also included in the theoretical aspects of these courses. (JQAC 2002). Requirements for training reflect expected standards of practice once trainees are qualified, and have been taken into account in the formulation of government documents such as the *Standards of Proficiency* (HPC 2003) and the *Benchmark Statement* (QAA 2004).

Although some important 'ingredients' of training courses have been established and reinforced by HPC monitoring processes, there are a number of areas that remain the subject of debate.

Examples of some of these disputed topics are:

- the overall character of the programme
- minimum exit qualification
- length of training
- commitment to personal therapy
- entry requirements for trainee arts therapists.

The overall character of the programme

Course components listed above are not implemented in the same way across different arts therapies programmes; for example, the overall ethos and philosophy of the courses may vary. The AT course at Goldsmiths college has a preference for using the term 'art psychotherapy' which reflects the psychodynamic bias of the training, while the equivalent Hertfordshire training has a reputation for a more art-based orientation. Similarly, the MT training course based in Cardiff has an explicit psychodynamic orientation, while the Nordoff–Robbins programme is clearly more art-based. Furthermore, the most appropriate balance between experiential and academic components of arts therapies training continues to generate discussion with some courses highlighting the experiential over the academic learning and vice versa. Whatever the emphasis of the course, written work in the form of case studies, presentations and/or essays, is required in all courses, even within those with a more experiential/artistic bias.

The degree to which research components are incorporated within existing training schemes also varies. Some claim that research work should be pursued only after basic professional training has been completed and sufficient clinical experience has been gained (Gilroy 1992). Others insist that research skills should be an integral part of the basic professional training (Edwards 2004, Wigram et al 2002). The supporters of the latter view seem to be gaining ground in the debate since basic research competencies are expected from the newly qualified arts therapist (QAA 2004). Closely connected with the discussion about the role of research in training is the idea of evidence-based practice. Evidence-based practice can be defined as the use of the best available information for making clinical decisions (Sackett et al 2000). It assumes that clinicians are good/intelligent consumers of existing research, if not researchers themselves. An evidence-based National Service Framework has been introduced within the NHS for all areas of health care including mental health (DoH 1999). Within the same NHS framework, and as a result of gathering research evidence of clinical effectiveness, guidelines have been published on treatment choices for psychological therapies including arts therapies (DoH 2001). It is expected that changes of this kind in the work environment will have a strong impact upon the shape and content of training programmes in arts therapies. Furthermore, it is expected that increased research activity will take place in HE institutions and new collaborations will be attempted, for example with local or national trusts or charities.

Minimum exit qualification

All training courses in arts therapies are at postgraduate level, in terms of both time and level. All of them are regarded as offering training at a 'Master's level' whether the exit point for trainees is a Diploma or a Master's qualification. At the moment, both exit points are in operation and in a number of different courses. Lengthy discussions are now underway regarding whether the minimum qualification for arts therapists should move from the minimum of a postgraduate Diploma to a minimum of a Master's degree. The latter type of qualification seems to be gaining in the debate, especially with the introduction of the Agenda for Change policy in which nationalised standards of payment are introduced for employees in the NHS. Arts therapies associations are making a case for the NHS to regard Arts therapists as qualified practitioners at a Master's level who carry high responsibility and deserve respective payment.

Length of training

The length of arts therapies training in the UK varies; the minimum is currently 1 year full-time (e.g. for MT), with part-time options also available. A tendency to develop training courses that are a minimum of 2 years in duration on a full-time basis is currently emerging. For several years, AT was the only field that required this length of training from its professional members. However, the extension of training into a 2-year period received heated debate that in some disciplines is still ongoing (Payne 1996/97). For example, in DMT those opposing such a change are primarily concerned with losing the support of the validating institution by creating courses that are at odds with other postgraduate courses which have a purely academic rather than training character. Waller (2001) in describing similar debates within the AT field when such a change was first implemented, argues that there have been a number of positive outcomes from the shift into 2-year training. There was financial commitment for both students and validating university, parity with other academic and/or psychotherapeutic courses, improved position of qualified art therapists within the wider health professions' picture, and implications for payment and professional status once qualified.

Commitment to personal therapy

A commitment to personal therapy for successful completion of training has become a requirement for all arts therapies training courses. The duration of personal therapy is often similar to that of the course. However, the type of therapy that should be pursued is still highly debatable.

Entry requirements for trainee arts therapists

Waller (1991) reports on the debate about entry requirements during the early days of the development of AT postgraduate training. 'To be first and foremost artists' was the main premise of many art therapists during that time. This debate ended with the agreement that AT courses should not only consider applicants with degrees in fine arts but also art experience or attendance at appropriate short courses. Similar discussions took place within the other arts therapies. Currently, artistic qualifications are preferred for entry to arts therapies courses (ADMT UK 2004, BAAT 2004, BADth 2004,

BSMT 2004). Applicants with other relevant qualifications such as in psychology or those of the health professions (e.g. nursing, occupational therapy and physiotherapy) might convince course convenors of their experience in the appropriate art form and consequently gain entry. Additional requirements for entering arts therapies training are: demonstration of personal maturity, relevant practical experience and possession of a clean police record. If applicants do not meet one or more of the entry requirements, they have the option to attend arts therapies foundation courses and join formal professional training at a later stage.

Table 1.1: Qualifications and backgrounds of respondents

Most of the arts therapists participating in our study (81.3%) were qualified practitioners with a *postgraduate diploma in a type of art therapy*. The table shows that 14.2% of the participants had more than just their postgraduate diploma, i.e. the minimum requirement expected for registration as an arts therapist up to this date. Almost 15% of our sample had qualifications at a *Masters level* and above *(MPhil and PhD)*. The few participants with *no qualifications* were possibly those who became involved with the field before the beginning of arts therapies training courses in the UK. It is also apparent from the table that artistic qualifications were an important part of arts therapists' professional identity with almost half of the respondents having a *BA in an art form*. Furthermore, it is shown that respondents to the survey had other relevant experiences and/or qualifications; as expected the largest percentage (27.6%) recorded *psychotherapy/counselling training*, but arts therapists also had experience in *further artistic work, social/community work* and *education*.

Arts therapies qualifications (%)		Artistic qualifications (%)	
Postgraduate diploma	81.3	BA	47.5
Masters	11.8	No qualifications	24.4
No qualifications	4.5	Short courses/certificate	22.9
MPhil/PhD	2.4	Postgraduate studies	5.2
Total	100.0	Total	100.0
Other relevant experiences			
Psychotherapy/counselling	27.6		
Artistic	21.7		
Social/community work	18.4		
Education	16.9		
Neighbouring areas	8.0		
Nursing	6.3		
Other	1.1		
Total	100.0		

Some of the backgrounds that arts therapists in the UK have are presented in Table 1.1. Artistic qualifications at a BA level are evident for almost half of these practitioners, while additional training in psychotherapy or counselling is fairly common. This can be attributed to the need for further professional development and recognition. It is worth adding that, given recent changes in arts therapies training programmes, the figure for people acquiring a Master's degree in arts therapies (as well as MPhil and PhD qualifications) is fairly high and is currently rising. It appears that arts therapies practitioners are responding to calls for increasing research activity in the field and providing evidence for effective practice. It is hoped that, alongside CPD development schemes, new training programmes will offer further support for professional development.

Areas of work

Arts therapists work with clients (the term 'client' is preferred to 'patient' throughout the book) with a wide variety of difficulties, ranging from those with severe mental health problems such as schizophrenia to those with stress, and from those with severe learning difficulties to those considered to have 'mild' difficulties. Specifically, difficulties that are frequently addressed by arts therapists are:

- mental health problems such as schizophrenia, depression, bipolar disorders, personality disorders, self-harm, eating disorders, anxiety and panic attacks, post-traumatic stress disorder, dementia
- learning difficulties that can be mild, moderate or profound, autism, Asperger's syndrome, attention deficit hyperactivity disorder (ADHD), language and communication problems
- social deprivation and isolation due to imprisonment, confinement or social exclusion, e.g. offenders, refugees, homeless
- medical problems such as cancer, human immunodeficiency syndrome (HIV) and acquired immunodeficiency syndrome (AIDS), strokes and/or heart attacks, chronic pain
- sensory and/or physical problems
- stress, low self-esteem, and emotional or social problems.
  (Odell-Miller et al 2003, QAA 2004)

Research studies (some of which adopted randomised controlled trial [RCT] designs) offer evidence for the efficacy of arts therapies with a number of the above client groups such as: those suffering from severe and enduring mental health problems, people with autism, with Asperger's syndrome, with ADHD and profound learning disabilities. Arts therapies are also shown to be effective for those with dementia, people who self-harm, have suffered trauma and who have survived physical, sexual and emotional abuse. Finally, there are a number of studies that support the value of arts therapies for dealing with issues of self-esteem and anxiety with a number of different client groups. References to some of the above studies can be found in research reviews and research registers published in the field, either in books, reports or arts therapies websites, such as Dent-Brown (2004), Karkou (2003), Odell-Miller et al 2003, Payne (1993) and Wigram et al (2002).

Overall, arts therapists in the UK avoid using diagnostic labels to refer to their clients. The use of medical terminology is met with discomfort. Medical terminology can be regarded as questioning the individuality of each client and as blinding the practitioner from seeing what the client's needs really are (Woddis, 1986). In our study we have also avoided medical labels. Instead we focused on clients' difficulties and adopted educational terminology to describe these difficulties (see Fig. 1.4). We found that emotional/behavioural difficulties (i.e. mental health issues) and learning difficulties were the most frequently cited difficulties of the main client groups of arts therapies practitioners, while the age of clients varied from young children to the elderly.

Our findings also suggest that most arts therapists tend to work with a number of different client groups at the same time (see Fig. 1.4). Arts therapies is still a fairly new profession and keen to grow and develop. It is possible that working with different client groups at present reflects such growth. However, this finding can also be indicative of professional instability; for example, arts therapists may work with a range of client groups as a means of professional survival rather than out of choice.

Arts therapists work in a variety of settings in the private and/or public sector. For example, they can be found in:

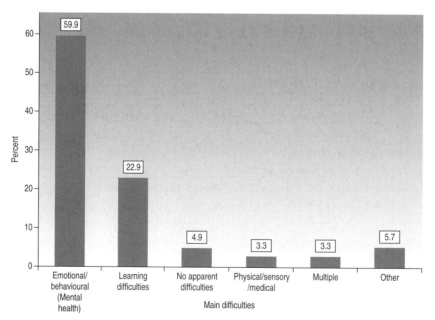

Figure 1.4: *Main client group: difficulties.* Emotional/behavioural *and* learning difficulties *were most frequently mentioned when respondents were asked to state the type of difficulty of their* main client group. No apparent difficulties received only 5% response rate. However, respondents were working with more than one client group. Higher percentages were found when they were asked to state the difficulties of all the client groups with whom they were working. Emotional/behavioural and learning difficulties, social deprivation, multiple difficulties, medical problems and physical/sensory difficulties were mentioned by more than 30% of the respondents.*

- *hospitals*: adult mental health services, child and adolescent services, services for older people with mental health problems, services for people with learning difficulties, special hospitals, children's hospitals and hospices
- *education*: special and/or mainstream schools, referral units, learning support services
- *community-based settings*: social services, voluntary and private organisations, community mental health and learning disability teams
- *Home Office settings*: prisons, secure units and detention centres
- *private practice*: senior arts therapists may also work in private practice. (Odell-Miller et al 2003, QAA 2004)

Health services, and the NHS in particular, are areas where established posts exist for arts therapists. The fact that arts therapies are currently recognised allied health professions within the NHS and are regulated by the HPC has an impact upon a respective professional recognition within the NHS, and also explains the relatively high numbers of arts therapists working in such settings (see Fig. 1.5).

It is less common for arts therapists to work in education, although a respectable number of practitioners appear to be employed there too as Figure 1.5 shows. Despite the fact that many of the pioneers of arts therapies in the UK have had an educational background (Jennings 1987, Payne 1992, Waller 1991), the relatively high proportion of arts therapists currently working in such environments was unexpected. This was mainly because overall, there is

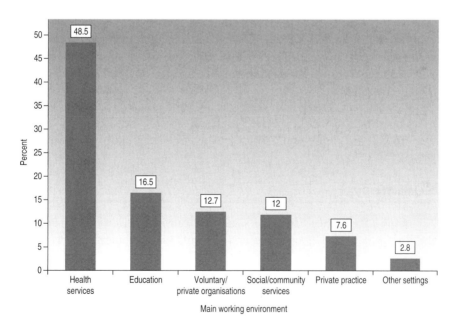

Figure 1.5: *Main working environments. Almost half of the respondents to the questionnaire regarded health services as their main working environment as shown in the figure. Educational settings, voluntary/private organisations and social/community work were, respectively, the second, third and fourth main areas of work for arts therapists in the UK. It is notable that when arts therapists were asked to give all the places in which they work, the percentages were significantly higher: 64% for health services, 31% for education, 29% for voluntary and private organisations, 26% for social/community work and 23% for private practice. The higher percentages in this second question suggest that arts therapists were working in more than just one place.*

no formal recognition of arts therapists within the British educational system. It is suspected that partly, this finding reflects work undertaken at independent schools and/or on a sessional basis. It is also possible that several of these practitioners are employed as teachers rather than as arts therapists, and that at times they may incorporate arts therapies practice alongside other, educational, duties (Sanderson & Karkou 2000).

Alongside the NHS and education, community-based work is growing, especially since the shift of care from large institutions to the community in the 1990s (Karkou, in press). Arts therapists who work in the community are often employed on short-term contracts or offer sessional or 'freelance' work. Overall, stable posts for arts therapists are rare. This can be seen as a characteristic of the employment situation for the field as a whole that can be confirmed by an APMT survey of 1990 (Bunt 1994), the BADth Membership list of 1991 (Meldrum 1994), and a survey undertaken by McNab & Edwards (1988). Findings from our study (see Fig. 1.5) suggest that, several years later, the number of stable full-time posts remains limited and possibly the conditions of employment largely unchanged.

Problems arising from this type of work are not just problems for the profession, but also for the potential users of arts therapies services. In a recent publication produced by the Department of Health (DoH 2004), there is a clear acknowledgement that despite the fact that psychological therapies, including arts therapies, are essential parts of healthcare, existing provision remains inadequate. There are long waiting times, unclear care pathways and limited accessibility. The document refers to consistent complaints by users of mental health services on this account and refers to existing services as: 'patchy, uncoordinated, idiosyncratic ... and not fully integrated into management systems' (p. 1). This is even truer for arts therapies that have a much shorter duration of recognition within healthcare provision than other therapies and up to now very unstable patterns of employment. As long as employment remains the same, accessibility to many arts therapies services relies on the good will of isolated professionals, the persistence of service users to practise choice and a lot of hard work on the part of arts therapies practitioners.

Summary

Arts therapies practice has made significant progress since the formation of the first professional associations and the initial development of arts therapies training. Each of the existing associations has promoted the arts therapies disciplines and expanded their work to include clients of different ages, with a wide range of difficulties such as mental health and learning disabilities. Cooperation is evident in the pursuit of the common goal of official recognition as a profession and in working together in various arts therapies committees and conferences. Similar patterns exist in relation to the training courses established. Common standards are negotiated between these courses, with professional associations playing leading roles.

The practitioners currently registered as arts therapists are members of separate professional bodies and have been trained in either AT, MT, DT or

DMT postgraduate courses at a Master's level (i.e. qualified with a minimum of a Diploma or recently a Master). These qualifications have often been gained in addition to artistic or psychotherapeutic/counselling qualifications. Their working environments are predominantly the NHS and to a lesser extent educational settings, voluntary/private agencies and social/community services. Despite the high qualifications of arts therapists, and the complex and diverse issues of their clients, employment and career structures for arts therapists remain erratic.

References

- Aristotle (Butcher S H, trans.) 1961 Aristotle's poetics. Hill and Wang, New York
- Association for Dance Movement Therapy UK (ADMT UK) 2004 Training. Online. Available: http://www.admt.org.uk/training.html 11 Dec 2004
- Association for Dance Movement Therapy (ADMT UK) 2004/2005 Register of members. ADMT UK
- Attenborough Report 1985 Arts and disabled people. Carnegie UK Trust, London
- Berne E 1961 Transactional analysis in psychotherapy: a systematic individual and social psychiatry. Souvenir Press, London
- Biley F 2000 The effects on patient well-being of music listening as a nursing intervention: a review of the literature. Journal of Clinical Nursing 9:668–677
- British Association of Art Therapists (BAAT) 2004 Training. Online. Available: http://www.baat.org/training.html 11 Dec 2004
- British Association of Dramatherapists (BADth) 2004 Training. Online. Available: http://www.badth.org.uk/training.html 11 Dec 2004
- British Society for Music Therapy (BSMT) 2004 Music therapy training courses in the UK. Online. Available: http://www.bsmt.org/train.html 16 Mar 2004
- Bunt L 1994 Music therapy: an art beyond words. Routledge, London
- Cambrera I N, Lee M H M 2000 Reducing noise pollution in the hospital setting by establishing a department of sound: a survey of recent research on the effects of noise and music in health care. Preventive Medicine 30:339–345
- Chilvers I, Osborne H, Farr D 1988 The Oxford dictionary of art. Oxford University Press, Oxford
- Clark K 1966 Civilisation. Harper and Row, New York
- Dent-Brown K 2004 UK research register for DT. Online. Available: http://www.badth.org.uk/register.html 8 Oct 2004
- Department of Health (DoH) 1999 A national service framework for mental health. Department of Health, London
- Department of Health (DoH) 2001 Clinical guidelines for treatment choice decision in psychological therapies and counselling. Department of Health, London
- Department of Health (DoH) 2004 Organising and delivering psychological therapies. Department of Health, London
- Descartes R (Valery P, trans.) 1947 Discourse on the method. In: Valery P (ed.) The living thoughts of Descartes. David McKay, Philadelphia, p 41–110
- DHSS 1982 Personal memorandum PM (82) 6 March 1982
- Edwards D 2004 Art therapy. Sage, London
- Feder E, Feder B 1981 The expressive arts therapies. Prentice-Hall, Englewood Cliffs, NJ
- Fleshman B, Fryrear J L 1981 The arts in therapy. Nelson Hall, Chicago
- Gilroy A 1992 Research in art therapy. In: Waller D, Gilroy A (eds) Art therapy: a handbook. Open University Press, Buckingham, p 229–247
- Hacking S, Foreman D 2001 Psychopathology in paintings: a meta-analysis of studies using paintings by psychiatric patients. British Journal of Medical Psychology 74:35–45
- Health Professions Council (HPC) 2003 Standards of proficiency – arts therapies. HPC, London
- Hogan H 2001 Healing arts: the history of art therapy. Jessica Kingsley, London
- Jennings S 1987 Introduction. In: Jennings S (ed.) Dramatherapy: theory and practice 1. Routledge, London, p xv–xx

- Joint Quality Assurance Committee (JQAC) 2002 Handbook. Unpublished document produced by the Arts Therapies Board, APMT, BAAT and BADth
- Jones P 1996 Drama as therapy: theatre as living. Routledge, London
- Jung C G (ed.) 1990 Man and his symbols. Arkana, Penguin Group, London (first published by Aldus Books, 1964)
- Karkou V 2003 UK research register for DMT. Online. Available: http://www.admt.org.uk/res_research.html 11 Dec 2004
- Karkou V in press. Dance movement therapy in the community: group work with people with enduring mental health difficulties. In: Payne H (ed) Dance movement therapy: theory, practice and research. Routledge, London
- Karkou V, Burchell H, Warren V et al 2002 Supporting student placement learning: the tutor's role. Presented at the Hertfordshire Integrated Learning Project (HILP) Annual Conference, July 2002
- Klein M 1975 Collected works of Melanie Klein, vol. I, II, III and IV. Hogarth Press and Institute of Psychoanalysis, London
- Kneafsey R 1997 The therapeutic use of music in a care of the elderly setting: a literature review. Journal of Clinical Nursing 6:341–346
- Levy F 1992 Dance movement therapy: a healing art. American Alliance for Health, Physical Education, Recreation and Dance, Reston
- McNab D, Edwards D 1988 Private AT. Inscape (summer):14–19
- McNiff S 1986 Educating the creative arts therapist. Charles C Thomas, Springfield, IL
- Meldrum B 1994 Historical background and overview of dramatherapy. In: Jennings S, Cattanach A, Mitchell S et al (eds) The handbook of dramatherapy. Routledge, London, p. 12–27
- Odell-Miller H, Learmonth M, Pembrooke C 2003 The arts and arts therapists. Scoping Paper Commissioned by Nuffield Foundation
- Payne H 1992 Introduction. In: Payne H (ed.) Dance movement therapy: theory and practice. Tavistock/Routledge, London, p 1–17
- Payne H (ed.) 1993 Handbook of inquiry in the arts therapies: one river, many currents. Jessica Kingsley, London
- Payne H 1996/1997 Definition of DMT (letter). ADMT Newsletter VIII(4):18
- Payne H 2001 Arts therapies and psychotherapy training: an international survey. Virtual International Arts Therapies Journal 1(Dec): The Virtual Arts Therapies Network. Online. Available: http://www.derby.ac.uk/research/vart/journal/archives/2002/articles/intsurvey/index.html 2 Mar 2002
- Perls F, Hefferline R, Goodman P 1969 Gestalt therapy: excitement and growth in the human personality. Julian Press, New York
- Plato (Lindsay A D, trans.) 1957 The republic of Plato. E P Dutton, New York
- Quality Assurance Agency (QAA) 2004 Benchmark statement: healthcare programme – arts therapies. QAA, Gloucester
- Rogers C 1951 Client-centered therapy: its current practise, implications and theory. Constable, London
- Sackett D L, Strauss S E, Richardson W S et al 2000 Evidence-based medicine: how to practice and teach EBM, 2nd edn. Churchill Livingstone, Oxford
- Sanderson P, Karkou V 2000 Art therapy in mainstream education: a case study. Research report. The University of Manchester, School of Education
- Thomas G V, Jolly R P 1998 Drawing conclusions: a re-examination of empirical and conceptual bases for psychological evaluation of children from their drawings. British Journal of Clinical Psychology 37:27–39
- Waller D 1991 Becoming a profession: the history of art therapy in Britain 1940–1982. Tavistock/Routledge, London
- Waller D 1992 Different things to different people: art therapy in Britain – a brief survey of its history and current development. The Arts in Psychotherapy 19:87–92
- Waller D 2001 Come back Professor Higgins – arts therapists need you! The importance of clear communication for arts therapists. In: Kossolapow, L Scoble, S, Waller D (eds) Arts – therapies – communication: on the way to a communicative European arts therapy, vol. 1. Lit Verlag, Munster, p 244–256
- Wigram T, Pederson I N, Bonde L O 2002 A comprehensive guide to music therapy: theory, clinical practice, research and training. Jessica Kingsley, London
- Winnicott D W 1971 Playing and reality. Routledge, London
- Woddis J 1986 Reflections: judging from appearances. The Arts in Psychotherapy 13:147–149

Chapter 2

Defining Arts Therapies

Key issues:

- Arts therapies should be distinguished from the therapeutic use of the arts. Unlike arts therapies the latter does not target therapeutic change directly, but considers the process of art making and the production of an artefact as a therapeutic experience. Therapy training is not essential for therapeutic arts practitioners.

- The aims of arts education are different from those of arts therapies. Arts education involves developing creative artistic and aesthetic skills and the production of an artwork that can be evaluated.

- Although the arts therapies are closely associated with psychotherapeutic thinking, they differ from verbal therapies in the following ways: arts therapies involve the arts and creativity in the centre of their practice, and emphasise the 'doing' and the non-verbal over the 'talking'. They also differ in professional requirements and in some cases in duration of training.

- Arts therapies are currently recognised as health professions, having developed professional alliances with occupational therapy, physiotherapy, and speech and language therapy. Despite these alliances, a number of substantial differences exist between these fields and arts therapies.

- There are lengthy debates about the nature of arts therapies, which highlight either the psychotherapeutic or the artistic aspects of the work. The most recent definitions, with few exceptions, accept diversity as a characteristic of the field and avoid explicitly aligning with either psychotherapy or the arts.

Introduction

In the previous chapter we looked at ways in which arts therapies emerged, acquired professional shape, and how they are currently developing. However, the question still remains: what are 'arts therapies'? Deconstructing the term into its components 'arts' and 'therapy' immediately raises numerous and often complex issues. For example, the term 'arts' can refer to many different art forms with distinctive characteristics, traditions, practices and status. 'Therapy' can refer to numerous schools of psychotherapy and counselling, complementary therapies, and health professions such as occupational therapy, physiotherapy, speech and language therapy. Finally, used in its everyday sense, 'therapy' can be associated with virtually anything that makes one feel better. Both 'arts' and 'therapy' can become words that are too elusive to assist with defining arts therapies.

Furthermore, as Gestalt and many arts therapists would argue, the term 'arts therapies' can stand for more than just the sum of the parts (i.e. 'arts' and 'therapy'). Or more precisely it stands for something different, a separate field. In this chapter we will begin with outlining some of the differences of arts therapies from disciplines with which there have been historical connections. This discussion will offer a first sketch of the boundaries of the field. We will then look at definitions of arts therapies given by official arts therapies sources. Our analyses of these definitions will enable us to identify important aspects of arts therapies and to suggest our own definition.

Arts therapies and therapeutic arts

As we discussed in Chapter 1, historically, movements such as 'the arts for all' and 'the arts for health' have contributed to the emergence of arts therapies. Community and hospital artists led these movements and created a type of work we broadly term 'therapeutic arts' (this type of work can also be found with the name 'arts for health'). The professional origins of many of the pioneers of arts therapies can be found in this work, especially before training courses were developed (Waller 1991). Although the two fields are now perceived as different, it was not until the Attenborough report (1985) that any official document acknowledged these differences. In subsequent years, arts therapists and artists continued to be employed in similar environments and with similar client groups. On many occasions, artists offered a cheaper option for employers and on the basis of cost they were preferred to arts therapists. As a result, for most people, confusion still remains as to what are arts therapies and what are therapeutic arts.

There is indeed a common ground shared by both arts therapies and therapeutic arts. In both cases the emphasis is around using the arts in a *therapeutic* way. However, while arts therapists claim that their practice is a form of *therapy*, those who are not trained in arts therapies cannot claim to offer therapy. Important distinctions in the meanings of the two words 'therapy' and 'therapeutic' can further explain the differences between the two fields.

Therapy is often connected with the intentional targeting of psychological change. In the case of arts therapies it involves the intentional use of the arts for psychological change (Meldrum 1994). On the other hand, something may be *therapeutic* without directly setting out to be so, and without a clear articulation of what is, or is not, responsible for psychological change. In arts therapies, both intentional and unintentional psychological change can take place.

We believe that the arts have indeed great therapeutic *potential*. Several sources provide evidence of a number of therapeutic benefits for participants in arts projects. Such benefits are outlined, for example, in a study by the Health Development Agency (2000) as: development of interpersonal skills, opportunities for making friends and increased involvement. Therapeutic benefits of this kind are often the result of setting up a performance, organising an exhibition, etc., depending on the artistic interests of the facilitators. The artistic outcome often remains of primary importance while therapeutic outcomes can be seen as byproducts of the artwork, e.g. a performance. As the aim is to achieve therapeutic change, participating in arts projects cannot guarantee therapeutic outcomes, although the potential to arrive at such outcomes might be considerably high.

As Bunt (1994) states, in arts therapies the arts are used as a means to an end; the artistic product may or may not be an outcome in arts therapies. Consequently, in arts therapies we have a shift of focus from the art *product* to the *process* (Stanton-Jones 1992, Waller & Dalley 1992). Processes within arts therapies can be quite complex, incorporating art-making, the client–therapist interaction, therapeutically-sound interventions and so on. The arts therapist talks about such processes as vital for achieving change. Similar considerations are not necessarily relevant to the practitioner who uses the arts in a therapeutic way.

According to Waller (1992), this shift of focus from the art product to the therapeutic process does not remove the centrality of the artistic aspect from arts therapies. Arts therapists remain 'first and foremost artists' (Waller 1992, p. 90). As we have seen in the previous chapter, many arts therapists hold a first degree in an art form. However, our study revealed (Karkou & Sanderson 1997), that for the vast majority of arts therapists, their specific artistic interests are not reflected in an arts therapies session; the client's artistic interests are much more important. Furthermore, therapy training becomes an important characteristic of the arts therapies field and is acquired *in addition* to relevant artistic skills. Arguments for the need for therapy training stem primarily from the belief that the arts can have a strong impact upon the individual and as such, if not appropriately used, can be dangerous. Therapy training can safeguard against potential harm or unintentional abuse. As part of additional professional obligations towards the clients and assurance of quality of service, arts therapists practise within a strict code of ethics, are committed to clinical supervision and undertake continuing professional development. They are registered with one of the arts therapies professional associations and are regulated by the Health Professions Council (HPC). In contrast, those practising therapeutic arts may work with vulnerable clients without necessarily possessing any therapeutic training, without having any professional obligations and without monitoring procedures in place. Artistic ability and experience is often the only requirement.

At first glance, there are several similarities between arts therapies and therapeutic arts. Closer examination of these two fields however, reveals that there are differences in skills, professionalism and overall philosophical assumptions and orientation. These differences are summarised as follows:

- Arts therapies are therapies, while therapeutic arts are not classified as a form of therapy; they are artistic activities with a therapeutic potential.
- Within arts therapies there is an intentional use of the arts to target therapeutic change, while therapeutic arts use the arts to offer primarily artistic experiences.
- Artistic products may or may not be part of arts therapies, but in therapeutic arts the artistic product is the main focus.
- Therapeutic arts place a primary emphasis upon artistic considerations influenced by the artistic interests of the facilitator. Arts therapies, on the other hand, may include an emphasis upon both therapeutic and artistic elements of the work. However, the artistic interests of the therapist remain insignificant.
- In the therapeutic use of the arts, practitioners must have facility with their arts media. For arts therapies, both artistic and therapy training are necessary.
- Arts therapists are registered with an arts therapies professional association, are compelled to practise within specific codes of ethics, and are regulated by the HPC. To date, professional registration for those practising therapeutic arts is not in place.

Arts therapies and arts education

The distinction between arts therapies and arts education can also be confusing and from an historical point of view this is not surprising. As we discussed in the previous chapter, arts education has made significant contributions to the emergence of arts therapies in the UK. Indeed, the level of this contribution has been such that in the early days, arts therapies were often regarded as 'a sensitive form of arts teaching' (Waller 1992, p. 88). Child-centred perspectives held within education (including arts education) until recently, highlighted the emotional and social aspects of schooling as major intended outcomes of the learning process (Sanderson 1996a, 2002).

Major differences are more easily revealed when arts therapies are compared with mainstream arts education and national curriculum requirements; for example, the arts teacher is now compelled to concentrate on the aesthetic and artistic merits of the arts (QCA 2004). Arts education is therefore seen as primarily promoting pupils' knowledge, skills and understanding of art-making, and developing skills in appraising completed arts products (Sanderson 1984). The aims of arts therapies in contrast, are ultimately to achieve therapeutic (e.g. personal or social) goals (Karkou & Sanderson 2001a,b). *Difference of intention* is therefore one significant distinguishing factor between arts education and arts therapies.

Furthermore, according to the current national curriculum (QCA 2004), exposure to a number of different genres and traditions is an essential component of arts teaching in the UK. The arts therapist, however, does not follow a prescribed artistic agenda. Although both the teacher and the therapist might share a similar artistic training and similar belief in the arts, the latter has a 'therapeutic' agenda shaped by a client's preferences, psychological needs and the overall therapeutic framework the practitioner follows (Peter 1998). The *'aesthetic and artistic'* agenda of the teacher is different from the *'helping and healing'* agenda of the therapist.

Our study revealed that the vast majority of arts therapists agree that they do not teach anyone how to play, act, move or paint (Karkou 1999, Karkou & Sanderson 1997, 2001a,b). According to Peter (1998) good arts teaching has a strong interactive character, and in that respect it can resemble arts therapies practice. However, even if interactive or non-directive methods are employed, arts instruction remains an integral part of the role of the arts teacher. Therefore, the *presence or absence of arts instruction* is another major difference between arts therapies and arts teaching.

Artistic achievement plays an important role in arts teaching, and assessment of levels of achievement is an integral part of the teaching process. If students demonstrate high levels of aesthetic or artistic achievement, teachers may be confident that their approaches are working (Sanderson & Savva 2004). However, it is not unusual to find high levels of artistic quality within arts therapies, for mere exposure to the artistic media may also contribute towards the development of artistic skills (Byrne 1995). Nevertheless, for the arts therapist, it is not the artistic or aesthetic skills that are of major importance. Interest is more likely to be focused on *any change* in artistic or aesthetic skills, rather than on whether or not the *quality of the artefact* has improved. Artistic change is of interest because it might be an indication of a parallel psychological change.

For example, students showing skill in reciting parts of a Shakespearean dialogue may be highly rated within a drama session for their theatrical prowess. If the same incident happens within a dramatherapeutic context, emphasis might be placed on:

- the fact that the client chose to recite a specific text in preference to another
- the meaning of this text for a client within the specific time in the therapeutic process, in the context of relationships with the therapist and/or the group or in relation to the client's life outside the therapeutic context
- any transformational function of this dramatic activity.

Recent literature in arts therapies and art therapy (AT) in particular, acknowledges that aesthetic quality has an impact on the client, the therapist and the therapeutic process (e.g. Case 1996, Maclagan 2001, Schaverien 2000). However, the major premise remains that the aesthetic and artistic qualities of whatever is produced within arts therapies are not of primary importance. This, therefore, constitutes another main difference between arts therapies and arts teaching.

Many of the issues already covered in the discussion of differences between arts therapies and therapeutic arts are also relevant here. There are differences of classification, education versus therapy; differences in training; and differences in professional registration.

The arts education and therapies literature presents a lengthy list of other distinctions and differences between the two modalities (e.g. Bunt 1994, Jordan 1988, Meier 1997, Payne 1992, Sanderson 1996b, Valente 1991, Valente & Fontana 1991, Warwick 1995). Some of these differences including those already discussed are summarised below:

- The arts teacher aims towards the development of the pupil's artistic knowledge and skills; the arts therapist targets personal and social goals.
- The teacher has an 'artistic' agenda; the therapist has a 'therapeutic' agenda.
- Arts education involves specific teaching; arts therapists do not teach anyone how to paint, act, sing, play, move or dance.
- The arts teacher focuses on aesthetic and artistic components of art-making, but for arts therapists such considerations are not of primary importance.
- Teaching focuses on specific learning outcomes; therapy focuses on inward processes.
- In arts teaching, the specific art forms are focal points; in arts therapies the clients are the subjects of attention.
- Arts teachers often use open spaces, while arts therapists need private spaces.
- Arts teachers work with large groups of pupils, while arts therapists work mainly on a one-to-one basis and/or with small groups.
- There are differences in training, qualifications and professional registration.

Further discussion about similarities and differences between arts therapies, and either arts education or therapeutic arts can be found in Karkou & Glasman (2004).

Arts therapies and other therapies

Psychotherapy and counselling

The relationship of arts therapies with counselling and psychotherapy is complex. As we have already described, two of the three main schools of thought within psychotherapy, psychoanalytic thinking and humanistic therapies, have played important roles in the emergence of arts therapies, and today they remain significant. Consequently there are a number of similarities in current practice between psychotherapy and arts therapies, which we will discuss in more depth in Chapter 4 and subsequent chapters. Briefly here we can say that psychotherapists practising within a psychoanalytic or object relations framework may use the arts as tools for accessing unconscious material or for understanding the client–therapist relationship. Within humanistic psychotherapies there is a strong emphasis upon self-expression and a high value placed on creativity, aspects also pertinent to arts therapies. However, in the majority of psychotherapeutic practices, when the arts are involved, they play a peripheral role to the main verbal emphasis of the work. It can be argued that, in comparison with arts therapies, verbal therapies give a similarly peripheral role to creativity, non-verbal communication and the value of 'doing' over 'talking'.

The length of basic training for practitioners in the two fields is also substantially different. Although attempts have been made to change the content and length of arts therapies training to match psychotherapeutic standards, currently the training for psychotherapists in the UK can be as long as 7 years, several more years than the minimum requirement for arts therapies qualifications, as the discussion in Chapter 1 confirmed. Such differences do not exist between some arts therapies training courses and those of counsellors; each is of a similar length. Furthermore, there are a number of arts therapists who also possess either counselling or psychotherapy qualifications. In our survey of arts therapies practitioners in the UK, more than 27% of arts therapists possessed such additional qualifications (see 'Training Courses' in Ch. 1).

Regarding professional development, separate registration is the norm for both psychotherapists and counsellors. These practitioners are eligible to register either with the UKCP (UK Chartered Psychotherapists) or the BACP (British Association for Counsellors and Psychotherapists). Unlike arts therapists their registers remain voluntary and as such neither their title nor the public are protected. Recently, negotiations have started between psychotherapy bodies and the HPC. If counsellors/psychotherapists come under HPC jurisdiction, a number of possibilities for cross-fertilisations across disciplines open up.

Body therapies

Body therapies cover a wide range of therapeutic interventions that can fall under a broad humanistic classification and have names such as bioenergetics, biofeedback, autogenic training, rebirthing and structural integration. Most of these therapies stem from the contribution of Reich to psychotherapy. Gestalt therapy may also be regarded as a form of body psychotherapy. Arts therapies present close links with some of these therapies. Reichian therapy, for example, is frequently reported as connected with the emergence of drama movement therapy (DMT). Gestalt therapy is often referred to within the drama therapy (DT) literature. Relaxation training for example is frequently used as an adjunct to arts therapies practice particularly with reference to DMT, DT and music therapy (MT). The main premise of body therapies, to re-address the body–mind connection and bridge the split between the two, is in philosophical alliance with the holistic rationale held by many arts therapists. However, following registration with the HPC, arts therapies have been established as a health profession and in consequence, close working relationships with body therapy practitioners have neither been sufficiently explored nor systematically encouraged. The new international journal on DMT and body psychotherapy (*Body, Movement, Dance in Psychotherapy*) to be published by the Taylor & Francis Group and co-edited by one of the authors of this book is expected to be one step closer towards strengthening the links between the two fields and identifying important differences.

Complementary/alternative therapies

Therapies such as acupuncture, Chinese herbalism, reflexology, Shiatsu and aromatherapy are based upon traditional healing practices and are currently gaining increased attention and respect amongst the general public. Although both arts therapies and these practices are often perceived as falling under the same umbrella of complementary or alternative approaches to medicine, there is a main difference between the two fields – that of origin. As we have already discussed, arts therapies are the product of a western society, while complementary/alternative therapies derive mainly from eastern healing practices. The rationale of these two fields is therefore fundamentally different with consequent differences in the way therapeutic work is understood and implemented. Further differences exist in terms of professional development, with arts therapies being more closely aligned to health professions.

Arts therapies and other health professions

When arts therapies were granted state registration in the UK within the National Health Service and the HPC took over the regulation of the field, arts therapies achieved parity with other health professions. The distinctive nature of arts therapies was also officially acknowledged through setting up a distinctive arts therapies board that was separate from other health professions. However, professional boundaries between arts therapies and other types of therapies are not always clear. For instance, there can be confusion over the relationship between arts therapies and occupational therapy in particular, as well as with physiotherapy or speech and language therapy.

Occupational therapy (OT)

The important role played by OT in the emergence of arts therapies in the UK has already been acknowledged in the previous chapter and in fact, the first state recognition of arts therapies in 1982 was within the realms of OT (Bunt 1994). Although arts therapies are currently recognised as separate professions, and there are increasing numbers of arts therapies units across the country, many arts therapists are still based within OT departments and under OT administration.

Misconceptions regarding professional boundaries between the two fields may also be due to similarities in subject matter. As Lloyd & Papas (1999) report, OT has a long tradition of using the arts in therapy. In the late 1950s, there was a strong trend within OT towards using the arts as diagnostic tools. Specific projective techniques were employed in order to gather information about underlying personality traits and structures. Over time, greater emphasis was placed on using the arts to develop the therapeutic relationship, self-awareness and communication (Lloyd & Papas 1999). However, according to the same authors, since the 1980s there has been a decline in the incidence of publications regarding the use of the arts within OT. The main reason for this is the separate development of the arts therapies profession. Occupational therapists are currently more reluctant to use the arts as therapy unless they have additional arts therapies training, which involves specific therapy skills and a psychological understanding of the use of the arts. Difference in *training* is therefore a first important difference between the two fields. Level of training is also different: for OT it is primarily at an undergraduate level, while for arts therapies it is at a postgraduate level.

Another important distinction between the two fields is that when the arts are used within OT they usually refer to structured *activities*. These activities are closely connected with very specific aims (e.g. the use of woodwork to increase muscle power). According to Atkinson & Wells (2000) activities form the basis of the work of occupational therapists. In arts therapies such preoccupation with activities does not exist; furthermore the term 'activities' can have derogative connotations, mainly because it suggests a high degree of direction imposed on the client by the professional. When highly structured activities are used, many arts therapists question the therapeutic value of the work. From an arts therapies perspective, the way the arts are used within OT does not refer to therapy but rather to a therapeutic use of the arts (see earlier discussion on arts therapies and therapeutic arts).

The *range and type of media* used also varies between the two modalities. Occupational therapists readily utilise a number of different media such as paper and paint, sound and rhythm, body and movement, clay and sculpture. Arts therapists on the other hand, often specialise in one art form; dance, music, drama or visual arts. Although arts therapists may also use mixed media when this is seen as appropriate, artistic expertise in their own speciality is of paramount importance. For occupational therapists, technical and artistic skills are not that important or furthermore, as Atkinson & Wells (2000) claim, they are 'neither necessary nor desirable' (p. 20).

The two modalities also differ on *contextual issues*. For example, OT often takes place in open spaces, while privacy is important for arts therapies in order to assure safety, and enable the development of the client–therapist relationship and/or group dynamics. Artefacts produced in OT are often destroyed after the completion of the task, while in arts therapies the client generally makes choices regarding end-products such as: who retains them (the client or the therapist) and whether they are shared with others outside the therapy session through, for instance, performance work or exhibitions.

In summary, some of the main differences that can be found between the two fields are:

- Differences in the level and type of training: OT requires primarily undergraduate and arts therapies always postgraduate training. The latter stresses both the artistic and psychotherapeutic aspects of the work to a degree that is not apparent in OT.
- Differences in the degree of direction and structure of the interventions; OT values activities and tends to be more structured than arts therapies.
- OT utilises a number of different media, while arts therapies are specialised in one specific type of art.
- OT uses open spaces, while in arts therapies, privacy is safeguarded.

■ In arts therapies any end-product of the therapy process is given very carefully consideration. Clients are often encouraged to make choices concerning what should happen to their artistic products on completion of the therapy. In OT, agreement exists beforehand that end-products will be eventually destroyed.

Physiotherapy

The focus on the body through physiotherapy and some types of arts therapies can be another source of confusion. For example, working alliances between physiotherapy and MT are extensively discussed by Bunt (1994), although the closest link is generally accorded to DMT. Payne (1992) claims that some of the main areas of overlap between DMT and physiotherapy are the following:

■ Both fields utilise movement exercises. In DMT such exercises might be part of the warm-up for instance, and can be seen from a holistic perspective as a means of mobilising the body and mind of the client. Physical responses to verbal stimuli are often the main emphases of the physiotherapist; movement is valued for its quantifiable qualities and is perceived in a fairly reductive way. In contrast, the dance movement therapist emphasises the qualitative aspects of movement and makes a number of connections: between movement and the overall well-being of the individual; between movement and the client–therapist dance or the group dance, and the type of relationship that they reflect.

■ Increasing the movement range might be a common aim of the two modalities, albeit for different reasons. While the physiotherapist focuses on physical health, the dance movement therapist regards physical well-being as a fair reflection of psychological health. The way such aims can be achieved is also different: the physiotherapist stresses increasing movement effort, while the dance movement therapist encourages the development of relevant imagery, symbolism and dance-like work as a means of achieving the same target.

Speech and language therapy

Finally, there is a potential overlap between arts therapies and speech and language therapy. Although the development of speech is the clear target of speech therapists, arts therapists working with children or adults with speech or other communication problems, may also contribute to the development of such skills. For example Bunt (1994) discusses how MT might prepare the ground for speech therapy through the development of prelinguistic skills such as vocalisation, articulation and intonation. Emphasis in arts therapies on non-verbal skills may develop motivation, awareness of self and others, and may also contribute towards listening, attention and concentration, all of which are important qualities for improving communication. Parallels between language development and artistic development are frequently referred to in the arts therapies literature (Bunt 1994, Dubowski 1990, Payne 1990). The two fields can work in a complementary way with arts therapists focusing more on preverbal and emotional issues surrounding communication, and speech and language therapists offering specialised interventions that target direct improvement of speech and language skills.

Although there are clear differences between arts therapies and other health professions, it is not unusual to find cooperation across these disciplines. Arts therapists often work with other health professionals within a multidisciplinary team context. Increased clarity of professional identity and boundaries will probably enable the arts therapist to enter the multidisciplinary dialogue with more confidence, and allow further collaborative endeavours between arts therapies and other health professions.

Definitions and descriptions found within arts therapies publications

So far we have established that arts therapies are different from therapeutic arts, arts education, other types of therapy and other health professions. In order to now define the field in its own terms we will turn to statements provided by arts therapies professional associations or arts therapies committees in the UK. Overall, there are very few attempts to define arts therapies as a whole, mainly due to the fact that professional effort has primarily been focused on defining separate disciplines (i.e. AT, MT, DT and DMT). An early attempt to describe the field as a whole comes from the Standing Committee for Arts Therapies Professions (1989, cited in Dokter 1994):

> Arts therapists provide for their patients an environment, arts media and very importantly, themselves – in terms of time, attention and a clearly defined relationship. The aim of the session or sessions is to develop a symbolic language which can provide access to unacknowledged feelings and a means of integrating them creatively into the personality, enabling therapeutic change to take place. The therapist's focus is not particularly on the aesthetic merits of the art work (be this dance, drama, painting, music, etc) but on the therapeutic process – that is, the patient's involvement in the work, their perception of it, and on the possibility of sharing this experience with the arts therapist (p. 3)

In the above description emphasis is given to the provision of the place, the artistic medium and the therapist's self in such a way that a client can engage in a therapeutic process and eventually achieve therapeutic change. It is interesting that there are also attempts to clarify differences from other fields (e.g. therapeutic arts) and alleviate potential misconceptions. References, for example, are made to the therapeutic process as more important than the aesthetic merits of the artwork produced within sessions.

Descriptions of the separate arts therapies have also been provided by the same Committee. These and current definitions of the arts therapies separate disciplines are included in Table 2.1.

Looking at these definitions closely, a number of issues become apparent: a prescription to one or more than one psychotherapeutic school of thought, the stronger or less strong emphasis upon the use of the art form central to each modality, and the different use of language over time. For example, the 1989 definition of AT emphasises facilitating the expression of 'unconscious' feelings through focusing on images which will subsequently be explored

Table 2.1: Definitions and descriptions of arts therapies 1989–2004

AT 1989	MT 1989	DT 1991	DMT 1989
'The focus of AT is the image, and the process involves a transaction between the creator (the patient), the artefact and the therapist. As in all therapies, bringing unconscious feelings to a conscious level and thereafter exploring them holds true for Art Therapy, but here the richness of artistic symbol and metaphor illuminates the process. . .' (Standing Committee for Arts Therapies Professions 1989, quoted by Waller & Dalley 1992, p. 4)	'. . . [MT provides] a framework for the building of a mutual relationship between client and therapist through which the music therapist will communicate with the client, finding a musical idiom . . . [which] . . . enables change to occur, both in the condition of the client and in the form the therapy takes. . .' (Standing Committee for Arts Therapies Professions 1989, Quoted by Gilroy & Lee 1995, p. 3)	'. . . the intentional (planned) use of the healing aspects of drama in the therapeutic process' (BADth 1991, cited by Meldrum 1994, p. 45)	'DMT is the use of expressive movement and dance as a vehicle through which an individual can engage in the process of personal integration and growth. It is founded on the principle that there is a relationship between motion and emotion and that by exploring a more varied vocabulary of movement, people experience the possibility of becoming more securely balanced yet increasingly spontaneous and adaptable . . . The dance movement therapist creates a holding environment in which such feelings can be safely expressed, acknowledged and communicated.' (Standing Committee for Arts Therapies Professions 1989, quoted by Payne 1992, p. 4)

2004	2004	2004	2004
'AT is the use of art materials for self-expression and reflection in the presence of a trained art therapist. . . The overall aim of its practitioners is to enable a client to effect change and growth on a personal level through the use of art materials in a safe and facilitating environment. The relationship between the therapist and the client is of central importance . . .' (BAAT 2004, p. 1)	'There are different approaches to the use of music in therapy . . . . Fundamental to all approaches, however, is the development of a relationship between the client and therapist. Music-making forms the basis for communication in this relationship . . .' (BSMT 2004, p. 1)	'DT has as its main focus the intentional use of healing aspects of drama and theatre as the therapeutic process. It is a method of working and playing that uses action methods to facilitate creativity, imagination, learning, insight and growth.' (BADth 2004, p. 1)	'DMT is the psychotherapeutic use of movement and dance through which a person can engage creatively in a process to further their emotional, cognitive, physical and social integration.' (ADMT UK 2004, p. 1)

(Table 2.1). The centrality of the unconscious processes gives a strong indication of the importance attached to psychoanalytic and psychodynamic psychotherapy. However, this same psychoanalytic language is not retained in the latest description of AT from the British Association of Arts Therapists (BAAT) Reference to the image as central to AT practice is now extended to include the artefact, while diversity of theoretical stances is explicitly acknowledged: 'AT is a diverse profession. . .' (BAAT 2004, p. 1) (see Box 2.1).

Box 2.1: Changes in AT definitions and descriptions

1989: utilising psychoanalytic/ psychodynamic language/ thinking

2004: accepting diversity of approaches and theoretical bases

---

A similar change of emphasis is apparent in the two MT definitions/descriptions presented (Table 2.1). For example, although both descriptions/definitions acknowledge the central role of the needs of the client, the first MT definition refers to a 'mutual' relationship as important to the process. 'Mutuality' suggests an equal relationship in which both client and therapist are fully engaged in the process with their whole selves. This type of therapeutic relationship can easily refer to the idea of the 'real' relationship advocated by humanistic psychotherapists. We therefore see this first definition of MT as presenting a bias towards a humanistic rationale that is not apparent in the latest definition of the field. A diversity of approaches (and consequently types of relationships) is currently accepted as a feature of the MT field. Similarly, searching for a 'musical idiom' is acknowledged within the first definition of MT as an important part of the MT process. In the latest definition the 'musical idiom' is substituted with a number of examples of musical techniques that may be found within MT sessions. In summary, the latest description is less precise and therefore, more open to different MT approaches (see Box 2.2).

The healing aspects of drama are highlighted in the first definition of DT presented in Table 2.1. DT is seen as the intentional use of such healing qualities. However, this definition is particularly brief and general, raising questions about the content of the therapeutic process and the outcome of the therapy. It also raises questions about which aspects of drama are healing and whether there could be other aspects which may be less healing and/or even damaging. The current official definition of DT is not dissimilar to the 1991 version. The healing aspects of drama are still highlighted but there is more information about the aims of the work; DT is regarded as facilitating cre-

---

Box 2.2: Changes in MT definitions and descriptions

1989: humanistic connotations, references to specific theoretical bases

2004: accepting diversity of approaches and practices

---

ativity, imagination, learning, insight and growth. There is also more information about the art form. There are references to the use of action methods, while theatre has been added to drama as a potential therapeutic technique. However, the field is described as a method rather than as a type of therapy, something that is a significant departure from other definitions such as the following:

> Drama Therapy, like the other creative arts therapies (art, music and dance), is the application of a creative medium to psychotherapy. Specifically, Drama Therapy refers to those activities in which there is an established therapeutic understanding between client and therapist and where the therapeutic goals are primary and not incidental to the ongoing activity (Johnson 1982, p. 83)

This definition was devised by Johnson (1982), and it originated in the USA (note: in the USA, DT is represented by two distinct words 'drama therapy', whereas in the UK a single word 'dramatherapy' is more usual). In this definition, arts therapies in general, and DT in particular, are interpreted as the application of a creative medium to psychotherapy. Regarding arts therapies as a form of psychotherapy is a prevailing view in American practice. Despite its American origins, this definition has also been fairly popular among British dramatherapists. For example, it has been used by the British DT professional association (BADth) in their application for state registration as a health profession in the UK (Jenkyns & Barham 1991 cited by Meldrum 1994). In summary, it appears that there are different ways in which DT can be defined; currently both artistic and psychotherapeutic definitions co-exist in parallel (Box 2.3).

The DMT case presents a slightly different picture (Table 2.1). For example, there are differences between older and current definitions in the emphasis placed upon the therapeutic relationship. In the 1989 description of the field, the therapeutic relationship is not acknowledged. It is the engagement in expressive dance and movement that is important. Several 'movement-related' principles are also mentioned such as the motion–emotion connection, the increased range of movement having a positive impact on the clients' personality balance, spontaneity and adaptability, and the benefits that movement experiences bring to the clients' inner world, personal symbolism and relationships. Although the therapist is regarded as offering a 'holding environment' for the expression and exploration of feelings, the major emphasis of the process and the main agent for therapeutic change remains the engagement with the movement/dance.

Box 2.3: Changes in DT definitions and descriptions

	2004: healing aspects of drama and theatre (official)
1991: healing aspects of drama	or
	2004: a type of psychotherapy (unofficial)

It is interesting that the latest attempts to re-define DMT in the UK, initiated by ADMT UK (the DMT association) (Table 2.1), echo an American understanding of the field. DMT is seen as the psychotherapeutic use of movement and dance. This is almost a complete turning away from the earlier DMT definition that emphasised the artistic aspects of the work. At the moment DMT is the only art therapy in the UK that officially ties itself so closely to psychotherapy. It is possible that DMT, which is currently seeking wider recognition as a health profession, is tightening its focus and aligning itself with the more established field of psychotherapy, a stage that AT and MT went through earlier in their development (e.g. during the 1980s as their 1989 definitions suggest). The changes that have taken place within DMT regarding definitions/descriptions of this modality are summarised in Box 2.4.

Box 2.4: Changes in DMT descriptions and definitions

1989: emphasis on movement/dance   *2004*: utilising psychotherapeutic language

Our definition of arts therapies

The debate about whether or not arts therapies are primarily forms of psychotherapy or artistic modalities is ongoing, as are the attempts to successfully define the arts therapies field. Figure 2.1 illustrates our understanding of the range of existing arts therapies definitions regarding the arts–psychotherapy continuum.

Arts therapies definitions vary from those that regard the field as a type of applied arts with selected concepts borrowed from psychotherapy, to those that see it as a type of psychotherapy with the addition of the arts. As a type of applied arts, the artistic modality plays an important role and inputs from the art world and artistic traditions are highlighted. The theatre model in DT (see Ch. 7) and the creative MT approach (Ch. 5) are good examples of arts therapies practices firmly rooted within the arts. As a type of psychotherapy, arts therapies largely borrow concepts or adopt whole frameworks from existing schools of psychotherapy in order to offer justifications and/or explanations for their work and/or guide practices. Arts therapists who regard their work as a type of psychotherapy, may call their practice art, music, drama or dance 'psychotherapy'. Arts psychotherapy has not been adequately charted, but as the title suggests, arts therapists who prefer to refer to their work with this name either have come out of an arts psychotherapy training as is the case with some of the courses in AT (e.g. Goldsmith's College offers an arts psychotherapy programme) or have completed psychotherapeutic training in addition to their arts therapies training (e.g. Payne 1996/1997). Examples of this type of arts therapies practice with strong psychotherapeutic focus can be found in Section 2 of this book in all discipline-specific chapters.

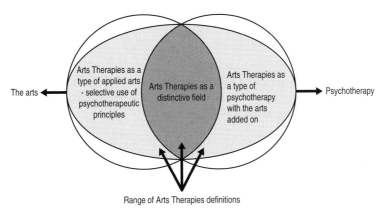

Figure 2.1: *Range of arts therapies definitions.*

Within the descriptions and definitions discussed earlier, diversity is acknowledged as an important feature of the field, either explicitly (as with MT and AT current definitions) or implicitly (as in the presence of a number of definitions in DT). This follows a wider sociological trend towards accepting diversity, strongly advocated by post-modern thinkers (Gergen 1991, Grentz 1996, Lyotard 1984) and endorsed by a number of arts therapists (e.g. Best 2000, Byrne 1995). However, within this diversity we believe that there are a number of commonalties binding the field together, even if this is done in a fairly loose way. These commonalties define the field as a distinctive profession and, while not departing entirely from either the arts or psychotherapy, attach a fairly unique character to arts therapies. Common factors may be found in the overlap between psychotherapy and the arts. Some of the common themes, revealed in the descriptions and definitions presented in Table 2.1 include:

- the use of the artistic medium, in terms of the image (AT), the music idiom (MT), the movement and/or dance (DMT) and the dramatic or theatrical structure (DT), as a vehicle for non-verbal communication
- facilitation of a trusting, safe environment in which creative processes can take place
- the pertinence of imagery, symbols and metaphors within the therapeutic process
- focus on non-verbal communication
- the establishment of a client–therapist relationship, interpreted as a transaction between client–artefact–therapist (AT), a relationship via music-making (MT), a supportive therapist and a self-responsible individual (DMT), or an established therapeutic understanding (DT)
- the pursuit of therapeutic aims. These may be very individually-based (MT), refer to change and growth (AT) or to personal and social integration (DMT), but therapeutic aims are always primary and not incidental to the ongoing activity (DT).

Based on the important themes outlined above, we suggest a new definition for the field, which is given in Box 2.5.

> **Box 2.5:** Definition of arts therapies
>
> Arts therapies are the creative use of the artistic media as vehicles for non-verbal and/or symbolic communication, within a holding environment, encouraged by a well-defined client–therapist relationship, in order to achieve personal and/or social therapeutic goals appropriate for the individual.

Summary

Similarities and differences between arts therapies and a number of neighbouring fields have been identified in order to clarify ambiguities and eliminate misconceptions. For example, arts therapies were discussed as different from the therapeutic arts and arts education; both of these fields played important roles during the early days of the arts therapies profession. Similarly, arts therapies were presented as different from psychotherapy and counselling, areas that still remain particularly influential upon arts therapies practice. Finally, although arts therapies are currently regarded as health professions, some of their differences from other health professions were outlined, for example in relation to occupational therapy, physiotherapy and speech and language therapy.

In order to define the field as a whole the definitions and description articulated by each of the four arts therapies professional associations have been presented and discussed. Important changes over time were highlighted, current tendencies were outlined and common themes were extracted. We believe that the definition we offer is, on the one hand, specific enough to distinguish the field from any other neighbouring fields and clarify professional identity, and on the other, generic enough to embrace all the different types of work found within arts therapies. In the following chapter some of the important themes upon which this definition is based will be presented and discussed in more depth.

References

* Association for Dance Movement Therapy (ADMT UK) 2004 What is DMT? Online. Available: http://www.admt.org.uk/whatis.html 11 Dec 2004
* Atkinson K, Wells C 2000 Creative therapies: a psychodynamic approach within occupational therapy. Stanley Thornes, Cheltenham
* Attenborough Report 1985 Arts and disabled people. Carnegie UK Trust, London
* Best P 2000 Theoretical diversity and clinical collaboration: reflections by a dance/movement therapist, The Arts in Psychotherapy 27(3):197–211
* British Association of Art Therapists (BAAT) 2004 What is art therapy? Online. Available: http://www.baat.org/art_therapy.html 11 Dec 2004
* British Association of Dramatherapists (BADth) 2004 About dramatherapy. Online. Available: http://www.badth.org.uk/therapy.html 11 Dec 2004
* British Society for Music Therapy (BSMT) 2004 What is music therapy? Online. Available: http://www.bsmt.org/what_is_mt.html 11 Dec 2004
* Bunt L 1994 Music therapy: an art beyond words. Routledge, London
* Byrne P 1995 From the depths to the surface: art therapy as a discursive practice in the post-modern era, The Arts in Psychotherapy 22(3):235–239
* Case C 1996 On the aesthetic moment in the transference. Inscape 1(2):39–45

- Dokter D 1994 Introduction. In: Dokter D (ed.) Arts therapies and clients with eating disorders: fragile board. Jessica Kingsley, London, p 1–4
- Dubowski J 1990 Art versus language: separate development during childhood. In: Case C, Dalley T (eds) Working with children in art therapy. Tavistock/Routledge, London, p 7–22
- Gergen K J 1991 The saturated self. Basic Books, New York
- Gilroy A, Lee C 1995 Juxtapositions in art therapy and music therapy research. In: Gilroy A, Lee C (eds) Art and music: therapy and research. Routledge, London, p 1–20
- Grentz S 1996 A primer on postmodernism. William B Eermans, Grand Rapids, MI
- Health Development Agency (HDA) 2000 Art for health: a review of good practice in community-based arts projects and initiatives which impact on health and wellbeing. Health Development Agency, London
- Johnson D R 1982 Principles and techniques of drama therapy. The Arts in Psychotherapy 9:83–90
- Jordan L 1988 A comparison between the aims and objectives of the dance therapist and the dance educationalist. Unpublished MEd dissertation, University of Manchester, UK
- Karkou V 1999 Art therapy in education: findings from a nation-wide survey in arts therapies. Inscape 4(2):62–70
- Karkou V, Glasman J 2004 Arts, education and society: the role of the arts in promoting the emotional well-being and social inclusion of young people. Support for Learning 19(2): 56–64
- Karkou V, Sanderson P 1997 Dance movement therapy approaches with particular reference to children with special needs. In: Anttila E (ed.) Proceedings of the 1997 (7th) Conference of Dance and the Child international (daCi), The Call of Forests and Lakes, Kuopio, Finland
- Karkou V, Sanderson P 2001a Dance movement therapy in the UK: a field emerging from dance education. European Physical Education Review 7(2):137–155
- Karkou V, Sanderson P 2001b Report: theories and assessment procedures used by dance movement therapists in the UK. The Arts in Psychotherapy. 28:13–20
- Lloyd C, Papas V 1999 Art as therapy within occupational therapy in mental health settings: a review of the literature. British Journal of Occupational Therapy 62(1):31–35
- Lyotard J F 1984 The postmodern condition. Manchester University Press, Manchester
- Maclagan D 2001 Psychological aesthetics: painting, feeling and making sense. Jessica Kingsley, London
- Meier W 1997 The teacher and the therapist. E-motion ADMT UK Quarterly IX(1):7–9
- Meldrum B 1994 Historical background and overview of dramatherapy. In: Jennings S, Cattanach A, Mitchell S et al (eds) The handbook of dramatherapy. Routledge, London, p 12–27
- Payne H 1990 Creative movement and dance in groupwork. Winslow, Oxon
- Payne H 1992 Introduction. In: Payne H (ed.) Dance movement therapy: theory and practice. Tavistock/Routledge, London, p 1–17
- Payne H 1996/1997 Definition of DMT (letter). ADMT Newsletter VIII(4):18
- Peter M 1998 'Good for them, or what?' The arts and pupils with SEN. British Journal of Special Education 25(4):168–172
- Qualifications and Curriculum Authority (QCA) 2004 National curriculum. Online. Available: http://www.nc.uk.net/index.html 11 Dec 2004
- Sanderson P 1984 Dance, art and aesthetics. Physical Education Review 7(2):160–164
- Sanderson P 1996a Dance within the national PE curriculum of England and Wales. The European Physical Education Review 2(1):54–63
- Sanderson P 1996b Physical education and dance. In: Piotrowski J (ed.) The expressive arts in primary schools. Special Needs in Ordinary Schools Series. Cassell, London, p 65–98
- Sanderson P 2002 An appreciation of the life of Irene Dilks, dancer and educator. Research in Dance Education 2(1): 103–105
- Sanderson P, Savva A 2004 Artists in Cypriot primary schools: the pupils' perspective. Music Education Research 6(1): 1–21
- Schaverien J 2000 The triangular relationship and the aesthetic countertrasference in analytic art psychotherapy. In: Gilroy A, McNeilly G (eds) The changing shape of art therapy: new developments in theory and practice. Jessica Kingsley, London, p 55–83
- Stanton-Jones K 1992 An introduction to dance movement therapy in psychiatry. Tavistock/Routledge, London
- Valente L 1991 Therapeutic drama and psychological health: an examination of theory and practice in dramatherapy. Unpublished PhD thesis, University of Wales, College of Cardiff, UK

- Valente L, Fontana D 1991 Dramatherapy and psychological change. In: Wilson G D (ed.) Psychology and performing arts. Swets, Amsterdam, p 121–131
- Waller D 1991 Becoming a profession: the history of art therapy in Britain 1940–1982. Tavistock/Routledge, London
- Waller D 1992 Different things to different people: art therapy in Britain – a brief survey of its history and current development. The Arts in Psychotherapy 19:87–92
- Waller D, Dalley T 1992 Art therapy: a theoretical perspective. In: Waller D, Gilroy A (eds) Art therapy: a handbook. Open University Press, Buckingham, p 3–24
- Warwick A 1995 Music therapy in the education service: research with autistic children and their mothers In: Wigram T, Saperston B, West R (eds) The art and science of music therapy: a handbook. Harwood Academic Publications, Switzerland, p 209–225

Chapter 3

Important Features of Arts Therapies

Key issues:

- There are a number of assumptions associated with the use of the arts within arts therapies, such as the lack of emphasis upon the artistic or aesthetic qualities, focus on process rather than outcome, the belief that the arts address preverbal levels of functioning, and the concept of a person as a whole being. The belief in the therapeutic potential of the arts is also discussed.

- The concept of creativity is highly regarded amongst arts therapists as contributing towards therapeutic transformation. The meaning of creativity is explored and ways of facilitating creative processes within arts therapies are mentioned.

- Arts therapies rely heavily upon non-verbal communication. This type of communication can take place on three levels: internal, dyadic and group.

- Imagery, symbolism, metaphors, and the artistic medium per se constitute the content of non-verbal communication. Additional information is gained through looking at how images, symbols and so on, are created. The 'how' often provides important information about relational aspects.

- The client–therapist relationship within arts therapies often takes the form of a triangular relationship with the arts at the third corner of this triangle. Many variations of this relationship can be found within arts therapies practice.

- Arts therapists' aims vary in terms of intended depth of intervention and type of issues targeted; the specific needs of the client often determine the selection of aims.

Introduction

Because we are describing arts therapies as a distinctive field from other neighbouring professional areas, it is important to look more closely at the special features that make the field unique. For example, in the previous chapter we identified some important aspects of arts therapies definitions such as the role of the arts, creativity, imagery, symbolism and metaphor, non-verbal communication, the client–therapist relationship and therapeutic aims. Given their relevance to the arts therapies field, in this chapter we will discuss these concepts in more depth, attempting to unfold their meaning, and present some of their uses within arts therapies. For the discussion of these concepts we draw primarily upon the arts therapies literature, although at times, we also make references to relevant sources in the arts, psychotherapy or psychology.

Assumptions about the role of the arts within arts therapies

There are a number of assumptions surrounding the use of the arts within arts therapies. Some of them have been raised in the previous chapter, especially when discussing differences between arts therapies and other modalities. The most important of these assumptions are that:

- a wide definition for the word 'arts' is retained
- attention shifts from the artistic product to the process of art-making
- engagement in the arts develops on a preverbal level
- every art modality involves the person as a whole, including sensori-motor, perceptual, cognitive, emotional, social and spiritual aspects
- the arts have a healing or therapeutic potential.

Retaining a wide definition for the word 'arts'

Music-making, for instance, may refer to repetitive banging on a drum and loud chaotic use of instruments, as well as to pieces of music with attractive tonal colour, clear duration (pulse or rhythm) and defined dynamics or structure. Artwork may refer to scribbling as well as to something with a defined pattern or interesting texture. Dance may be about a minimal gesture, a foot movement or 'jerky' uncoordinated movement, as well as a highly choreographed piece that involves the whole body, a range of actions or clear use of space.

'Permission' to widen the definition of the arts has been granted to arts therapies by initiatives such as 'arts for all' and 'arts for health' as we have already seen, as well as by numerous movements in the wider artistic community. Halprin (2003), for example, argues that with modernism, there was a first shift from stylised to more natural artistic expressions: the impressionists emphasised light; Klee, Kandinsky and Picasso emphasized line and shape; the surrealists stressed automatic expression; Isadora Duncan introduced natural movement as a new way of looking at dance; and later on the composer John Cage experimented with random sound and silence. With the emergence of postmodernism, grand narratives including 'high art' (i.e. what is often associated with classical arts) have become even more questionable and have encouraged, yet again, the development of new definitions of what the arts stand for. Diversity and difference have been valued and emphasis has been placed upon the significance of the context within which new definitions can be formulated.

Within an arts therapies context, the wide definitions with which the arts have been used, have allowed for a range of actions to be considered as 'artistic', while artistic/aesthetic value judgments are removed and consequently pressures to create something 'good' are withdrawn. With such an understanding of the meaning of the word 'arts', the level of skill becomes irrelevant – all can make music, draw, act or dance – while engagement in the artistic process is encouraged.

Shifting attention from the artistic product to the process of art-making

The emphasis during an arts therapies session is not just on what has been produced, but also how it has been produced. Although an end-product may convey interesting information about the artist/client, the arts therapist's interest expands to also attend to the meaning of the process of art making. Clients will be encouraged to adopt a similar attitude.

Similarly to the previous assumption, focusing on process over product challenges the notion that engagement with the arts is open only to the gifted few. According to the dramatherapist Landy (2001), while producing high quality artistic products is the domain of the artists, the process of art-making is democratic and therefore available to everyone. Even from within the arts world, and postmodernism in particular, the primacy of the artistic product is questioned in favour of the artistic process and spontaneous expressions. One such example can be found in the American avant-garde performance art, where art events in the form of happenings attempted to bridge the gap between art and daily life (Halprin 2003).

In a similar way as performance art focused on the mundane and common objects as part of the art event, in arts therapies, everyday human expressions (e.g. sounds, gestures, colours or shapes) can become part of the artistic process. And as with many other art-making processes, these expressions do not always develop into a final artistic product. Within arts therapies therefore, the arts may or may not refer to complete arts products.

Regarding engagement in the arts as developing on a preverbal level

Arts therapists believe that the capacity for art-making begins to develop before verbal skills and as such, early arts experiences, in an audio, movement or visual form, are stored in each one of us as preverbal memories and are carried throughout our adult lives (Payne 1990). Artistic expression is therefore, seen as a manifestation of deeper hidden structures, a means of accessing personal and/or cultural history that would not be available through verbal means. With the capacity of artwork to communicate meaning that originates from the depths of human existence, arts therapies become an appropriate intervention for a number of clients who would not necessarily receive as many benefits from other therapies. For example, arts therapies become useful for clients who may be highly verbal (and may hide behind words) or have limited verbal skills (and are therefore difficult to reach verbally). Although, when possible, both verbal and non-verbal communication is encouraged as a way of acquiring new and more comprehensive understandings of what is being expressed, the arts remain highly valued as agents of deep personal meaning.

Every art modality involves the person as a whole, including sensori-motor, perceptual, cognitive, emotional, social and spiritual aspects

Or as Bruscia (1988) put it, the arts reflect 'multifaceted dimensions of human experience'. This idea is consistent with the belief in the body–mind connection and holistic perspectives to therapy. It is also in accordance with the belief that growth within the arts is a sign of growth in the person as a whole. Arts therapists, therefore, place confidence in changes in art-making and/or arts products as important sources of information about therapeutic change. Given the multiplicity of human experience that is reflected through the arts, understanding the meaning of the arts within therapy becomes particularly complex. Unfolding these experiences and making meaningful connections is a major part of the work undertaken within arts therapies.

The arts have a healing or therapeutic potential

The role of the arts as a healing/therapeutic agent is a highly debated idea amongst health professionals. Unlike beliefs shared by some members of the medical profession for example, arts therapists rarely regard finished art products as a type of medicine that may alleviate pain, whether physical or emotional. Similarly, unlike beliefs held by, for example, some practitioners in therapeutic arts, arts therapists do not regard mere participation in art-making as sufficient for therapeutic change, nor art-making on its own as sufficient to describe their work as 'therapy'. Still, arts therapists in the UK have faith in the arts as having an important healing role to play within therapy. They believe however that art-making needs to be contextually located. They see art-making as a process that, given the circumstances surrounding its use, may become a powerfully positive or powerfully destructive force. The way the arts are used is a crucial factor that determines whether or not therapeutic transformation can occur. 'Therapeutic potential' rather than a universal and acontextual 'healing power' is largely attributed to the arts within the arts therapies field.

Creativity

The concept of 'creativity' is central to arts therapies. It is so central that arts therapies are often referred to by the generic term: 'creative arts therapies'. However, creativity is a complex concept that has generated a great deal of debate, theoretical exploration and psychological experimentation. What follows here is an outline of some ideas that are relevant to understanding the *concept* of creativity within arts therapies. Further discussion of creativity, and the *creative process* in particular, can be found in the next chapter (see 'The Artistic/Creative Trend' in Ch. 4).

Earlier psychotherapeutic literature did not seem to place as much value on creativity as more recent psychotherapists and arts therapists tend to do. Freud (1953) for example, regarded creativity as a form of neurosis or obsession, which attempts to compensate for inadequacies of personality and unresolved inner conflicts. Creativity, according to Freud, is something similar to daydreams or fantasies disguised to cover frustrations, unfulfilled wishes or unhappiness. Some contemporary psychoanalysts may continue to perceive creativity as a defence mechanism. However, overall, the negative connotations associated with creativity are reduced: creativity is now perceived as a useful defence mechanism that protects the 'self' against overwhelming feelings. Thus, a degree of control may be retained, while access to difficult unconscious material becomes possible. Other psychotherapists diverge even further from Freudian thinking. For instance:

- Winnicott (1971) values creativity as an indicator of mental health. He perceives his work as dealing with individuals who have lost 'the creative entry into life'
- for Rogers (1961), creativity is the emergence in action of a novel relational product, growing out of the uniqueness of the individual
- for Fromm (1959), it is the ability to see (or be aware) and to respond
- for May (1975), creativity is the process of bringing something into birth.

Although these perspectives highlight different aspects of creativity, all of them attach a positive interpretation to the meaning of the word. Creativity is seen as an expression of emotional health and maturity rather than as a sign of pathology as Freudian writings might suggest.

Our definition of creativity is presented in Box 3.1. This definition suggests that creativity refers to something new. However, unlike beliefs for the need of something entirely original, 'newness' is based on what is already there: the discovery of new connections, new relationships and new meanings. Understanding creativity in this way makes it useful for therapy work and arts therapies work in particular. First of all, it makes creativity a useful concept for arts therapies because it can become relevant to all aspects of life. Moreover, it makes it relevant to all individuals. Jung's (1961) understanding of creativity can help us unfold these ideas further.

Jung (1961) has argued that there are two types of creativity: the 'psychological' and the 'visionary'. The psychological comes from the realms of human consciousness and as such, reflects our environment. It is the creativity of the musician who plays a sonata written by Bach and that of the painter who records a landscape. The visionary aspects of creativity, however, come from the depths of human existence. According to Jung (1961) visionary creativity is not something all individuals are likely to achieve but only the talented few.

Although Jung has had a great impact upon arts therapies, the above typology of creativity can be strongly criticised. For example, the assumption that

Box 3.1: Definition of creativity (adapted from Stanton-Jones 1992 and Smitskamp 1995)

Creativity is the capacity to find new and unexpected connections, new relationships and therefore new meanings.

conscious art-making is equivalent to 'psychological' creativity cannot always be supported. Within an arts therapies context, the arts can be used both as a way of making something new, as well as something that follows formulaic styles and reproduces as closely as possible pre-existing art forms. For example, a client may attempt to copy an existing painting/song focusing on the correct style of the art genre. Another client may spend a number of arts therapies sessions reproducing the same drawing or movement over and over again. If the arts are used in the latter way, they are not equivalent to creativity; 'newness' is not demonstrated.

The implication of referring to creative and non-creative uses of the arts is that the meaning of the word 'creativity' becomes broader than that of 'the arts'. It is indeed common to refer to creativity as something that can be traced in bodies of knowledge outside the arts (e.g. in the sciences) as well as everyday life (e.g. in gardening, cooking and other leisure pursuits). Within an arts therapies context, acquiring such a broad definition for the word creativity can translate to clients also becoming creative in other parts of their lives beyond the arts and beyond the therapeutic session. Once their creativity is mobilised, clients can become creative in the way they perceive themselves, run their own lives and/or relate to others.

From an arts therapies perspective, Jung's second type of creativity, the 'visionary' creativity, can also be debated. This idea can be seen as elitist and as clashing with the belief in the democratisation of the arts to which, as we have already seen, arts therapists subscribe. Getting in touch with the depths of human existence is an aspect of arts therapies work that does not require exceptional artistic talents. Questioning elitist ideas of creativity means that, at least as far as arts therapies are concerned, creativity is a capacity which, when appropriately cultivated, can be demonstrated in varying degrees by all.

In contrast to the Jungian typology of creativity, the idea introduced by May (1975), that it takes a great deal of courage to be creative, is particularly relevant to arts therapies. According to May (1975), courage is necessary in order to 'let go' of existing inner boundaries and so be free to make something new. Accepting the limitations of one's own thinking process is not easy, letting go of old beliefs and values can be risky. As such, special attention is needed to mobilise creativity in a way that remains safe for the individuals involved. Our understanding of creativity, as defined above, suggests that using what is already known and familiar is essential for the new to emerge and is an important safeguard for clients. Existing building blocks are not to be abandoned but reviewed and reconnected in new ways. The arts therapist's task is to prepare the ground for the process to start and then to facilitate the continuation of this process. According to Malchiodi (1998), creativity is mobilised within arts therapies by providing a safe environment and a non-judgemental atmosphere. It also requires a clear intention to make something and draws heavily upon openness, spontaneity and playfulness (Malchiodi 1998).

Creativity is also closely linked with important psychological functions such as imagery and fantasy, symbolism and metaphor. These concepts are particularly relevant and extensively used within arts therapies practice, as we will see in the following section.

Imagery, symbolism and metaphor

Imagery, symbolism and metaphor are concepts that are highly valued by a number of different arts therapists with diverse orientations. However, they are often used without clear definitions of what they stand for. Our understanding of these terms and some of their uses within arts therapies is as follows.

Imagery often refers to a cluster of images, i.e. objects or events, as the definition in Box 3.2 describes. According to this definition, imagery takes place within the boundaries of an individual body ('inner representation') in the absence of an actual stimulus (i.e. imagery is created 'at will'). The starting point for creating these inner representations can be traced back to the person's senses. Imagery can therefore be seen as being multimodal in that it may have, for example, a visual, audio and/or kinaesthetic character. Furthermore, in the same way as primary imagery is facilitated by the interaction with the primary carer and the environment, exposure to arts material and other artistic stimuli can facilitate this process further, i.e. activate the person's awareness of existing inner representation of 'objects' and 'events' or create new inner representation of 'objects' and 'events'.

When imagery is dealt with in association with other mental processes such as emotions, thoughts, memories and wishes then imagination comes into action. In general, images/imagery are perceived as the raw material of imagination. Or as Gordon (1987), a Jungian dramatherapist, has put it, imagery relates to imagination in the same way as photographs and still pictures relate to the moving picture, the film.

According to the same author, imagination has two characteristics: (1) It allows the individual to look at, experience and enjoy his or her inner 'film'. (2) Similar to watching a movie, the person may also critically assess the products of his or her imagination in terms of fact, reality, truth, consistency and so on. These two characteristics make imagination different from other psychological processes. For example, the ability of the individual to take a critical stance, while imagining, makes this process different from hallucinations; hallucinating does not allow for critical self-assessment. Imagination is also different from fantasy. Despite the fact that both address unconscious aspects of the self and allow explorations into the unknown, imagination – more than fantasy – also incorporates conscious, cognitive thinking. Thus, bridges are built between the conscious and the unconscious, the known and the unknown and this results in creating unifying experiences for the individual.

Although a number of therapeutic approaches acknowledge the value of imagination (e.g. Jungian therapy, psycho-imagination therapy, eidetic psychotherapy) and several others use imagery within their practice as a useful

---

Box 3.2: Definition of imagery (adapted from Walrond-Skinner 1986)

Imagery often refers to inner representations of objects and events created at will.

technique (e.g. cognitive therapies and systematic desensitisation), within arts therapies, imagery and imagination are placed in the centre of the therapeutic process. For example, with clients who tend to stay in the fantasy world, the arts therapies process may involve altering fantasy into imagination through highlighting critical self-assessment. For clients who are stuck and unable to imagine, the arts therapist can offer help in the form of introducing gradual steps. For example, Dosamantes-Alperson (1981), an American dance movement therapist, talks about such steps in order to activate kinetic imagination. Similar processes can take place with other artistic media (if other artistic media are concerned, in the following list references to the body and physical experiences can be substituted with auditory/musical experiences or visual/artistic experiences):

1. becoming receptive (the person needs to be relaxed and to pay attention to internal events)
2. focusing on the body as a whole, identifying subtle sensory feelings and discriminating between experiences (in other words, paying attention to the body and looking at subtle clues)
3. matching the physical experience with images (images can be selected on the basis of sharing some of the qualities of the physical experience)
4. following the emergent physical-image interaction (i.e. unfolding imagery and crystallising content)
5. making obvious the salient features of the interaction between the body and the image through movement as well as through subsequent articulation of aspects of this experience through words.

The experience of expressing one's imagination during physical work or any other art-making process and the ability to self-assess the products of this process (e.g. artistic products) allow for new meaning to emerge and changes to take place. The links between imagination and creativity are apparent (see definition of creativity in the previous section as the capacity to make new connections and find new meanings; this capacity is increased through activating imaginative processes). There are also close links between imagery/imagination and internal communication, as we will see in the following section.

Symbolism and metaphor are other important concepts central to the arts therapies practice and are often used interchangeably within associated literature. However, they refer to slightly different processes. Symbolism for example is often defined as the representation of an idea or a wish by something else (Box 3.3).

The definition presented in Box 3.3 reveals two processes: (1) creating representations of something else because of the similar qualities shared

> **Box 3.3:** Definition of symbolism (Walrond-Skinner 1986, p. 338)
>
> Symbolism is the representation of an . . . idea or wish . . . by something else that either possesses analogous qualities or comes to stand for this idea or wish due to consistent associations.

between the representation and the thing represented (e.g. a wavy line may represent sea water because its shape looks like sea water, a drawing of a picture of a person to represent this person, the sound of a cat to stand for a cat, etc) and (2) representing an idea or wish which has nothing to do with the thing they represent (e.g. a flag standing for a nation, a pair of scales that represents the concept of justice, a star standing for the concept of self, a fist gesture standing for power or a loud sound for anger, etc).

In the arts therapies literature, a number of different frameworks are used to offer further explanations of the role of symbolism within practice. For example, Pavlicevic (1997), a music therapist, refers to the field of semiotics and discusses the arts in arts therapies as 'signs'. Saussure (1969), the founder of semiotics, argues that a 'sign' consists of the signifier (i.e. representation) and the signified (i.e. the thing represented). In the first process described above (i.e. creating representations with similar qualities to what is represented), the sign is known as the 'icon', and in the second process (representations of something that does not share similar qualities) as the 'symbol'. Schaverien (2000) discusses similar symbolic processes in relation to pictures created within an AT context. She refers for example to 'diagrammatic' and 'embodied' pictures. In the former type there is a one-to-one link between the picture and what it represents, while in the latter, the meaning of the picture is rich and unexpected. We see the former type of artwork as an example of an icon, while the latter as an example of a symbol.

However, not all types of artistic expression are necessarily symbolic. According to the field of semiotics, there is a third type of sign that can become relevant to the use of the arts within arts therapies: signs as 'index' (Pavlicevic 1997). In this case, the arts can have a direct and natural effect, can create an 'organic pair', without necessarily representing anything else (e.g. a scribble created without any reference outside itself, a sound made merely for making it, moving for its own sake, etc). While in the first two cases (i.e. the case of an icon and the case of a symbol) symbolic action takes place, in the case of the arts as index, symbolic processes cannot be claimed. For example, with people with severe learning difficulties, artistic exploration might stand for a mere sensation of moving the body, playing with the material or creating sounds. In this case, the arts are used primarily as index.

Within an arts therapies context, the arts can therefore be seen as concrete objects that are created as part of a symbolic process and get expressed as icons or symbols as well as non-symbolic objects, i.e. as index. In all cases, semioticians claim that the meaning of the arts as signs is created within a cultural context and due to cultural conventions, and may reflect structures underlying the society from which they originate. As Pavlicevic (1997) argues, in arts therapies, meaning can also be entirely personal and may reflect internal psychological structures. We can add that their meaning can also reflect the quality of the interaction with the therapist and other members in a session.

In the case of symbol formation, Jones (1996) claims that the process can be either intentional or spontaneous. In the first case (i.e. intentional creation of symbols), a forest might be chosen by a DT group as a symbol to be explored in terms of discovering the role of each individual within this group. In the second case (i.e. spontaneous creation), a forest might be part of a DT enactment that eventually acquires symbolic meaning beyond its original insubstantial function as merely a component of a story.

Overall, symbols are simpler forms compared to what they refer to. Consequently, the referent is not always easily or linearly readable. Furthermore, as Pavlicevic (1997) points out, symbols can grow and transform; the process can involve drawing from older symbols to creating new ones. However, as Pavlicevic (1997) also notices, once the association between the symbol and its meaning is made, this association remains stable enough for symbolic meaning to be discovered. In order to understand this meaning, the arts therapist may use:

1. Social and/or cultural conventions (e.g. certain colours will refer to certain feelings within a specific culture, and myths and folk stories carry associated meaning). Within this category we will also include what are often perceived as 'universal' symbols such as Freudian psychosexual symbols (e.g. snakes, fishes and snails), Jungian archetypes (e.g. the self, the shadow, magna mater and the wise old man) or Winnicott's emphasis upon 'transitional objects' (e.g. comfort blankets and teddy bears).

2. What Jones (1996) calls the 'local dictionary'. This dictionary is context specific and is therefore based upon the experience of a certain vocabulary used by the client within the arts therapies sessions. For example, the use of an imaginary ball within DMT may equally represent 'a burden' as well as 'playful game'. For some clients this imaginary ball may represent the same thing every time. For other clients it may have a changeable meaning. Understanding the 'what' and the 'how' of the client's symbolic language is essential for subsequent therapeutic work.

The role of the client within this process as the main contributor to unfolding symbolic meaning for him/herself is highly valued within the arts therapies literature. On the other hand, the role of the therapist in terms of articulating interpretations is highly debated. The more art-oriented practitioners within the field claim that symbols communicate meaning to the individual without the need for verbal translations. Those with a stronger psychoanalytic/psychodynamic orientation emphasise the therapeutic value of appropriate and timely verbal interpretations (Payne 1992, Jones 1996).

Similar to symbolism, metaphor enables connections with other elements (Box 3.4). However, as Box 3.4 suggests, metaphor does not represent something else but actually is this other thing. Metaphor therefore, goes beyond

> **Box 3.4:** Definition of metaphor (Walrond-Skinner 1986, p. 213)
>
> Metaphor is an indirect method of communication by which two discrete elements are juxtaposed, the comparison between the two serving to create new meanings. . .
>
> With symbolism, the symbol represents something else; with a metaphor it is said to be something else.

representation to the actual merging between two different things. In addition, metaphor does not have to take the form of a concrete object as a symbol does. It might equally be a situation or activity within the arts therapies work that will stand for something else in the client's life. For example, being unable to keep a drawing within the boundaries of the paper in AT may stand for impulsivity or lack of self-control. Consistently being unable to move within a specific corner of the DMT room may stand for difficulties in moving on in a certain area of one's life. Feeling a sense of coldness when trying to enter a castle within a dramatic enactment in DT may stand for similar difficulties to communicate with ('get through to') one's own parental figure.

Within arts therapies, metaphors may appear as the result of improvised and/or spontaneous arts engagement. For clients who are less able to engage spontaneously in the artistic process, setting up artistic metaphors for them may be part of the arts therapies process. For example, a dance movement therapist may suggest a structure in which clients may explore moving in and out of the therapeutic circle in order to explore issues of inclusion and exclusion.

Both symbolism and metaphor are highly valued amongst arts therapies practitioners because:

- They enable an 'as if' situation to be created between the client and the therapist. According to Jennings (1996), Stanislavski was the first to introduce this idea in the theatre. However, this idea is now valued by many arts therapists as creating distance from overwhelming feelings, avoiding direct confrontation and offering safety.
- Due to this sense of safety they enable the discovery of deeply-rooted problems, which otherwise would not be identified and brought to the surface. This idea is closely linked with psychoanalytic/psychodynamic perceptions of the unconscious (e.g. Waller & Dalley 1992).
- For some clients who are only able to deal with the concrete, symbolism and metaphor may enable them to become familiar with the abstract and the elusive. According to Jones (1996) this can be therapeutic in itself.
- Both symbolism and metaphor enable multiple readings. Byrne (2001) drawing upon Heidegger and his hermeneutic phenomenology claims that the arts open up to the 'hermeneutic circle'. Thus, the same thing can be read and re-read with new layers of meaning attached to these readings every time.
- As a result of this, symbolism and metaphor offer many more possibilities for creative solutions compared with solutions found from direct articulation of problems. Thus, both concepts are regarded as closely linked with creativity and as being another way of enhancing well-being.

Summarising this section we will agree with Gordon (1987) who states that imagery is part of the 'furniture' of the mind while symbolism and metaphor is the powerful 'content' that connects the self with the other or others. Consequently, while imagery primarily rests with the client's inner make-up, symbolism and metaphor are processes with relational capacity. In the following section these concepts will be placed within the wider field of arts therapies non-verbal communication.

Non-verbal communication

Non-verbal communication has been studied extensively in a number of different fields (e.g. social psychology, counselling and psychotherapies) and is an important tool for the arts therapist. Although non-verbal communication is often interpreted as referring primarily to body language, i.e. facial expressions, eye contact, proximics, body posture, gesture, movement type and movement quality, our understanding of the term embraces all human expressions that do not fall under the realms of a strict linguistic structure (Box 3.5).

In arts therapies, non-verbal communication can be based on voice and sounds, the body and its movement, visual media, costume, objects or rituals. For example:

- human voice and musical sound are media used within MT, and may develop into advanced musical communication
- DMT practitioners pay attention primarily to the body and movement; communication can take the form of a meaningful dance improvisation
- in AT, media such as paint, papers and pens are some of the 'tools' of a visual communication
- a combination of all of these can be utilised within DT, which may also include objects, costumes or rituals, alongside the verbal or written word.

The above can be associated (but not always) with processes such as imagery, symbolism and metaphor as described in the previous section.

It is commonplace to say that non-verbal communication utilises 'non-verbal language' or, in the case of arts therapies, an 'artistic or aesthetic language'. Although parallels between non-verbal and verbal language have been discussed (e.g. Bunt 1994, Dubowski 1990, Payne 1990), artistic language is significantly different from other forms of language. Referring to visual arts, Case & Dalley (1992) claim that 'no picture can be fully explained in words; if it could, there would be no need to make it' (p. 55). This seems to be true for all art forms. Artistic language is rich in expressiveness and can have many layers of meaning that do not necessarily correspond to a verbal language. Thus, just as translating from Chinese to English misses out a lot of subtleties and cultural connotations, translating from the non-verbal to the verbal can become even more difficult and at times impossible. This difficulty turns a number of arts therapists towards the idea that non-verbal communication is adequately located within artistic media without the need

---

Box 3.5: Definition of non-verbal communication

Non-verbal communication is any meaningful interaction that does not involve verbal or written words[1] and provides information concerning the psychological state of the individual or individuals involved.

[1] Sign language is also excluded.

for verbal translations. Although this is not the case for all arts therapies practices, this tendency highlights both the difficulty of translating from one medium to another, as well as the value of communicating through an artistic 'language'.

Our understanding of non-verbal communication is influenced by Breunlin (1979) (a communication theorist), in that we find that there are three main levels upon which non-verbal communication takes place in arts therapies:

- An *internal level*, i.e. an internal dialogue, which addresses emotions, intrapsychic processes or psychopathology (Bruenlin calls this level the 'organismic').
- A *dyadic level*, i.e. non-verbal communication that involves two people. During this communication, emotions, affect and contextual aspects become important (Bruenlin 1979 refers to this level as the interpersonal level).
- The level that refers to the group, i.e. non-verbal communication between more than two people. In this case, non-verbal communication is seen as a function of the group itself: in order to regulate activities, to preserve the group's life or to achieve the group's aims, for instance (Bruenlin 1979 refers to this level as the family/group level).

While the first level is primarily an intrapersonal one, both the dyadic and the group level are interpersonal.

Internal level

A large part of arts therapies work involves non-verbal communication within the person. This is a type of communication that is not necessarily apparent to an observer, since it takes place within the self. It might happen when: listening to a favourite piece of music, and at times during music making; when becoming aware of body sensations and/or moving with closed eyes; when contemplating an image during or after a drawing has been completed. The common factor in all these cases is that the client's focus of attention is internal and information may or may not be conveyed to the therapist. Communication theorists argue that when the environment provides favourable stimuli, there is a favourable response from the person concerned through eye contact. In arts therapies, this can be expressed in a wide variety of ways, but in most cases, responses remain of minimal size and quality. Figure 3.1 illustrates the type of non-verbal communication that focuses on the client's internal processes.

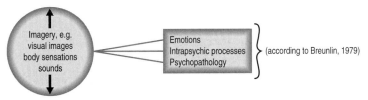

Figure 3.1: *Internal level. (Adapted from Breunlin 1979, with permission of Taylor & Francis.)*

According to Breunlin (1979), this level addresses the individual's emotions, intrapsychic processes (i.e. process that occurs within the psyche, between the ego, id or superego, or between the conscious, unconscious or preconscious) and/or their own psychopathology. The arts may mobilise imagery (i.e. inner representations of objects or events created at will) and thus awaken parts of the client's self, which have remained immobile for some time. They may also enable imagination, and thus allow the person to enjoy an internal 'film', making links with different parts of the self and making self-assessments. At the same time, they may mobilise dysfunctional parts of the self, encourage hallucinations and/or fantasy depending on the clients' psychopathology. Given the ability of the arts to evoke imagination as well as fantasies and hallucinations, especially where vulnerable clients are concerned, safeguarding this process becomes of paramount importance.

Dyadic level

In contrast to the esoteric character of the internal level of non-verbal communication, interpersonal non-verbal communication is behaviourally more explicit. In arts therapies the dyadic level, in particular, refers to the communication between the client and the therapist. Reading the client's non-verbal cues and responding appropriately varies depending on the conceptual frame utilised by the therapist (see Ch. 4). In all cases however, the client's non-verbal signs are hardly ever seen in isolation but rather within the context that these signs have been expressed (see Fig. 3.2).

Dyadic non-verbal communication has a content or topic that is equivalent to words in verbal communication (or what communication theorists refer to as the 'digital' mode of communication, e.g. Bateson 2000, Watzlawick et al 1967). As with words in verbal language, imagery, symbolism and metaphors provide some of the topics for this communication. Personal imagery can be shared with the therapist, symbolism can be expressed as icons or symbols, and events with a metaphoric meaning can be enacted. Another topic for this communication can be artistic expressions in the form of colours or shapes, sounds or movements, that do not represent anything else outside themselves (what we have already termed as arts as index).

However, a very important aspect of non-verbal communication within arts therapies is how the interaction (or what communication theorists call the 'analogic' mode of communication) takes place. The quality of the interaction provides important additional information about what is going on between the client and the therapist. Here is a hypothetical interaction between a client and a therapist:

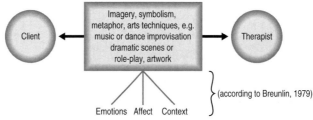

Figure 3.2: *Dyadic level. (Adapted from Breunlin 1979, with permission of Taylor & Francis.)*

Scenario

The client gives a ball to the therapist; the therapist takes the ball and places it on the floor.

This same interaction can take place in a number of different ways as the following examples illustrate.

Example 1

The client gives the ball to the therapist *in a direct and efficient way, leaning forward and half standing up while doing so.* The therapist takes the ball in time and places it *quickly on the ground but without looking at the client.*

Example 2

The client gives the ball to the therapist *in a hesitant way, leaning back and forth while doing so and making no eye contact.* The therapist takes the ball and after pausing for a second places the ball *carefully on the floor and facing the client continuously.*

The initial, basic scenario offers the subject matter; however, it does not say much about the interaction, other that there has been an exchange of a ball. When additional information is given, emotional atmosphere is added to the description. It is apparent that the atmosphere in the two examples is significantly different with the greater emotional loading present in the second case. In other words, the 'how' of the interaction offers supplementary information about emotional states. When therapists recognise that they are 'about right' in 'reading' the signs, and can enter into non-verbal dialogue with their clients, we may say that successful communication is taking place.

Group level

Finally, non-verbal communication within arts therapies might take place in groups (see Fig. 3.3). According to Breunlin (1979), non-verbal communication within groups has a number of different functions such as regulating activities, preserving the group's life or achieving the group's aims. Communication in groups can be quite complex and can be seen in many different ways, for example, from the point of view of the individual within the group or from the point of view of the group as a whole. Theories of group dynamics offer substantial support to understanding group interactions and group processes

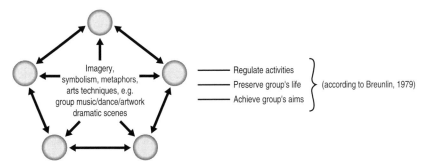

Figure 3.3: *Group level. (Adapted from Breunlin 1979, with permission of Taylor & Francis.)*

(e.g. Bion 1961, Foulkes 1964, Yalom 1970). Despite the value of these theories in understanding group processes, they have emerged primarily from verbal groups. Arts therapists are currently conceptualising their own models to view group interactions that place a more central role on the use of the arts (e.g. McNeilly 2000, Sandel & Johnson 1983, Schmais 1985).

Client—therapist relationship

Unlike communication and non-verbal communication that describe primarily exchanges of information and meaning on an internal, dyadic or group level, the client–therapist relationship is regarded as referring directly to the agent of therapeutic change. The client–therapist relationship is an extension of the dyadic communication described before but may also include communication that takes place internally as well as in relation to a group.

Research in psychotherapy stresses that the client, the therapist and their relationship are closely connected to the outcome of the therapy (Frank 1979, Hynan 1981). Arts therapists also seem to greatly value this relationship, either explicitly or implicitly, as evident in the definitions of arts therapies (see Ch. 2). This relationship starts with the initial contact with the client and develops in line with the development of the therapeutic process. The arts medium plays an important role within this relationship, since it is often through this medium that the relationship is formed, established or worked through.

Arts therapies have made extensive use of psychotherapeutic thinking in order to conceptualise the most important issues surrounding the client–therapist relationship. Confidentiality and therapeutic boundaries are, for example, frequently discussed. The client and the therapist are not involved in a social interaction and it is important that both parties have a mutual understanding at the outset, of the nature of the client–therapist relationship. Clarkson (1994) calls this the 'working alliance'. Within arts therapies, this alliance may be translated as a verbal or written contract, or a less formal but clear agreement that client and therapist will work together with the single aim of benefiting the client. The working alliance may also involve an understanding that the work will be carried out within a specific arts therapies modality. Finally, it is important that client and therapist share some common ground, so that both feel they can connect at some level. Common goals, bonds and tasks are therefore, some of the constituent elements of a working alliance.

Other types of therapeutic relationships that are coloured by psychotherapeutic thinking are: the 'transferential' relationship and the 'real' (or 'I-you' or 'core') relationship (Clarkson 1994, Greenson 1967). The former emphasises the process whereby the client displaces onto the therapist, feelings, attributes and attitudes that properly belong to a significant figure from the client's past (e.g. a parent) and responds to the therapist accordingly. This relationship is encouraged through frequent meetings with the therapist, long-term work and, often, a therapist's attitude that entails a degree of distance and the absence of personal disclosures. The therapist acts as a mirror in which the clients will re-experience and re-work relationships with significant people from their past lives. This relationship is particularly emphasised amongst arts therapists with psychoanalytically-informed practice (for more on this type of practice, see 'The Psychoanalytic/Psychodynamic Trend' in Ch. 4). The 'real' relationship, on the other hand, takes place in the here-and-now of the interaction. It is regarded as entailing mutual participation, with the therapist wholly present, showing empathy, warmth, positive regard and genuineness. The therapeutic change comes from the moments of 'real' meetings between client and therapist. There is recognition that not only the client but also the therapist is changed by the other. What is going on in the therapy may often go beyond the expectations and understanding of the therapist. This relationship is more often present within arts therapies practice that is influenced by humanistic thinking (see 'The Humanistic Trend' in Ch. 4).

Although these relationships are particularly popular among arts therapists, many argue that conceptualisation borrowed from psychotherapeutic thinking is not sufficient for understanding the client–therapist relationship within arts therapies. One of the main reasons for this is the presence of the arts as part of this relationship. Some would claim that the arts constitute the third corner in a 'triangular relationship' between the therapist and the client (see Fig. 3.4). This model has been extensively discussed in AT (Case 1990, 1996, 2000, Wood 1984, 1990, Schaverien 1990, 1992, 1994, 1997, 2000). We propose that this model can also be a useful way of looking at relationships beyond AT, for example in MT, DT and DMT.

Within an arts therapies context, for example, there can be many variations on the above model, which are not necessarily exclusive of one another. In some cases, despite the significance placed upon the arts, their actual use may remain peripheral to the process. The relationship can be visualised as shown in Figure 3.5.

This is characteristic of an arts therapies practice at the margins between psychotherapy and arts therapies. This type of relationship can be found at various stages in the therapeutic process and bears similarities to traditional

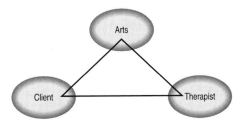

Figure 3.4: *The triangular relationship.*

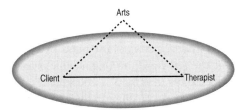

Figure 3.5: *The client–therapist relationship.*

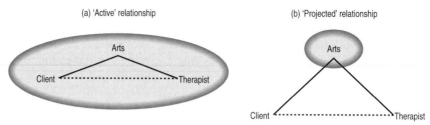

Figure 3.6: *The artistic relationship.*

verbal psychotherapy or counselling. Given that the arts do not play an important role, this relationship can be understood in terms of relationships described in psychotherapeutic literature (e.g. the transferential or real relationship).

More often, however, the arts therapist relates to the client predominantly via the arts. This type of relationship celebrates the arts as the main feature of the therapeutic process and may take the form of either (a) or (b) as presented in Figure 3.6. It can be seen that the client–therapist axis becomes less important (interrupted line), distinguishing it from the client–therapist relationship described previously.

The relationship in Figure 3.6a refers to an active engagement in the art-making process for both the therapist and the client. This type of relationship closely resembles the 'real' relationship as conceptualised in the psychotherapeutic literature, with the important difference that the arts play a central role. Although the significance of the engagement in the artistic process is emphasised amongst the majority of arts therapists, caution is also expressed concerning the level of involvement of the therapist; full engagement for instance, could mean missing important messages sent out by the client. The art-making itself might become seductive for the artist within the therapist and artistic preferences may take over. In order to ensure safe practice, Johnson (1992), for example, suggests that therapists should keep a part of themselves back. The relationship in Figure 3.6b, or what we call the 'projected' relationship, when used in conjunction with the 'active' relationship, offers an additional safeguard for practice. The 'projected' relationship refers to the time within the therapeutic process when there is more distance between therapist and client on the one hand and the arts on the other. It is the time of reflection on what has happened within one session or over a number of sessions, the time when both client and therapist may be engaged in looking at a drawing, watching a performance or just remembering what took place. The focus remains on the arts but there is an important difference in terms of the degree of active involvement in art-making for both the client and the therapist. In the 'projected' relationship, active involvement in the art-making is substantially reduced. This relationship resembles the idea of the dramatic and aesthetic distance discussed extensively within the DT and to a lesser extent the AT literature (e.g. Jennings 1994, Jones 1996).

Another set of relationships that may be found within arts therapies refers to whether it is the therapist or the client who is acting as the artist. In these relationships there is no mutuality of roles in the way they were described before. The triangular relationship is therefore represented with different

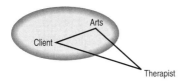

(a) Relationship with the client as the artist

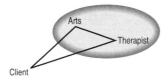

(b) Relationship with the therapist as the artist

Figure 3.7: *The client or the therapist as the artist.*

geometrical proportions: from an isosceles to a scalene triangle (Fig. 3.7). Given these non-mutual relationships, issues of unequal power and the potential abuse of this power become particularly relevant and are discussed in the recent arts therapies literature (e.g. Bunt 1994, Hogan 1997, Jennings 1996).

In the relationship in Figure 3.7a the therapist might play a more distant role (e.g. be an observer), while the client will be the one mainly involved in the art-making. This type of relationship seems equivalent to the 'transferential' relationship described earlier with the important difference of the presence of the arts. This type of relationship is extensively used within AT practice, when the client is engaged in drawing or painting in the presence of the observing therapist, in DMT, when the client moves in the presence of the non-moving therapist, and so on. Less often, the therapist will be involved in the art-making process and the client will be an observer as in the relationship in Figure 3.7b. Active involvement from the part of the client is less important; his/her role might be one of an observer. The therapist's self-perception is often that of the shaman or the healer (Johnson 1992). It can also be one that refers to the 'knowledgeable expert' who follows an educative or behavioural model. Uneasiness has been expressed amongst British arts therapists with practices in which the client does not have enough control over the art-making process (e.g. Meldrum 1994). The therapist as the sole artist in the therapeutic relationship is seen as potentially acting out their own rather than the client's needs. Despite criticisms, this kind of relationship can be found at different times in MT and DT when, for example, the therapist is playing music and the client listens (Alvin 1978, refers to this as one of the 'receptive' techniques in MT) or the therapist is telling a story to the client (as part, for example, of Gersie's 1991 story-making method in DT). In most of these cases the clients are encouraged to make choices and intervene or even reject the therapist's suggestions and/or artistic input as a way of avoiding client disempowerment and increasing the therapeutic value of the intervention.

Therapeutic aims

Numerous aims have been reported in the arts therapies literature. The wide range of aims is also reflected in findings from our survey. To a great extent these aims vary depending on the client involved. When possible, the aims are agreed in collaboration with the client, with those associated with the client and/or with other therapists. Arts therapists claim that they do not attempt to make clients 'normal'. The notion of 'normality' has negative connotations such as the client being 'abnormal' prior to treatment, and opposes deeply-rooted beliefs in the uniqueness of the individual.

Liebmann (1981), in an attempt to categorise aims held by art therapists, refers to specific purposes relating to single clients/groups as well as 'general personal' purposes and 'general social' purposes. We suggest that this categorisation may be applicable to all arts therapies disciplines. Dokter (1993), reporting on her anthropological study of the different DT practices across Europe, found that in northern Mediterranean countries, there is a physiological orientation within therapy alongside psychological, social and supernatural orientations, whereas the British DT practice is described as holding mainly psychological and social orientations. This position seems to add further support to the categorisation of aims into personal and social (see Table 3.1).

Often these aims are influenced by the overall theoretical model held by practitioners or by the client group with whom they work. However, there are only a few studies that look specifically at the aims of arts therapies. One such piece of research work comes from the USA and is based on a survey of music therapists (Wheeler 1987). According to this study, there are three sets of aims corresponding to three levels of therapy work: the first level is called activity therapy, the second re-educative, and the third reconstructive. According to Wheeler (1987) there are connections between clients' diffi-

Table 3.1: General therapeutic aims (adapted from Liebmann 1981)

General personal purposes (not in order of priority)	General social purposes (not in order of priority)
• Creativity and spontaneity	• Awareness, recognition and appreciation of others
• Confidence-building, self-validation, realisation of own potential	• Co-operation, involvement in group activity
• Increased personal autonomy and motivation, development as an individual	• Communication
• Freedom to make decisions, experiment, test out ideas	• Sharing of problems, experiences and insights
• Express feelings, emotions, conflicts	• Discovery of universality of experience/uniqueness of individual
• Work with fantasy and the unconscious	• Relating to others in a group, understanding of the effect of self on others, and on relationships
• Develop insight, self-awareness, reflection	• Social support and trust
• Promote ordering of experience	• Cohesion of group
• Aid relaxation	• Examination of group issues

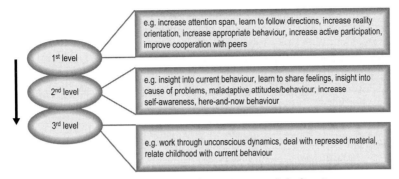

Figure 3.8: *Levels of therapy. (Based on Wheeler's 1987 research findings.)*

culties and these different sets of aims and levels. For example, music therapists working with clients with schizophrenia tend to work on the first level, while with clients with issues of substance abuse, affective disorders, neurosis or personality disorders work can take place on either level two or three. Situational disturbances are the one type of difficulty that is primarily addressed on level three. We suggest that these different levels of work may also reflect overall psychotherapeutic orientations, for example, the first loosely connects with behavioural work, the second with humanistic thinking and the last with a psychoanalytic orientation (Fig. 3.8).

Summary

In this chapter we have discussed some important features that are responsible for the unique character of the arts therapies field. We identified for example, a number of assumptions regarding the use of the arts that are common across arts therapies disciplines: democratic uses of the arts that validate natural human expressions and art-making processes; beliefs in the preverbal development of the arts and their reference to the person as a whole; emphasis upon the healing or therapeutic potential of the arts.

'Creativity' is considered to have a crucially important role in the arts therapies process, and so this highly complex and contested concept has been scrutinized and meanings elucidated. The internal, dyadic and group levels of non-verbal communication in arts therapies were also presented and discussed, revealing the complexity of such processes as well as the extensive knowledge and experience necessary for interpretation by therapists. An exploration of non-verbal communication suggested that the *content* of non-verbal communication consists of imagery, symbolism, metaphors and concrete artistic expressions (artistic expressions without symbolic meaning). Further information was gained, including important details on relational aspects, from considering *how* these symbols, metaphors and so on, are created.

Variations on the client–therapist–arts triangular relationship have also been discussed. For example, we referred to the triangular relationship and relationships such as the active and projected relationships. This chapter finished with a brief discussion of therapeutic aims relevant to arts therapies. We talked about personal and social purposes as well as aims that correspond to different types ('levels') of therapy. Further discussion of different types of therapy is included in the following chapter.

References

- Alvin J 1978 Music therapy for the autistic child. Oxford University Press, London
- Bateson G 2000 Steps to an ecology of mind: collected essays in anthropology, psychiatry, evolution, and epistemology. University of Chicago Press, New York
- Bion W R 1961 Experiences in groups. Tavistock/Routledge, London and New York
- Breunlin D 1979 Non-verbal communication in family therapy. In: Walrond-Skinner S (ed) Family and marital psychotherapy. Routledge and Kegan Paul, London
- Bruscia K E 1988 Perspective: standards for clinical assessment in the arts therapies. The Arts in Psychotherapy 15:5–10
- Bunt L 1994 Music therapy: an art beyond words. Routledge, London
- Byrne P 2001 Proposed new identities. In: Kossolapow L, Scoble S, Waller D (eds) Arts–therapies–communication: on the way to a communicative European arts therapy, vol. 1. Lit Verlag, Munster, p 251–265
- Case C 1990 The triangular relationship (3): the image as mediator. Inscape (winter):20–26
- Case C 1996 On the aesthetic moment in the transference. Inscape 1(2):39–45
- Case C 2000 'Our lady of the Queen', journeys around the maternal object. In: Gilroy A, McNeilly G (eds) The changing shape of art therapy: new developments in theory and practice, p 15–54
- Case C, Dalley T 1992 The handbook of art therapy. Routledge, London
- Clarkson P 1994 The psychotherapeutic relationship. In: Clarkson P, Pokorny M (eds) The handbook of psychotherapy. Routledge, London, p 3–27
- Dokter D 1993 Dramatherapy across Europe: cultural contradictions. In: Payne H (ed.) Handbook of inquiry in the arts therapies: one river many currents. Jessica Kingsley, London p 79–90
- Dosamantes-Alperson E 1981 Experiencing in movement therapy. American Journal of Dance Therapy 4(2):33–44
- Dubowski J 1990 Art versus language: separate development during childhood. In: Case C, Dalley T (eds) Working with children in art therapy. Tavistock/Routledge, London, p 7–22
- Foulkes S H 1964 Therapeutic group analysis. Allen and Unwin, London
- Frank J D 1979 The present status of outcome research. Journal of Counsulting and Clinical Psychology 47:310–316
- Freud S 1953 On creativity and the unconscious. Harper and Row, New York
- Fromm E 1959 The creative attitude. In: Anderson H (ed) Creativity and its cultivation. Harper and Row, New York
- Gersie A 1991 Storymaking in bereavement: dragons fight in the meadow. Jessica Kingsley, London
- Gordon R 1987 Playing on many stages: DT and the individual. In: Jennings S (ed) DT: theory and practice 1. Routledge, London, p 119–145
- Greenson R R 1967 The technique and practice of psychoanalysis, vol 1. International University Press, New York
- Halprin D 2003 The expressive body in life, art and therapy: working with movement, metaphor and meaning. Jessica Kingsley, London
- Hogan S (ed) 1997 Feminist approaches to art therapy. Routledge, London
- Hynan M T 1981 On the advantages of assuming that the techniques of psychotherapy are ineffective. Psychotherapy: Theory and Practice 18:11–13
- Jennings S 1994 The theatre of healing: metaphor & metaphysics in the healing process. In: Jennings S, Cattanach A, Mitchell S et al (eds) The handbook of dramatherapy. Routledge, London, p 93–113
- Jennings S 1996 Brief DT: the healing power of the dramatised here and now. In: Gersie A (ed) Dramatic approaches to brief therapy. Jessica Kingsley, London, p 201–215
- Johnson D R 1992 The dramatherapist in role. In: Jennings S (ed) Dramatherapy: theory and practice 2. Routledge, London, p 112–136
- Jones P 1996 Drama as therapy: theatre as living. Routledge, London
- Jung C G 1961 Memories, dreams, reflections. Pantheon, New York
- Landy R 2001 Establishing a model of communication between an arts-based discipline and its applied creative art therapy. In: Kossolapow L, Scoble S, Waller D (eds) Arts – therapies –

communication: on a way to a communicative European arts therapy, vol 1. Lit Verlag, Munster, p 305–310

- Liebmann M 1981 The many purposes of art therapy. Inscape 5(1):26–28
- McNeilly G 2000 Failure in group analytic art therapy. In: Gilroy A, McNeilly G (eds)The changing shape of art therapy: new developments in theory and practice. Jessica Kingsley, London, p 143–171
- Malchiodi C 1998 The art therapy sourcebook. Lowell House, Los Angeles
- May R 1975 The courage to create. Norton, New York
- Meldrum B 1994 Historical background and overview of dramatherapy. In: Jennings S, Cattanach A, Mitchell S (eds) The handbook of dramatherapy. Routledge, London, p 12–27
- Pavlicevic M 1997 Music therapy in context: music, meaning and relationship. Jessica Kingsley, London
- Payne H 1990 Creative movement and dance in groupwork. Winslow, Oxon
- Payne H 1992 Shut in, shut out: dance movement therapy with children and adolescents. In: Payne H (ed) Dance movement therapy: theory and practice. Tavistock/Routledge, London and New York, p 39–80
- Rogers C 1961 On becoming a person. Houghton Mifflin, Boston
- Sandel S, Johnson D 1983 Structure and process of the nascent group: dance movement therapy with chronic patients. The Arts in Psychotherapy 10:131–140
- Saussure F de 1969 Course in general linguistics. McGraw-Hill, New York (first edition 1911).
- Schaverien J 1990 The triangular relationship (2): desire, alchemy and the picture. Inscape 1(winter):14–19
- Schaverien J 1992 The revealing image. Routledge, London
- Schaverien J 1994 Analytical art psychotherapy: further reflections on theory and practice. Inscape 2:41–49
- Schaverien J 1997 Transference and transactional objects in the treatment of psychosis. In: Killick K, Schaverien J (eds) Art, psychotherapy and psychosis. Routledge, London, p 13–37
- Schaverien J 2000 The triangular relationship and the aesthetic countertransference in analytical art psychotherapy. In: Gilroy A, McNeilly G (eds) The changing shape of art therapy: new developments in theory and practice. Jessica Kingsley, London, p 55–83
- Schmais C 1985 Healing processes in group dance/movement therapy. American Journal of Dance Therapy 8:17–36
- Smitskamp H 1995 The problem of professional diagnosis in the arts therapies. The Arts in Psychotherapy 22(3):181–187
- Stanton-Jones K 1992 An introduction to dance movement therapy in psychiatry. Tavistock/Routledge, London
- Waller D, Dalley T 1992 Art therapy: a theoretical perspective. In: Waller D, Gilroy A (eds) Art therapy: a handbook. Open University Press, Buckingham and Philadelphia, p 3–24
- Walrond-Skinner S 1986 Dictionary of psychotherapy. Routledge and Kegan Paul, London
- Wheeler B 1987 Levels of therapy: the classification of music therapy goals. Music Therapy 6(2):39–49
- Watzlawick P, Beavin-Bavalas J, Jackson D D 1967 Pragmatics of human communication: a study of interactional patterns, pathologies and paradoxes. W W Norton, New York
- Winnicott D W 1971 Playing and reality. Routledge, London
- Wood C 1984 The child and art therapy: a psychodynamic viewpoint. In: Dalley T (ed) Art as therapy. Tavistock, London, p 85–103
- Wood C 1990 The triangular relationship (1): the beginnings and endings of art therapy. Inscape (winter): 7–13
- Yalom I D 1970 The theory and practice of group psychotherapy. Basic Books, New York

Chapter 4

Therapeutic Trends across Arts Therapies

Key issues:

- In order to acquire an overall conceptualisation for their work, arts therapists have drawn upon neighbouring fields such as humanistic psychotherapy, eclectic approaches, psychoanalytic/psychodynamic psychotherapy, developmental models, artistic/creative and active/directive approaches. Principles and overall frameworks from these fields have been adapted and further developed within arts therapies to varying degrees; we refer to these sets of different influences as 'therapeutic trends'.

- The humanistic trend is very strong within arts therapies to such a degree that humanistic principles are incorporated within 'mainstream' practice without always a direct acknowledgement of this being the case. When arts therapists follow an explicit humanistic orientation, they often claim that they follow a model of growth.

- The psychoanalytic/psychodynamic trend is also important for arts-therapies practice, especially because it offers a rich conceptual frame for understanding practices. Arts therapies practices with such an orientation pay attention to unconscious processes, the client–therapist relationship and the interplay between internal and external realities. From an object relations perspective the arts are often seen as transitional objects that lie between the self and the other.

- Developmental models are extensively used within arts therapies practice, especially where children are concerned. The theory of development stems either from (1) psychotherapeutic thinking or (2) psychology/education. The former focuses more on emotional processes, while the latter focuses more on cognitive processes.

- The artistic/creative trend is characteristic of the arts therapies field but does not always fully explain practices theoretically. This trend can often be found in conjunction with psychotherapeutic frameworks. When it stands on its own, the therapeutic process is very similar to the artistic process, and the ultimate aim of the therapy is to strengthen the artistic/creative self.

- The active/directive trend is closely linked with the fact that arts therapies are action therapies. However, the degree of direction and structure appropriate for clients has been extensively debated. Links between this trend and psychoeducative, behavioural models and brief therapy are made, and caution is raised regarding unquestionable usage of activities in a reductive or a-theoretical way.

- The eclectic/integrative trend is the second most important trend within arts therapies and consists of the combination of all of the other therapeutic trends. Although it links well with current post-modern thinking and the need to accommodate diverse client needs in a flexible way, careful selection of principles/approaches should be made in order to avoid amorphous and ill-defined practices.

- Emphasis upon one therapeutic trend over another varies depending on a number of factors such as the client group, working environment and practitioner's age and background.

- For example, with clients with mental health problems, there is a stronger psychoanalytic/psychodynamic preference; for clients with learning disabilities, ideas and practices from developmental, active/directive and artistic/creative trends can be used; while with people with no apparent difficulties, it is common to draw upon either humanistic or artistic/directive principles.

- In health services, psychoanalytic/psychodynamic thinking prevails; in education, art therapists prefer to work within humanistic frameworks and to a lesser extent through developmental and active/directive perspectives; while in private practice there is strong emphasis upon humanistic practices.

- Older arts therapists draw more heavily upon a number of different models; the middle-aged group (40–50 years) shows a stronger preoccupation with psychoanalytic/psychodynamic thinking; while the younger generation of arts therapists has a stronger faith in eclectic/integrative thinking. These tendencies may correspond to different stages of professional development of the therapists and/or different strands valued over time from the point of view of the overall development of the four professions.

Introduction

Issues covered in the previous chapter refer to important features of the field but do not give a comprehensive picture of arts therapies processes. In arts therapies there are a number of therapeutic frameworks that conceptualise and guide these processes. In this chapter we will present some of these frameworks as they were revealed in our empirical study. Initial findings consisted of statements from expert practitioners regarding theory and clinical methodology (interviews – stage 1). These statements were tested with as many practising arts therapists in the UK as possible for degree of agreement (survey – stage 2) and were eventually grouped together statistically (details on methodology of the study are included in Appendix 1). All of these categories received a fairly strong agreement amongst arts therapies practitioners and are listed from the most to least important:

1. humanistic
2. eclectic/integrative
3. psychoanalytic/psychodynamic
4. developmental
5. artistic/creative
6. active/directive.

In this chapter, we will therefore present these groups of statements, highlight overall theoretical and methodological principles that go across the different arts therapies disciplines and contribute towards some first broad descriptions of the field. We refer to these findings as trends in order to suggest the diversity with which therapeutic frameworks are applied in practice.

We need to make two points here:

- Despite the fact that the eclectic/integrative trend received strong agreement amongst practitioners (it was the second most popular group) we decided to present it last, believing that it consists of the other therapeutic trends combined together in one way or another.
- We found that the background, training and age of the practitioner, as well as the client group and setting determined to a great extent the choice of one therapeutic framework over another. Towards the end of this chapter we will therefore discuss these factors further and consider some ways in which they distinguish arts therapies practices.

The humanistic trend

'Humanistic' is a generic term used to refer to a number of different, although related, approaches to psychotherapy. This group of approaches is generally regarded as a main force within psychotherapy and its relative importance for arts therapies is confirmed by the results of our study. Some of the approaches generally regarded as falling under the humanistic umbrella include: client-centred therapy (Rogers 1951), Gestalt therapy (Perls et al 1969), transactional analysis (Berne 1961), existential therapy (May 1961) and interpersonal individual/group therapies (Laing 1959, Sullivan 1955, Yalom 1970). Maslow (1968) is also associated with this school of thought but is also regarded as a founder of transpersonal therapy, i.e. a group of therapeutic approaches that are often regarded as the fourth force in psychotherapy, next to behavioural, psychodynamic and humanistic thinking.

In humanistic psychotherapy there is a preoccupation with the development of the person (the person 'becoming') and human potential. Frequently cited goals for therapy are self-realisation (or self-actualisation) and self-responsibility. During the course of therapy, the whole person is engaged, while self-expression and creativity are highlighted. The therapist is active during the sessions, stresses the here-and-now of the interaction and encourages the discovery of personal meaning (often in a non-interpretive way). The humanistic perspective values a close relationship between the therapist and the client, otherwise called the 'real' relationship, and both are seen as equal partners on the therapeutic journey.

We have already discussed that humanistic thinking with the contribution of Moreno, the founder of this movement, and the booming of humanistic approaches in the 1960s and 1970s, has contributed to the emergence and development of the arts therapies field (see 'The Emergence of Arts Therapies in the 20th Century' in Ch. 1). We have also suggested that Wheeler's (1987) discussion of the second 'level' of arts therapies can be associated with this type of work with a range of client groups (see 'Therapeutic Aims' in Ch. 3). Consequently, principles from humanistic approaches can be found in many arts therapies practices. To start with, there is a strong impact upon dramatherapy (DT) from psychodrama, Moreno's creative approach to groups, as we will see more closely in Chapter 7. References to Roger's (1951) client-centred therapy and/or his core conditions of psychological contact, empathy, congruence and can be found in Section 2; Ansdell (G. Ansdell, unpublished interview, 2002; Ch. 5), Silverstone (1993) and Thomas (D. Thomas, unpublished interview, 2002; Ch. 6). References to Gestalt therapy are made by Bonny (1994), Mottram (2000, 2001), Ford (J. Ford, unpublished interview, 2002; Ch. 6), and Penfield (1992). Inclusion of interpersonal theories in arts therapies practice is also relevant (see Odell-Miller 2000, Waller 1993, Karkou, in press). Studies such as those of Schmais (1985) and, Jones (1996) have elaborated upon Yalom's (1970) curative factors (i.e. instillation of hope, universality, imparting of information, altruism, corrective recapitulation of primary family group, development of socialising techniques, imitative behaviour, interpersonal learning, group cohesiveness, catharsis and existential factors) and have adapted them for different arts therapies practices.

Box 4.1 highlights some 'humanistic' beliefs, aims and techniques that are common amongst arts therapists in the UK. This group of statements, for example, consists of a number of 'humanistic' aims such as attempting to achieve *self-responsibility, self-actualisation,* and *facilitating awareness of another.* Box 4.1 also refers to a *holistic practice* that attempts to bring together different aspects of one's self. One of the statements clearly states that there is an underlying belief in a close body–mind connection. Finally, the humanistic bias towards valuing 'real' relationships is implicitly included through references to the role of the therapist; the therapist for example, is expected to *respond to the client with his or her whole self.* The 'real' relationship often takes place in the here-and-now of the interaction; there is mutual participation and also recognition that both the client and the therapist experience positive change.

> **Box 4.1:** Humanistic group of statements
>
> ## Statements
>
> - What I am working towards is a sense of self-responsibility.
> - The purpose of the therapy has to do with the 'wholeness'.
> - Arts therapies have to do with individuals becoming who they really are.
> - The aim is facilitating awareness of another.
> - One of my fundamental hypotheses is that there is a strong body–mind relationship.
> - I am trying to offer to clients a learning experience.
> - I am trying to respond with my whole self.
>
> (mean* = 3.89, standard deviation^f = 0.49, internal consistency$^\alpha$ = 0.66)
>
> *The higher the score, the stronger the agreement with this group of statements (a five-point scale was used ranging from strongly agree = 5 to strongly disagree = 1).
> ^{f}The higher the value, the higher average variation of this group of statements from the group mean score.
> $^\alpha$The higher the value, the more consistent the responses to different statements; for example, those who agreed with one also agreed with the other statements of this group.
> Humanistic principles are particularly relevant to the arts therapies practice as the high mean score suggests. This group of statements attracted the strongest agreement among arts therapies practitioners. Furthermore, the relatively high internal consistency of the group suggests that arts therapists who agreed with one of these principles tended to also agree with the rest of the principles in this group.

However, as we have already outlined, in arts therapies the therapeutic relationship can be seen as three-fold: it is a relationship between the client, the arts and the therapist (i.e. the 'triangular' relationship) in which different sides of the triangle are stressed each time (see the 'Client–Therapist Relationship' in Ch. 3). The 'real' relationship that is valued within humanistic approaches becomes equivalent to the 'active' relationship within arts therapies, during which both therapist and client are engaged in the art-making. To a lesser degree 'projected' relationships (in which the client and the therapist retain a distance from the artwork) are also present, next to relationships in which either the client or the therapist are primarily the artists. In all cases warmth and support from the part of the therapist are 'bottom-line' properties of the humanistic attitude.

Similar to counsellors and psychotherapists with a humanistic orientation, arts therapists with a humanistic perspective claim to follow a model of growth. This model is very different from other types of work such as the psychoanalytic/psychodynamic perspective or behavioural models described in later sections.

Figure 4.1 illustrates a way of conceptualising humanistic arts therapies approaches. As this figure shows, within the humanistic model the person is perceived as a whole and as such, problem areas are not necessarily focused upon. Indeed some humanistic arts therapists perceive focusing on the problem as disempowering for the client and furthermore, as diverting attention away from the 'healthy' self and its associated strengths. The underlying belief is that the healthier aspects of the person are able to contribute towards therapeutic change and so the therapy's attention is directed towards growth in these areas. The role of the artistic medium along with the therapist's positive, caring approach promotes positive change. Thus, the client may be 're-educated' and at the end of the intervention, may emerge enriched by these experiences. It is argued therefore, that through a humanistically-informed arts therapies approach problem areas become less important or even diminish.

Although this model has been criticised as bearing the danger of encouraging clients to act out without achieving deep personality changes and/or lasting effects, the impact of humanistic psychotherapy upon arts therapies is so important that different aspects of such frameworks are currently part of 'mainstream' arts therapies practice. It is often the case that humanistic principles are found in conjunction with other approaches including the developmental, the artistic/creative and/or the active/directive. Furthermore, principles traditionally associated with humanistic psychotherapy are often utilised by arts therapists who do not necessarily acknowledge a predominant humanistic orientation in their work. Such principles can act as a form of guidance for therapists in terms of how they can be in the session with clients even if conceptual understanding of the meaning of what has taken place can be gained by drawing upon other theoretical frameworks such as the psychoanalytic/psychodynamic perspective.

The psychoanalytic/psychodynamic trend

Psychoanalytic/psychodynamic theory is a major force within psychotherapy and consists of a number of related schools of thought. For example, the term 'psychoanalytic' is often associated with the theories and practices of Freudian psychoanalysis, while 'psychodynamic' is used in a much broader sense to include meta-Freudian thinking (e.g. Erikson 1959), Jung (1990), object relations theory (e.g. Klein 1975, Mahler et al 1975, Winnicott 1971), attachment theory (Bowlby 1969) and group analysis (Bion 1961, Foulkes 1964). We use the two terms together in order to indicate this set of wide-ranging approaches within psychotherapy and their respective range of uses within arts therapies.

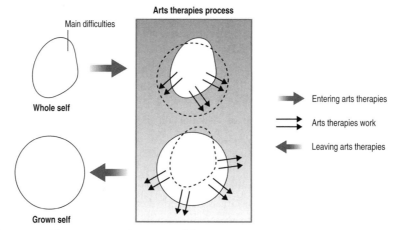

Figure 4.1: *A humanistic arts therapies model.*

One of the major combining elements of all these different schools of thought is the belief in the existence of the unconscious. The unconscious has been defined as anything that is not readily available to consciousness and that is manifested in products (e.g. dreams), processes (e.g. word associations, free associations and errors of speech or other errors) or behaviours (e.g. symptoms) (Walrond-Skinner 1986). Within an arts therapies context, the unconscious is seen as also manifested within the arts (the art-making process and/or artistic products). Similarly, arts therapists with a psychoanalytic/ psychodynamic perspective argue that their work involves deep therapeutic work that attempts to reconstruct clients' personalities. This is equivalent to Wheeler's (1987) third 'level' of arts therapies aims that again can be applied to a number of different client groups (see 'Therapeutic Aims' in Ch. 3). Given the argument for deep work, lengthy periods of client–therapist contact are usually preferred (e.g. 2 years or longer).

Psychoanalytic/psychodynamic theories have been particularly relevant to arts therapies since the emergence of the profession (see 'The Emergence of Arts Therapies in the 20th Century' in Ch. 1). Results from our study suggest that these theories are currently playing a major role in conceptualising practices within the field and/or informing clinical methodology. This is not surprising, given that psychoanalytic/psychodynamic thinking is very well articulated, its literature is rich and the field well established. Psychoanalytic/psychodynamic principles that have received strong agreement amongst practitioners are listed in Box 4.2.

Box 4.2 shows that arts therapists with a psychoanalytic/psychodynamic perspective use analytic thinking in their actual practice (they *analyse in a*

Box 4.2: Psychoanalytic/psychodynamic group of statements

Statements

- I do analyse in a psychoanalytic way.
- I am trying to link the clients' past with their present lives.
- I am looking at the transference between client and therapist.
- Psychoanalytic theory provides me an explanation of what is going on in the session.
- Therapeutic change is facilitated by achieving insight.
- I work quite hard verbally.

(mean* = 3.35, standard deviation^f = 0.44, internal consistency$^\alpha$ = 0.71)

*The higher the score, the stronger the agreement with this group of statements (a five-point scale was used ranging from strongly agree = 5 to strongly disagree = 1).

^{f}The higher the value, the higher average variation of this group of statements from the group mean score.

$^\alpha$The higher the value, the more consistent the responses to different statements; for example, those who agreed with one also agreed with the other statements in this group.

The mean score for this group of statements was relatively high, which suggests that psychoanalytic/psychodynamic theory was an important approach within arts therapies for the therapists. In addition, this group of statements presents the highest internal consistency, which implies that those whose practice is informed by psychoanalytic/psychodynamic theory are in general agreement with most of the principles stated above.

psychoanalytic way) and attempt to *make links with the past*. Artistic experiences are seen as initiated at preverbal stages, and as such can enable clients to return to early life experiences, re-work issues from their early development and acquire some understanding of their meaning for their current lives (i.e. *achieve insight*). In general, there is a tendency amongst such therapists to identify latent meaning in the 'there-and-then' in contrast to the 'here-and-now' of humanistic perspectives.

'Transferential' relationships are particularly relevant to psychoanalytic/ psychodynamic thinking, i.e. the process whereby the client displaces on to the therapist's feelings, attributes and attitudes that belong to a significant figure of the client's past (see the 'Client–Therapist Relationship' in Ch. 3). This type of relationship is often acknowledged within arts therapies with psychoanalytic/psychodynamic orientation, but the arts can also play an important role. Transferential relationships within arts therapies with a psychoanalytic/psychodynamic orientation can become present when arts therapists encourage the client to fully engage with the artwork, while they keep themselves in a more distant role. While the client is involved in the artistic process, issues of transference may become apparent and worked through within the art-making itself. Artistic or other forms of disclosure on the part of the therapist are often avoided. 'Projected' relationships are also found extensively within such approaches. Not only the arts therapist but also the client can, at times, be distanced from the artwork. Thus they both become able to reflect on the process of arts-making and/or the end-product, and the client–therapist relationship, can make links with the past, and understand issues pertinent to the client's current life.

The projected relationship enables links between what has been unconsciously expressed during the art-making process and the conscious understanding of this process. The link between the conscious and the unconscious self can be encouraged through *verbal communication*. Valuing verbal communication is common amongst arts therapists with a psychoanalytic/psychodynamic bias, which contrasts with the non-verbal bias of other arts therapies approaches. Verbal language is seen as closely linked with the conscious self, while artwork is perceived as readily revealing aspects of the unconscious. Consequently, verbalisation becomes an important component of the process of bringing the unconscious artistic expression into conscious awareness. Another reason why this approach favours verbalisations is practical: arts therapists adopting this approach often avoid direct artistic involvement. Therapeutic interventions are therefore not necessarily artistic but often of a verbal nature. Such verbal interventions can comprise descriptions of what has happened, suggestions for further work or interpretations of the underlying issues faced by the client (Payne 1992, Waller & Dalley 1992).

Within arts therapies, references to Freudian thinking are often found (see, e.g. Alvin 1975, Kestenberg 1975, Naumburg 1966, Odell-Miller 2000, Priestley 1995, Siegel 1985, Curtis, unpublished interview 2002, Ch. 8). However, object relations theory is even more popular within a British context and the art therapy (AT) discipline in particular (see Ch. 6). Theories developed by Klein (1975) and Winnicott (1971) are often perceived as able to offer close resonance to arts therapies practices. Winnicott's concept of the 'transitional object' for example (defined as a material possession that enables children to bridge their internal/subjective world and the external/objective world), gives direct justification for the use of the arts within arts therapies (see Byrne 1995, Case 1990, 2000, Levinge 1993, Meekums 2002). According to the dramatherapist Johnson (1998), within arts therapies with a Winnicottian perspective, the arts are important tools for exploring the space between the client and the therapist, the self and the other, the internal and the external, the literal and the metaphorical.

Another important approach traditionally categorised under the psychoanalytic/psychodynamic tradition is the work of Jung (1990). Jung (1990) introduces a fairly 'active' form of therapy with a strong emphasis upon the 'real' relationship between the client and the therapist/analyst. Unlike traditional psychoanalytic thinking, Jung (1990) focuses on the positive role of the unconscious and self-realisation. According to Clarkson (1994), these features place his approach much closer to humanistic than traditional psychoanalytic thinking. Irrespectively of categorisation, Jung's work has become very relevant to arts therapies practices. In Jungian thinking, the arts receive a valuable role as a means of accessing the 'shadow' self. His notion of the collective unconscious, which consists of 'archetypes' that are universally shared, offers fresh ways of looking at the arts and discovering meaning. It also offers a theoretical justification for studying and incorporating myths, legends and rituals within arts therapies (see Bonny 1994, Chodorow 1991, Schaverien 2000, Slade 1954, Whitehouse 1979, Lindqvist [Pearson 1996]).

Finally, a different type of work occurs when arts therapists with a psychoanalytic/psychodynamic perspective work with groups. Foulkes' (1964) contribution to group dynamics (e.g. the identification of different levels of communication within groups and the relevance of the group 'matrix') and Bion's (1961) discussion of primitive states (or 'basic assumptions', i.e. dependency, fight/flight, pairing) are often used to explain and guide practices. Within arts therapies group work, group dynamics become particularly important as we can see in Dokter (1994, 1998), McNeilly (2000), Odell-Miller (2000), Waller (1993), Papadopoulos (N. Papadopoulos, unpublished interview 2002; Ch. 8) and Sandel & Johnson (1983).

In Figure 4.2, there is a graphic representation of how arts therapies with a psychoanalytic/psychodynamic orientation might look. This example is a simplified version of Johnson's (1998) articulation of three stages of therapeutic action within psychoanalytic/psychodynamic arts therapies, that is the stage of externalisation, transformation and internalisation.

As Figure 4.2 suggests, the self is perceived as comprising both conscious and unconscious sides and as carrying a number of defences that compensate for unresolved internal conflicts ('the defensive self'). Initially, the client is encouraged to work with the artistic material. This work involves externalising unconscious aspects of the self and as loosening the client's defences. Issues identified during the art-making process are worked through; the relationship with the art-making process and the therapist enable changes to take place ('transformation'). Underlying issues are then brought into the client's consciousness and new experiences of being and relating are re-integrated within the client's psyche ('internalisation'). The client leaves arts therapies with much more knowledge about him or herself (the 'knowledgeable self')

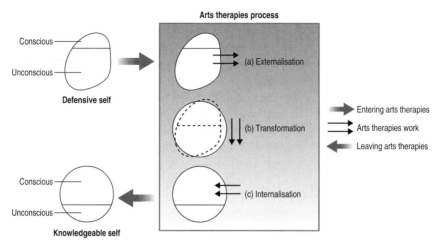

Figure 4.2: *An arts therapies model informed by psychoanalytic/psychodynamic thinking.*

and an ability to continue working toward self-discovery without the need of the arts therapies space.

Johnson (1998) clarifies that the process of externalisation is not equivalent to a behavioural expression of feelings and that similarly, internalisation is not the same as imitation. During both of these actions both expression of feelings and imitation can take place. On a psychological level, there is a movement out (externalisation) and in (internalisation) of the self and a concurrent movement from internalising to externalising 'objects' (i.e. inner representations of real or phantasised person or aspects of a person that either satisfies or frustrates individual needs). Transformation takes place within the arts/playspace (a space frequently referred to within arts therapies literature as a 'transitional space' to reflect influences from Winnicott's 1971 ideas of transitional phenomena and objects), often through empathetic but also through discrepant experiences with the arts or/and the therapist.

A strong influence from object relations theory is apparent in this model. For example, Johnson's (1998) therapeutic actions resemble closely Bion's (1964) notion of containment and the processes of projection, digestion and introjection. This theoretical orientation is also perceived as informing some of the developmental approaches followed within arts therapies and as such, we will discuss this further in the following section.

The developmental trend

Arts therapists often hold developmental perspectives, especially if they work with children. Some 'developmental' principles are outlined in Box 4.3. This box shows that a number of arts therapists view *development in terms of stages* and are often involved in *identifying these stages for their clients*. This enables them to *set appropriate objectives* at the onset of the work and to *evaluate the therapeutic work*. Ease with evaluations and use of *precise criteria* during this process is also indicated.

We believe that when it comes to developmental perspectives, there are two major sources of theories utilised within arts therapies: on one hand

Box 4.3: Developmental group of statements

Statements

- I hold developmental stages in mind most of the time.
- I am aware of the developmental stages my clients are at.
- The objectives are linked to the developmental stage the client is at.
- I use precise criteria when I evaluate.
- There is no resistance in me about evaluating therapy.

(mean* = 3.21, standard deviation^f = 0.50, internal consistency$^\alpha$ = 0.63)

*The higher the score, the stronger the agreement with this group of statements (a five-point scale was used ranging from strongly agree = 5 to strongly disagree = 1).

^{f}The higher the value, the higher average variation of this group of statements from the group mean score

$^\alpha$The higher the value, the more consistent the responses to different statements; for example, those who agreed with one also agreed with the other statements in this group.

The mean score for this group of statements is above 3 (i.e. neither agree/nor disagree), which suggests that generally, arts therapists agreed to such principles. Internal consistency remains at acceptable levels, showing that overall, arts therapies practitioners who agree with one of these statements possibly agree with most of them.

there are psychotherapeutically-derived models, on the other hand there are theories adapted from developmental psychology and educational theories. Depending on the specific developmental model followed, there is emphasis on different aspects of human development (e.g. cognitive, emotional, social and physical) and a range of links with the arts. Furthermore, it is often the case that with the use of the latter set of theories (theories from developmental psychology and education), there is indeed ease with conducting evaluations, using precise criteria and specific evaluative tools. In contrast, with the former set of theories, reflection and clinical supervision are two of the main tools for evaluation and there is a lot of scepticism about evaluating change in more concrete ways.

Developmental approaches from psychotherapy

Arts therapists with a psychoanalytic/psychodynamic approach often term their approach as being developmental, especially if their clients are children. We have already seen that the arts within arts therapies are seen as making links with unconscious processes and the client's past (see previous section). Overall, approaches of this kind discuss ways of forming personalities, highlight the emotional maturation of the individual and emphasise the developmental aspects of psychoanalytic/psychodynamic thinking. For example, practitioners with a Freudian perspective will perceive the client's work as representing psychosexual stages of development varying from the oral to the mature genital stage (see Table 4.1). Practitioners with an object-relations bias will draw directly upon theories of development articulated by Klein (1975), Mahler (Mahler et al 1975) or Winnicott (1971). For example, they may see development as moving from a paranoid/schizoid position to the depressive position (Klein), from the stage of normal autism to consolidation of individuation (Mahler), or from absolute dependence to relative independence (Winnicott) (see Table 4.1). References to such approaches within arts therapies can be found in Case (1990, 2000), Dokter (1994, 1998), Kestenberg (1975), Levinge (1993), Siegel (1984).

Most of the above theories acknowledge relational factors as affecting development. However, there are arts therapists who find that Bowlby's (1969) theory places a stronger emphasis upon the interpersonal aspects of emotional development than object relations theory (see Table 4.1) and because of this it offers a more useful model for their work. Others question the preoccupation of object relations with the early years of life and turn to Erikson (1959) for his understanding of development as extending throughout the life span (see Table 4.1). Finally, there is another group of arts therapists who criticise psychoanalytic/psychodynamic perceptions of development as limited in its articulation of associations with cognitive development. The theoretician most extensively associated with cognitive development is Piaget (1972), according to whom there are the following stages of cognitive development:

- Sensori-motor stage (infancy: intelligence is demonstrated through motor activity without the use of symbols).
- Preoperational stage (toddler and early childhood: intelligence is demonstrated through the use of symbols, but thinking is done in a non-logical, non-reversible manner).
- Concrete operational stage (elementary and early adolescence: intelligence is demonstrated through logical and systematic manipulation of symbols related to concrete objects, while mental actions that are reversible develop).
- Formal operational stage (adolescence and adulthood: intelligence is demonstrated through the logical use of symbols related to abstract concepts).

Arts therapists who value Piaget's contribution but at the same time hold an overall psychoanalytic/psychodynamic perspective may find particularly useful Stern's (1985) widely quoted model of the interpersonal world of the infant. Stern's model bridges the gap between cognitive and emotional development and portrays child development as moving from an emergent sense of self to a verbal sense of self (see Table 4.1 for domains of experience according to Stern). Much stronger cognitive emphasis is found in the following group of developmental approaches.

Developmental approaches from psychology and education

There are a number of development psychologists who deal with aesthetic/artistic development from a cognitive perspective (e.g. Duffy 1979, Housen 1983, Parsons et al 1978). Amongst them, the most frequently cited model in the arts therapies literature comes from the USA and has been developed by Gardner (1973) and his colleagues at Harvard University (most of their research work comes under the name 'Project Zero'). Their research on aesthetic development is based on Goodman's (1976) taxonomy of symbol systems and processes, and Piaget's (1972) theory of cognitive development,

Table 4.1: Examples of developmental models from psychotherapy

Psychosexual stages of development
Freud (1953)

Oral stage	Anal stage	Phallic stage	Latency stage	Mature genital stage
1 year of age	2–3 years of age	3–5 years of age	6–11 years of age	12 + years of age

Object relations theory
Klein (1975)

	Paranoid/schizoid position	Depressive position		
	Early life experience time not specified	Continues throughout one's life; beginning is not specified		

Mahler et al (1975)

Normal autistic phase	Normal symbiotic phase	Separation/individuation sub-phases: (i) differentiating phase, (ii) practising phase, (iii) rapprochement phase, (iv) object constancy phase		
1st month	2–5 months	6–36 months		

Winnicott (1971)

Absolute dependency		Relative dependency		Relative independence

Continued

Table 4.1: Examples of developmental models from psychotherapy—cont'd

Attachment theory, formation of attachments
Bowlby (1969)

Pre-attachment	Attachment-in-the-making	Clear-cut attachment	Post-attachment
Up to 6 weeks	6–6/8 weeks	6/8–18/24 months	18/24 months +

Psychosocial Development, life crises
Erikson (1959)

Basic trust vs basic mistrust despair	Autonomy vs shame and doubt	Initiative vs guilt	Industry vs inferiority	Identity vs identity confusion	Intimacy vs isolation	Generative vs stagnation	Integrity vs despair
1 year of age	2 years of age	3–6 years of age	7–10 years of age	11–20 years of age	Young adulthood	Childbearing period	Later life

Interpersonal model, domains of experience
Stern (1985)

The emergent self	The core self	The subjective self	The verbal self
1st month	2–5 months	6–9 months	10–18 months

with clearly defined stages in the development, use and understanding of symbols. According to the Project Zero team, there is a sequential development from one stage to another in at least music, painting and literature as described in Table 4.2.

Despite criticism of the neglect of affective and socio-cultural factors (Sanderson 1991), the well-researched character of some of these psychological models can help arts therapists to understand clients' cognitive needs, set objectives close to the developmental capacities of their clients and evaluate the degree to which such objectives have been achieved (see Box 4.3). For example, an arts therapist will be able to judge whether the artistic age of children scribbling is in accordance with their chronological age and when their drawings suggest development beyond a sensorimotor stage, e.g. into symbolic action.

Another important point of reference for a number of arts therapists has been the work completed within arts education. For example, Kellogg (1969) and Lowenfeld (1957) made extensive collections of children's drawings, which they subsequently studied from a developmental perspective. Links with Piaget's theory of cognitive development are once again apparent in these models (see Ch. 6 for further discussion of Lowenfeld's model). Developmental ideas and models have emerged from all arts education disciplines and have varied applicability to the current arts therapies practice; see for example: Moog (1976), Pflederer (1964) and Rider (1981) from music education, Courtney

---

Table 4.2: Examples of a linear and a spiral model of aesthetic/artistic development

Linear model
Gardner (1973)

Pre-symbolic period	Period of symbol use	Later artistic development
0–1 years of age	2–7 years of age	8 + years of age
Sensorimotor development	(i) Immersion in symbolic media (ii) Exploration and amplification of the symbol (iii) Sense of aesthetic form and familiarity with culture's code	Skill development, code undergoes familiarisation and manipulation

Spiral model
Swanwick and Tillman (1986)

Themes	Mastery	Imitation	Imaginative play	Meta-cognition
	0–4 years of age	5–9 years of age	10–15 years of age	15 + years of age
Individual features	Sensory	Personal	Speculative	Symbolic
Modes	**Materials**	**Expression**	**Form**	**Value**
Social features	Manipulative	Vernacular	Idiomatic	Systematic

(1974), Heathcote (1991) and Slade (1954) from drama education, and Laban (1975) and Sherborne (1990) from dance education.

Models of artistic development are often criticised for presenting a linear progression from infancy to maturity. Hargreaves (1982) for example, studied children's sensitivity to stylistic categories of music and found that although sensitivity increased with age, the patterns were complex. Bunt (1994), a music therapist, claims that a 'spiral' type of development is more persuasive than sequential/linear development and cites Swanwick & Tillman's (1986) model as an example. The advantages of this spiral model are an inherent flexibility in the developmental process, an acknowledgement of the complexity of such development, and recognition that the social context, i.e. environment, plays a crucial role in shaping such a process. This model consists of a number of themes (from mastery to meta-cognition) and modes (from sensory to systematic) and is relevant to children as well as adults (see Table 4.2). Developmental models articulated within the arts therapies field often acknowledge some of these characteristics. For example, the lack of linearity is emphasised within the DT developmental model of Jennings (1990) that sees embodiment, projection and role-play as three stages that people move between throughout their life span (see Ch. 7). Other references to this type of developmental thinking (as opposed to psychotherapeutically-informed models) that can be found in Section 2 of this book are Cattanach (1994a,b), Dubowski (1990), Johnson (2000), Lewis (2000), Payne (1990), Penfield (1992), and Sobey (K. Sobey, unpublished interview, 2002, Ch. 8). Spiral development can also be relevant to the process of arts therapies sessions as the following section discusses.

The artistic/creative trend

Artistic/creative approaches are another major trend within the arts therapies field. We have referred to the artistic versus psychotherapy debate when defining the arts therapies field in Chapter 2. For example, we talked about how practitioners primarily aligned to the arts regarding artistic rationales sufficient for guiding and explaining practices, while others either consider their work as a form of psychotherapy with the arts 'added on' or insist on an amalgam of approaches within which both artistic and therapeutic principles are valued. According to Gilroy (1989), the engagement of arts therapists with their own artistic practice varies in a similar way. Her survey of art therapists delineated three groups: (1) practitioners who consider themselves as predominantly artists; (2) those who consider the art as inseparable from therapy; (3) those with marginal involvement with the art. We think that this categorisation could apply to all arts therapies. It is also possible that the varied involvement of those practitioners with the arts also suggests a similarly varied degree of emphasis of the artistic and creative element within their arts therapies work.

Box 4.4 shows some important characteristics of artistic/creative approach. According to this box, arts therapists who value artistic practices perceive their work as being about *encouraging clients to do something*, to *get fully engaged in the artistic process* and to be *spontaneous*. This does not mean that arts therapies sessions entail constant activity. Part of art-making also involves

> **Box 4.4:** Artistic/creative group of statements
>
> ## Statements
>
> - The therapeutic process is always about encouraging clients to do something.
> - I try to enable clients to really engage with the art process as fully as possible.
> - I encourage clients to be as spontaneous as they could possibly be.
> - My artistic background determines the techniques I use.
> - I am much more active in the early stages of the therapy.
> - I am trying to set up a metaphor for something that might happen in real life.
>
> (mean* = 3.13, standard deviation^f = 0.59, internal consistency$^\alpha$ = 0.60)
>
> *The higher the score, the stronger the agreement with this group of statements (a five-point scale was used ranging from strongly agree = 5 to strongly disagree = 1).
> ^{f}The higher the value, the higher average variation of this group of statements from the group mean score.
> $^\alpha$The higher the value, the more consistent the responses to different statements; for example, those who agreed with one also agreed with the other statements of this group.
> Both the mean score and the standard deviation show that overall agreement with this group of statements was close to the middle point of the scale (3 = neither agree not disagree). Nevertheless, most of the statements concerned artistic/creative practices and responses presented a sufficient degree of internal consistency.

silences (we will call them 'artistic' silences) to permit the important processes of listening, observing, reflecting (Jones 1996, Schaverien 2000). Although the *therapist's artistic background* plays an important role in the choice of techniques brought to the session, this background does not necessarily restrict arts therapies content and the way clients' needs are addressed. The *therapist is often active during early stages* of the work in order to enable the client to become familiar with the process, but this is not always the case; it depends on the client group, the setting and/or the arts therapies approach followed.

Given the separate artistic traditions within music, visual arts, drama/theatre and dance and their multiple translations within each of the arts therapies subfields, discussing a common rationale for all arts therapies with a predominant artistic orientation is particularly difficult. Further exploration of art-based approaches can be found in Section 2 where arts therapies are seen as separate disciplines (see the creative MT model by Nordoff & Robbins 1971, 1977; the work of Hill 1941, 1951, Adamson 1970, 1984, and Liebmann 1986; the theatre-based approaches of Evrenov and Iljine [Jones 1996] and Jennings 1998; the movement-based approaches of Laban 1975 and North 1972). We can say here however, that in all of these approaches, the artistic/creative process appropriately modified for arts therapies, constitutes the therapeutic approach.

A popular model of creativity (Hadamard 1954, Wallas [Arieti 1976], Poincaré 1982) found with the arts therapies literature can provide us with an example of a truly artistic/creative perspective within arts therapies as a whole (Fig. 4.3). Both Mottram (2000, 2001) and Meekums (2000, 2002), for example, find this model particularly useful for their practice and argue that the model unfolds in a spiral rather than a linear way.

According to this model, creativity consists of the following stages:

1. *Preparation.* Familiarisation with artistic activities, and collection of information and materials are often explored in this first stage of the process. Direction, purpose and meaning are important aspects for starting the creative process.
2. *Incubation.* This stage is more difficult, mainly because it involves not only working but also not working (e.g. resting), and dealing with both what is known and the frustration of the unknown or undiscovered.
3. *Illumination.* Illumination is that part of the creative process when something new and meaningful is generated. Something that, although perhaps not complete, is satisfying and fulfilling. It is the 'aha' moment, the time of inspiration and enlightenment.
4. *Verification.* This is the final stage, during which the final clarifications and modifications are applied to what has been created.

Arts therapists aligned to an artistic/creative way of thinking may see that enabling clients to go through the whole artistic/creative process is the main therapeutic task. Furthermore, they perceive such models as explaining experiences and processes, and enabling therapeutic change. It is sometimes the case that artistic/creative models are associated with performances/exhibitions at the end of the therapeutic work that celebrate the new 'artistic' identity of the client. For such work, the therapist and/or the client often make artistic choices and have artistic concerns, often to an extent that is more pronounced than in other less art-based arts therapies practices.

The main criticism of these models is that they often have a weak explanation of the underlying therapeutic rationale. Thus, they are often perceived as ways of working (i.e. clinical methodology) rather than as therapeutic approaches on their own. Artistic/creative approaches can often be used in conjunction with other models, such as the eclectic/integrative, developmental, humanistic or psychoanalytic/psychodynamic.

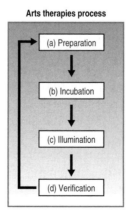

Arts therapies process

- (a) Preparation
- (b) Incubation
- (c) Illumination
- (d) Verification

Figure 4.3: *An artistic/creative perspective within arts therapies.*

The active/directive trend

According to Walrond-Skinner's (1986) dictionary of psychotherapy, arts therapies are regarded as action therapies. The same source claims that one of the main strengths of action therapies is their non-verbal emphasis. Looking at the artistic content as well as how this content is communicated (see Ch. 2 for more on non-verbal communication) offers potential for describing and understanding the meaning of the therapeutic process. In order to achieve such communication, both the client and the therapists are engaged in 'behavioural acts', which at some point may or may not be associated with words.

Arts therapies can therefore be seen as having an active as well as a directive nature in that: there is an expectation that clients, and at times also therapists: will use pens, paper, paint or clay; will make sounds or music; will move or dance; will engage in dramatic enactments or create stories. This expectation offers a first degree of direction as well as suggests action on the part of the client, the therapist and/or both (see Box 4.5).

The group of statements presented in Box 4.5 suggest that the arts therapist tends to:

- *be actively involved* within the session in a way that the artistic work is guided
- *make therapeutic choices* in terms of the use of appropriate techniques
- *hold aims* in mind that give an overall direction to the arts therapies work and enable the client to grow in a desirable area.

Box 4.5: Active/directive group of statements

Statements

- Sometimes I will actively do artwork myself during the session.
- I may concentrate my work on physical aspects.
- I do direct more than just for basic safety.
- I do have certain techniques that I bring out when it is appropriate.
- I may concentrate my work on helping a client with some intellectual/cognitive aspects.

(mean* = 3.08, standard deviation^f = 0.49, internal consistency$^\alpha$ = 0.56)

*The higher the score, the stronger the agreement with this group of statements (a five-point scale was used ranging from strongly agree = 5 to strongly disagree = 1).

^{f}The higher the value, the higher average variation of this group of statements from the group mean score.

$^\alpha$The higher the value, the more consistent the responses to different statements; for example, those who agreed with one also agreed with the other statements of this group.

The group mean score for this group is close to the middle point of the scale. Strong agreement with this group of statements cannot therefore be assumed. Furthermore, the low internal consistency of this group implies that arts therapists who agree with some of these statements do not necessarily show strong agreement with all of them.

Active/directive practices have received a number of criticisms from both psychoanalytic psychotherapists and certain psychoanalytically-informed arts therapists. For example, active therapies have been seen by psychoanalytic psychotherapists as encouraging the client to act out. According to this criticism, acting out refers to an unregulated expression of emotions, is a form of resistance and is a hindrance to the therapeutic work. Within a verbal psychotherapy context, Sandler et al (1970) talk about techniques such as containment, interpretation, prohibition and strengthening the client's ego for managing with unnecessary or dangerous acting out (e.g. aggressive and or sexual responses that can put in danger the client, others in the group and/or the therapist). Similar techniques can be applied in arts therapies, especially if the arts therapist has a psychodynamic orientation. For example, the client's aggressive impulses externalised upon the arts media and/or therapist can be re-introduced to the client either through the relationship with the therapist and/or the artistic work. The arts media and the therapist can function as a form of containment. The arts therapist with a psychoanalytic/psychodynamic orientation may also offer verbal interpretations. With the arts therapist making thoughtful therapeutic choices, unwanted behaviour can be diminished (prohibition). By holding aims in mind, the arts therapist can offer an overall direction to the arts therapies work and enable the client to grow in a desirable area (thus, potentially strengthening the client's ego).

References to directive practices have also raised heated discussions in arts therapies, especially within the art therapy discipline, between supporters of 'directive' versus 'non-directive' practices (see Liebmann 1986, McNeilly 1983). For example, one of the issues discussed within AT has been the introduction of themes from the therapist at the onset of the therapeutic work. The supporters of the directive approaches have claimed that such themes offer safety for the client and a rationale for beginning the therapeutic work. Their opponents (primarily art therapists with a strong psychoanalytic/psychodynamic bias) have argued that themes should be allowed to emerge from the clients themselves. During the process of this debate, there has been an extensive discussion of different types of practices and a final acknowledgement of the value of adapting practices to client needs. We regard thorough explanation of practices and flexibility as a useful outcome from this debate and relevant to more than just AT.

Another area that is closely connected with active/directive practices is the degree of structure within arts therapies sessions. While some arts therapists insist that there is a need for structure, others regard structure as a possible interruption to the therapeutic process. For example, dramatherapists such as Jones (1996) and Pearson (1996) (see Ch. 7), and dance movement therapists such as Chace (Chaiklin & Schmais 1986), North (1972) and Papadopoulos (N Papadopoulos, unpublished interview 2002; Ch. 8), make explicit references to following an explicit structure within their sessions. Practitioners with a strong psychoanalytic/psychodynamic orientation such as Curtis (S Curtis, unpublished interview, 2002; Ch. 8) and Sobey (K Sobey, unpublished interview, 2002; Ch. 5), or those following a Rogerian client-centred approach, e.g. Thomas (D Thomas, unpublished interview, 2002; Ch. 6) discuss the fact that there is very limited structure within their sessions with the client leading the process. Bruscia (1988), an American music therapist, discusses these two perspectives in more detail. He observes that within improvisational music therapy (MT) there are two types of sessions: 'free-flowing' and 'structured' sessions. With structured sessions there are 'procedural phases' sequenced in such a way that there is a movement towards and/or away from a focal activity or event, while within free-flowing sessions, phases are repeated and/or layered based on the client's recurring musical or emotional themes. The golden medium is suggested by those music therapists who are influenced primarily by Alvin (1978). These therapists refer to the need for both freedom and structure, e.g. Bunt (L Bunt, unpublished interview, 2002; Ch. 5) and Oldfield (1995). Again we see this feature of practice as potentially relevant to more than just MT and the debate about the degree to which arts therapies are active/directive as ongoing.

Although the active/directive trend can be a characteristic of many arts therapies practices, especially insofar as clinical methodology is concerned, theoretical articulation of why such methodology is followed varies considerably including humanistic, developmental or artistic rationales (see previous sections). Active/directive approaches can also be associated with an overall behavioural orientation. Behaviourism is an umbrella term that refers to a number of approaches ranging from the far end of objective behaviourism in which only what is observable is worthy of attention, e.g. Skinner's behaviour modification model (Skinner 1953), to the other, relatively more holistic, end of the spectrum of cognitive behaviour therapy (Meichenbaum 1977). All behavioural approaches are based on learning theory and are often considered as very technical interventions with a reductive character. They have been criticised as failing to understand underlying problems and to achieve 'real' change. Further criticism refers to them as focusing on the problem and pathologising the person.

As we have discussed in Chapter 1, there are limited applications of behavioural models with arts therapies practices in the UK. Nevertheless, few references to such models can be found in MT, particularly in American practice (Bunt 1994, Moreno et al 1990). There are also many arts therapists who have a history of using the arts in a task-oriented or educative way (e.g. many practising arts therapists were initially either artists or art teachers). Thus, they may either explicitly or implicitly draw upon learning theory and, at times, practise in ways that appear closer to behavioural models than openly acknowledged (see, e.g. North 1972).

The active/directive trend can also be associated with theoretical justifications offered by brief approaches to psychotherapy and counselling. Brief therapy draws upon a wide range of theoretical underpinnings including psychoanalytic/psychodynamic thinking (e.g. focal psychotherapy [Ballint et al 1972, Malan 1976], time-limited psychotherapy [Mann 1973]) and behavioural practices (e.g. solution-focused counselling [Miller et al 1996], strategic therapy [Haley & Rocheport-Haley 2003]). In all cases, Butcher & Koss (1978) argue that brief therapies share at least the following features:

1. They are time-limited (1–25 sessions)
2. They have limited goals (a focus is sought on specific symptoms and problems of areas of difficulty)

3. They present centredness (there is focus on current problems and immediate context).

4. They involve directiveness and activity on the part of the therapist.

These characteristics bear close resemblance to arts therapies principles outlined in Box 4.5. Furthermore, literature in arts therapies provides evidence of the relevance of such work for arts therapists. Woddis (1992), for example, has claimed that there is a need for AT to develop theoretical frameworks for focused interventions, while Mottram (2000, 2001) makes references to brief therapy as relevant to the time-limited aspect of her work (see Ch. 6). Other publications, such as Gersie's (1996) edited book, make specific suggestions as to how DT can be used as a brief intervention drawing upon a number of different theoretical perspectives. Gersie (A Gersie, unpublished interview, 2002) herself, for example, describes her work as a type of strategic DT (see Ch. 7).

Figure 4.4 offers a conceptual representation of active/directive approaches within arts therapies. Task-oriented, behaviourally-informed approaches and some types of brief arts therapies may look like this.

As Figure 4.4 shows, the client may be seen as presenting difficulties in a number of different areas. Therapeutic work often begins with identifying the client's most urgent and/or major problem/s. When possible, a therapeutic contract is established between the client and the therapist and exploration of the agreed issues begins. Unlike humanistic or psychoanalytic/psychodynamic arts therapies approaches that address the person in a more holistic way, interventions with a strong active/directive character are often targeted towards the most important difficulties of the client. At times, due to the nature of the art-making process, multiple issues can be concurrently addressed but not particularly focused upon. A number of variations of the client–art–therapist relationship are possible including one in which the therapist acts as the artist in the presence of the client (see the 'Client–therapist Relationship' in Ch. 3).

This type of work falls closely into what Wheeler (1987) refers to as the first level of therapeutic work (see 'Therapeutic Aims' in Ch. 3) and can be particularly relevant when there are time restrictions in the overall duration

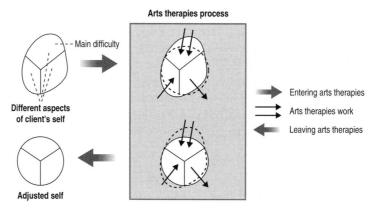

Figure 4.4: *An active/directive arts therapies model.*

of the therapeutic contact; increasing pressures for short-term interventions with quick outcomes and limited resources are currently the case in most places of employment. Stronger active/directive elements can also be found in group over individual work and with certain client groups over others (e.g. with clients with schizophrenia, learning difficulties, addiction and/or phobias). When the therapist is particularly active/directive, the need to articulate therapeutic rationales becomes even more important in order to avoid mere application of ad hoc arts therapies techniques with a potentially harmful effect on the clients. Further discussion on the need to conceptualise practices is included in the following section.

The eclectic/integrative trend

Eclectic/integrative trends advocate the selection of ideas and methods from a number of different schools of thought within one approach. In psychotherapy, such perspectives have been supported by people like Garfield (1980) and Thorne (1967) and extensively discussed by a number of others.

The arts therapies field has essentially an eclectic/integrative character. It consists of the overlap between the arts and psychotherapy (see 'Our Definition of Arts Therapies' in Ch. 2). Current practice bears memories of movements contributing to the emergence of the field such as those in the arts, psychoanalysis, humanistic psychotherapies, education and the input from other emerging professional groups such as occupational therapists and hospital artists (see 'The Emergence of the Profession in the 20th Century' in Ch. 1). Moreover, current definitions of the field accept diversity as an important characteristic of the field (see 'Definitions and descriptions found within arts therapies publications' in Ch. 2). Additional evidence for the presence of this tendency within the arts therapies field is the overall agreement of arts therapists with the group of eclectic/integrative statements presented in Box 4.6. This group of statements gained the second highest mean score (the first was the group of humanistic principles discussed earlier in this chapter) and thus showed strong relevance for the arts therapies practice.

Despite the prevalence of eclectic/integrative principles amongst arts therapists, there is an ambiguous position of many arts therapists regarding the degree to which they might call their practice an 'eclectic/integrative approach'. This is possibly due to the fact that there have been a lot of criticisms about such practices from psychotherapists and arts therapists themselves (see Abram 1992, Thorne 1967, Valente & Fontana 1993). Most of these criticisms are about eclectic rather than integrative approaches. The former term is often regarded as suggesting insufficient training and ill-defined therapeutic rationales, while the latter implies the existence of theoretical justification, research-based choices and the development of a coherent and consistent new therapeutic framework. Critics of eclecticism argue that certain such practices suggest a mere 'lumping' together of principles and methods without a clear rationale, some of which may be often conceptually contradictory. If practice is only loosely supported from theory, the value of therapeutic frameworks as a safeguard for practice becomes questionable; so is the safety of the client (Karkou & Sanderson 2000, 2001, Karkou 1999).

In response to such criticisms, several arts therapists argue that eclectic approaches offer *flexible perspectives* (Box 4.6). By adopting flexibility the client is not boxed in predetermined notions of human functioning or in fixed ideas about artistic expression. Thus, the arts therapist attempts to understand client issues in a number of different ways, to acknowledge such different perspectives and enable working through issues in an accepting and democratic manner. Emphasis on *the central role of the client* in forming the direction of the work and the most suited theoretical framework often translates to questioning the role of the therapist as the 'all-knowledgeable expert' and allowing the client to become a 'teacher' for the therapist.

In Section 2, there are examples of arts therapies work with either implicit or explicit references to the eclectic/integrative trend. For example, in Chapter 5, Alvin's work is perceived as integrating wide-ranging influences into a coherent interactive MT whole (Alvin 1975). Bunt (L Bunt, unpublished interview, 2002), closely connected with Alvin's interactive trend within MT, acknowledges a number of different theoretical underpinnings to his work. Ansdell (G Ansdell, unpublished interview, 2002) in discussing the creative MT approach, refers to artistic, as well as humanistic and psychoanalytic/psychodynamic principles. Priestley, although the founder of analytical music therapy, borrows principles and ideas from more than psychoanalysis (Scheiby 1999). Odell-Miller (H Odell Miller, unpublished interview, 2002), primarily a psychoanalytically-informed music therapist, also acknowledges the relevance of other psychotherapeutic explanations for her group MT practice.

Examples of eclectic/integrative practices can also be found in the AT field. Mottram (2000, 2001) for example, presents an art-based approach with

---

Box 4.6: Eclectic/integrative group of statements

Statements

- I use a number of different approaches for each client.
- It depends which population I am working with, what sort of theoretical approach I am adopting.
- I do not think I have got one model that I follow.
- The clients I work with have taught me most of what I know.
- My ideas are designed in collaboration with the clients.

(mean* = 3.69, standard deviation^f = 0.63, internal consistency$^\alpha$ = 0.62)

*The higher the score, the stronger the agreement with this group of statements (a five-point scale was used ranging from strongly agree = 5 to strongly disagree = 1).
^{f}The higher the value, the higher average variation of this group of statements from the group mean score.
$^\alpha$The higher the value, the more consistent the responses to different statements; for example, those who agreed with one also agreed with the other statements of this group.
It is apparent from the high mean of this group of statements that there is an overall agreement with eclectic/integrative statements. However, there is a range of opinions about this issue (high standard deviation) and responses are not necessarily consistent.

strong influences from Gestalt, brief therapy and conversation therapy. Waller (1993) talks about her group interactive AT as drawing upon group analysis and systemic thinking next to the prevalent interpersonal influences from Sullivan (1955) and Yalom (1970). DT, discussed in Chapter 7, shows a strong affiliation with eclectic/integrative models as expressed in the pioneering work in the field and subsequent developments. For example, Slade (1954) is presented as having drawn for his work primarily upon education, and child drama in particular, but also as influenced by Jungian thinking. Jennings' (1983, 1992, 1995, 1998) wide-ranging work also shows an eclectic/integrative rationale. Although a strong advocate of the theatre model in DT, she acknowledges strong influences from social anthropology and affiliation with humanistic and developmental ideas. Finally, in Chapter 8, the eclectic/integrative character of many dance movement therapy (DMT) approaches is apparent. For example, within a wide psychoanalytic/psychodynamic frame, there is a strong eclectic/integrative character in the work of both Curtis (S Curtis, unpublished interview, 2002) and Papadopoulos (N Papadopoulos, unpublished interview, 2002), while Payne's (1994) work is described as an integrative practice that stresses the value of different therapeutic principles depending on the client.

Further justifications of eclectic/integrative practices are currently increasingly drawn from post-modern thinking in sociology and the arts that question the relevance and usefulness of grand narratives within current thinking (e.g. Gergen 1985, 1991, Grentz 1996, Lyotard 1984). As a result, fixed notions of the self and the arts have been questioned. From a post-modern perspective, personal identity is understood as socially-constructed, the result of experiences which are not solely determined by the genes (biological perspectives), instincts and/or the result of the first years of one's life (psychoanalytic/psychodynamic perspectives). The self is seen as being in flux (some post-modern thinkers talk about the 'multiple self'), reflecting a similar state of flux on a societal level. Regarding the arts, divisions between high and popular art, and between the artist and the non-artist have been challenged. Similarly, divisions between different art forms are currently blurred. The visual, the musical, the dramatic/theatrical and the dance art forms have given their place to installations, performances, mixed media, video and electronic arts, i.e. artistic creations which cannot be clearly located in one or another art form (Waller 2001).

As notions of the self and the arts are changing, so is the arts therapies practice. Evidence of arts therapies practices that address such changes can be found in Section 2 of this book. Byrne (1995), for example, acknowledges the post-modern perspective of his practice. He finds the Winnicottian's concept of interaction as parallel to Foucault's (1967) notion of discourse and valuable for AT practice (Ch. 6). Jennings (S. Jennings, unpublished interview, 2002) refers to the value of artistic construction in DT as equivalent to post-modern notions of social construction (Ch. 7), while Allegranti (1997), Best (2000) and Best & Parker (2001) describe important features of their practice through the perspective of social construction theory (Ch. 8).

The effects of post-modernism on arts therapies are apparent, as are the problems deriving from such a shift. Some of these problems are:

- Post-modernism and its associated social construction theory lack a new therapeutic model or models that can guide arts therapies practice. Post-modern ideas have come from sociology and the arts and are not as yet fully explored and discussed within a therapy context.
- As a result of the critique on old practices and ideas, post-modern thinking does not necessarily suggest something new. Because of this, practitioners often revert to older therapeutic models, which, although perceived under the light of a post-modern criticism, offer sufficient guidelines and coherent rationales.
- Accepting diversity sets no limits on what may take place within the arts therapies space and during the arts therapies process and raises the danger of 'everything goes with everything'. A thorough articulation of all the principles utilised, the therapeutic approaches drawn upon and the links between them is not always available.

In an attempt to address the above issue (i.e. clarifying the nature of arts therapies practices), we suggest that the eclectic/integrative character of the arts therapies field consist of a dialogue among the main trends discussed earlier such as the humanistic, psychoanalytic/psychodynamic, developmental, artistic/creative and active/directive. Additional components of the eclectic/integrative trend can also be drawn from a number of other fields (e.g. family/systemic therapy, transpersonal psychology, personal construct theory, narrative therapy, anthropology, social psychology, neuroscience and so on), i.e. areas that are becoming increasingly relevant to arts therapies practices but are not as yet widely spread.

Furthermore, our study in the field has revealed that the eclectic/integrative practices are not used erratically but follow certain patterns. For example, particular therapeutic perspectives are preferred in certain settings and with certain client groups as Figure 4.5 suggests.

Other important factors that distinguish practices are the age of the arts therapist, professional qualifications and other relevant experience. We will look at these issues in more detail in the following sections. Finally, the specific type of arts therapies modality is another important factor that suggests specific ways of working. Prevailing differences between disciplines will be presented and discussed in Section 2.

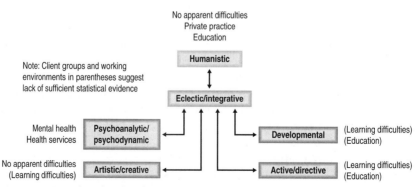

Figure 4.5: *Strands within the eclectic/integrative trend.*

Arts therapies trends and client groups

With clients who face mental health problems or learning difficulties, and clients with no apparent difficulties, certain arts therapies approaches are more highly regarded than others.

Clients with mental health issues

When working with different people with mental health problems, arts therapists show a higher preference for psychoanalytic/psychodynamic perspectives (see Fig. 4.5). John (1995), Killick & Greenwood (1995) and Levinge (1993) are just a few of a long list of arts therapists who have researched their own psychoanalytic/psychodynamic approach with this population. Compilations and reviews of research studies provided by arts therapies professional associations refer to working psychoanalytically/psychodynamically with people with a variety of mental health issues: those who have suffered trauma and/or survived physical, sexual and emotional abuse (e.g. Dent-Brown 2004, Karkou 2003, Odell-Miller et al 2003). Many more case studies from final year trainee arts therapists can also be found at higher education (HE) institutions that offer arts therapies training courses. The majority of these studies are clinical (rather than research) case studies that offer descriptions and explanations of the therapeutic process, often with a single client or a single group. Where clinical case studies are concerned, the focus is upon the client–therapist relationship over the duration of the therapeutic contact. Large-scale research studies that look at the efficacy of psychoanalytic/psychodynamic arts therapies with this client group are still very rare. Odell-Miller and her colleagues at the Addenbrooke's NHS Trust in Cambridge (Odell-Miller et al 2001) has offered one of the few examples of randomised control trials of primarily psychoanalytically-informed arts therapies with clients with continuing mental health issues. Although quantitative results from this study were not conclusive due to the high variability of interventions and client diagnosis (all types of arts therapies were included and a wide range of psychiatric diagnosis), and the small sample sizes, positive change was shown on most of the standardised mental health measures used. Furthermore, qualitative findings suggested that therapists' and clients' perceptions of the outcome of the treatment coincided in all treatment cases.

Further support for the value of psychoanalytic/psychodynamic orientation with this client group can be drawn from studies on verbal psychotherapies. For example, there is research evidence from studies with clients with depression, personality disorders, post-traumatic stress symptoms, children and adolescents with separation anxiety and older people with depression (Roth & Fonagy 1996, Department of Health 2001).

Given the wide range of symptoms included in this client group, arts therapists often adapt the psychoanalytic/psychodynamic underpinnings of their approach to the needs of their clients. For example, Killick & Greenwood (1995), referring to AT and clients with schizophrenia, talk about the need to focus on concrete art-making processes, suspend references to content and meaning, and avoid interpretations. Preliminary results from a randomised controlled study recently completed by Priebe & Röhricht (2001) supports the view that working in a concrete way with this client group can be useful.

Although in this study the therapeutic intervention moves further away from psychoanalytic/psychodynamic thinking to an activity-based treatment, results show that concrete body-based work has an effect upon the negative symptoms of schizophrenia. Other arts therapists discuss the need for a supportive approach when working with clients with schizophrenia, which does not attempt deep personality restructuring (e.g. John 1995, Stanton-Jones 1992, Wheeler 1987, Whitelock 1987) and/or may emphasise interpersonal arts therapies models, e.g. Chace (Chaiklin & Schmais 1986).

It appears that although, overall, psychoanalytic/psychodynamic arts therapies approaches predominate when working with clients with mental health issues, not all clients who fall into this category are perceived as readily benefiting from such frameworks. For example, according to the Department of Health (2001), cognitive/behavioural approaches and/or brief interventions are seen as more appropriate ways of working with people with anxiety disorders (e.g. phobias). This type of work is closely connected with the active/directive trend discussed before. With people with addictions, arts therapies can be applied as a form of insight psychotherapy as well as in a directive/educative way (the latter for example, can be particularly relevant during the early stages of abstinence [Karkou & Sanderson 1997]). Further study and research is needed in order to determine when psychoanalytically/psychodynamically-informed practices are useful with this client group, how they can be modified and/or when they should be completely abandoned.

Clients with learning difficulties

In our study we found that developmental ideas appear relevant to working with clients with learning difficulties, albeit with weak statistical support (Fig. 4.5). This result might be due to the fact that clients with learning difficulties often present an entirely different type of development from clients with no disability. There is not simply a delayed development as is popularly believed. Identifying appropriate developmental models that are relevant to such clients is therefore not necessarily an easy task. Furthermore, the arts therapies literature dealing with this client group is split between advocates of developmental theories drawn from the arts, psychology and education on the one hand and on the other those who adopt psychotherapeutic, and psychoanalytic/psychodynamic frameworks in particular. The former group of arts therapists favours active/directive practices, while the latter supports less directive interventions. When developmental perspectives with a psychoanalytic/psychodynamic orientation are adopted for this client group, the writings of Klein (1975) and Winnicott (1971) are extensively discussed within the arts therapies literature (Heal-Hughes 1995, Hughes 1988, Rabiger 1990, Tipple 1992). Furthermore, Sinason (1992), and her application of psychoanalytic/psychodynamic thinking to people with learning disabilities, becomes particularly relevant to arts therapies work (e.g. Sinason features in most contributions to Rees' edited book on AT and learning difficulties [Rees 1998]).

Others argue that psychoanalytic/psychodynamic approaches are potentially inappropriate ways of working with these clients. For example, Payne (1992) claims that group analytical DMT is not useful when working with people with severe learning disabilities. Instead developmental movement tasks provide focus for the therapeutic work and offer experiences that can meet developmental needs. Lawes & Woodcock (1995) make similar claims for MT regarding clients with dual diagnosis of learning difficulties and self-injurious behaviour. In their research study with this client group, Lawes & Woodcock (1995) perceived the psychoanalytically-informed MT intervention based on free improvisation as responsible for the lack of significant change in the clients' self-injurious behaviour. It is implied that a more focused intervention could have possibly produced more positive results regarding the reduction of self-harm.

Finally, with this client group, next to the developmental and the active/directive approaches, we can also find practices with a strong artistic/creative character. For example, extensive art-based work has been undertaken with people with learning disabilities by arts therapies pioneers in MT (e.g. Nordofff & Robbins 1971, 1977), pioneers in DT (e.g. Lindkvist [Pearson 1996]) and by some of the disciples of Laban in DMT (e.g. Meier 1997, Sherborne 1990).

It appears that, due to the wide diversity of needs of this client group, a wide diversity of therapeutic models is followed. Once a specific therapeutic perspective is selected the need to adapt it to the specific characteristic of the client/client group becomes also particularly important.

Clients with no apparent difficulties

Humanistic and artistic/creative perspectives are highly valued with this group of clients (Fig. 4.5). The use of the arts with this client group in the presence of a caring therapist can offer possibilities for dealing with everyday anxieties, encourage self-development and enable spiritual explorations. Furthermore, it is possible that people without serious psychological difficulties do not necessarily need lengthy support. Such interventions may therefore take the form of one-off workshops or a short number of sessions. Highlighting the artistic aspects of arts therapies and therapeutic principles such as the Rogerian 'core conditions' for example, can make the work interesting and valuable for the participants within a short period of time. Finally, it is possible that some of the clients who do not present apparent difficulties are seen in private practice where mainly humanistic, and to a lesser extent, artistic/creative practices, prevail (see discussion about arts therapies trends and private practice in the following section).

Arts therapies trends and working environments

The working environment is an additional factor responsible for the choice of an arts therapies approach. Although fundamental arts therapies principles and characteristics may remain the same in different settings, arts therapists tend to emphasise different approaches when working in health services compared with work situated in education or in private practice.

Health services

In health services, arts therapists work mainly within a psychoanalytic/psychodynamic framework (see Fig. 4.5). Hospital-based work for arts therapists was first established in 1982, at a time when psychoanalytic/psychodynamic practices became particularly influential for the arts therapies field (Waller 1991, Wood 1997). Within such settings arts therapies practitioners deal mostly with clients with mental health problems. We have seen before that psychoanalytic/psychodynamic approaches are generally perceived as more appropriate ways of working with this client group.

The overall culture of the setting is another reason that can explain the use of psychoanalytic/psychodynamic thinking amongst arts therapists working in health services. Although in the NHS the medical model is prevalent, we have seen how, soon after the Second World War, psychiatrists showed an increased interest in the use of the arts as a means of rehabilitation and began using the arts as an adjunct to psychoanalytically-oriented practices (Hogan 2001, Jones 1996, Waller 1991). As a result of this movement, within current psychiatric mental health teams there is often sufficient knowledge and understanding of psychoanalytic/psychodynamic principles. Furthermore, the culture of long-stay inpatient units and the presence of a well-defined structure within the NHS have allowed arts therapists to offer long-term therapeutic interventions within such settings. Long-term work is closely affiliated with psychoanalytic/psychodynamic thinking. Since the shift of care from the hospital to the community, arts therapists, in the same way as other professionals and patients, have had to make adjustments to accommodate much shorter patient–therapist contact time and much more flexible models of work. Although it appears that psychoanalytic/psychodynamic thinking persists in the work of arts therapists employed by the NHS, their work is often modified for brief therapy, work in the community and so on.

Education

Arts therapists working in schools show a clear preference for humanistic principles (see Figure 4.5). We have already discussed the contribution of child-centred education to the development of arts therapies and the fact that, as Waller (1991) states, during the early days of the arts therapies development the field was perceived as a sensitive type of teaching. We have seen that with the introduction in 1988 of the National Curriculum in England and Wales in 1988 there has been a shift within education from the original child-centred perspective to emphasising learning outcomes. However, many teachers today are still valuing child-centred principles and practices. It seems therefore reasonable for arts therapists working within such settings to utilise a type of work that is understood and valued by many of their colleagues.

We believe that within education, active/directive and developmental models are also incorporated next to a child-centred rationale. Although there are no statistically significant results to support this claim, active/directive and developmental models seem to fit with the overall culture of education. The current school philosophy favours knowledge and skills and values cognitive models of human development. For example, Piaget's (1972) theory of development is particularly popular amongst teachers. Furthermore, many arts therapists who are employed in schools work primarily with children with learning disabilities. For these children, as we have seen before, developmental models with or without an active/directive bias can be very relevant. Currently, arts therapies work is expanding towards working with children with emotional/behavioural difficulties and children with no apparent difficulties within mainstream school environments (Sanderson & Karkou 2000). This expansion is expected to also raise discussions about appropriate ways of working and relevant theoretical frameworks.

Private practice

Similar to education, arts therapists who work in private practice show high preference for humanistic approaches (see Fig. 4.5). Clients who attend private practice are often people who are relatively well-functioning, are able to work, live in the community and seek arts therapies as a way of self-development. Approaches that place clients in the centre of the therapeutic process, regarding them as their own experts and highlighting the artistic/creative components of arts therapies work, are possibly appropriate ways of working in private practice.

A number of ethical concerns are also associated with private practice. McNab & Edwards (1988) claim that problems might arise from the fact that the client is, in most cases, the person who also determines the continuation or not of the therapy, and consequently the payment or not of the therapist. In order to assure high standards of practice and avoid abuse or malpractice, arts therapies professional associations have adopted various policies. BAAT (the British Association of Art Therapists), for example, encourages only experienced art therapists to engage in private practice, while ADMT UK (the Association for Dance Movement Therapy UK) allows only senior registered dance movement therapists to practise privately.

Arts therapies trends and the arts therapist

The personal characteristics of the arts therapist play an important role in the choice of a specific approach. For example, we have found that age, level of professional qualifications and other relevant experiences are some important characteristics that determine whether a practitioner follows, for example, a humanistic, psychoanalytic/psychodynamic or an art-based arts therapies approach. It is interesting that gender, a personal characteristic that is frequently cited as determining a person's stance, has not been found as a distinguishing factor between practices. Like most other caring professions, there are many female arts therapists in the arts therapies field. This seems to create a predominantly female culture in itself, from which the fewer male voices (i.e. around 21%) do not divert significantly. Some of the characteristics of arts therapists that distinguish practices are further discussed below.

The age of the arts therapist

Older practitioners (over 50 years) tend to favour humanistic arts therapies approaches to a greater degree than do younger arts therapists. This is possibly a result of a direct involvement of such practitioners in the humanistic movements of the 1960s and 1970s, and the subsequent impact of these movements upon the field during this period and approximately a decade later. As we have already discussed, such movements had a direct impact upon the emergence of the arts therapies profession. It is also possible that many older practitioners work in private practice, as they have long experience and possibly fulfil the criteria for private practice set out by arts therapies professional associations. As we have seen, humanistic approaches are preferred in private practice.

Older practitioners favour developmental ideas more than younger generations of arts therapists. We have already noted that arts therapies partly emerged as the result of arts education. This finding can be explained as the result of the fact that a number of the first arts therapists in the UK were originally arts teachers who, along with child-centred principles, also valued developmental ideas. Despite the fact that recent thinking challenges ideas of linear development and questions neatly presented models (see 'The Developmental Trend' section in this chapter), developmental ideas are still pertinent within educational establishments.

Finally, older arts therapists are also keener than younger generations on artistic/creative practices. This result again can be explained due to historical reasons. For example, many of the first arts therapists were originally artists who shifted their attention from the artistic to the therapeutic aspects of their work, and contributed towards the emergence of the arts therapies field. The artistic/creative elements within arts therapies are possibly kept alive with these practitioners (as Waller [1992] stated, arts therapists are 'first and foremost artists'). Active/directive aspects of work also score higher amongst this group of arts therapists than amongst younger age groups. Overall, it is apparent that younger arts therapists are more sceptical than older arts therapists about principles that are added or borrowed from neighbouring fields.

Arts therapists aged 41–50 years are more in favour of psychoanalytic/psychodynamic frameworks than younger arts therapists. It is possible that this is the result of additional psychotherapeutic training acquired after the completion of their original training. It is also possible that this finding reflects the fact that during the late 1980s and early 1990s there was a significant turn towards justifying arts therapies through a psychoanalytic/psychodynamic perspective (Waller 1991, Wood 1997). Such an emphasis is not as apparent in more recent times, and with younger arts therapists. This youngest group of arts therapists seems sceptical of the humanistic, developmental, artistic/creative, active/directive and psychoanalytic/psychodynamic practices drawn upon by their older colleagues. They probably perceive arts therapies as a field with a distinctive, yet eclectic/integrative character. We have discussed how the eclectic/integrative character of arts therapies is increasingly addressed within contemporary definitions, diversity is accepted as an integral component of arts therapies and post-modernism offers direct resonance for the need to adapt perspectives to contexts and clients' individual realities (see Ch. 2, for more on defining arts therapies and 'The Eclectic/Integrative Trend' section in this chapter:). Figure 4.6 shows age groups of practitioners with associated preferences regarding arts therapies approaches. Figure 4.6 can also be viewed as a development of arts therapies, from the initial borrowing of ideas directly from neighbouring fields (during the 1970s and 1980s) to the incorporation of a strong psychoanalytic/psychodynamic bias (1980s and early 1990s) and finally to the acceptance of the the distinctive nature of arts therapies with an eclectic/integrative character (current trend).

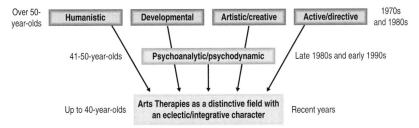

Figure 4.6: *Age of the arts therapist and preferred arts therapies trend.*

Professional qualifications and other relevant experiences

We have found that arts therapists who entered the arts therapies professions via the 'grandparent route' prefer practices that are more closely associated with their original training. For instance, arts therapists who were originally artists are stronger advocates of the artistic/creative approach. Arts therapists who have entered the profession through the 'grandparent route' are also keener on humanistic and active/directive approaches to arts therapies, reflecting original training in education or a related health profession. The impact of original training upon practice is acknowledged within the field. This is one of the reasons for the emphasis placed upon good training programmes in arts therapies in the UK: they are placed within higher institutions or are validated by higher institutions that guarantee a degree of quality of teaching, are accredited by the professional associations, and/or currently the Health Professions Council, that assure the quality of the content of the course and good standards of knowledge and skills for the qualified practitioner. Similarities and differences between courses, however, remain anecdotal. Further research is needed in order to identify the extent to which original arts therapies training affects subsequent practice and is responsible for either similarities or differences among graduates.

Summary

This chapter underlined the importance in practice, of consistent methodological principles based on well-founded theory, along with a clear understanding of the major therapeutic approaches. According to our research, there are important therapeutic trends such as the humanistic, eclectic/integrative, psychoanalytic/psychodynamic, developmental, the artistic/creative and active/directive. These were described and analysed in this chapter, and we came to the conclusion that while most have been adapted from the principles and frameworks of neighbouring fields, they have been further developed, and continue to be developed, within the arts therapies modalities. The therapeutic approach selected appears to vary according to a number of factors, notably the therapist's age, background, client group, the working environment and the arts therapies modality.

As the chapter dealt mainly with overall tendencies, specific approaches as found in each of the different arts therapies disciplines were not considered. Descriptions of such practices are presented in Section 2.

References

- Abram J 1992 Individual psychotherapy trainings: a guide. Free Association Books, London
- Adamson E 1970 Art and mental health. In: Creedy J (ed) The social context of art. Tavistock, London
- Adamson E (in association with Timlin J) 1984 Art as healing. Coventure, London
- Allegranti B 1997 Exploring the social construction of gender through movement improvisation. Unpublished Masters dissertation, University of Surrey-Roehampton
- Alvin J 1975 Music therapy. John Clare Books, London
- Alvin J 1978 Music therapy for the autistic child. Oxford University Press, London
- Arieti S 1976 Creativity and magic synthesis. Basic Books, London
- Balint M, Ornstein P, Balint E 1972 Focal psychotherapy. London, Tavistock
- Berne E 1961 Transactional analysis in psychotherapy: a systematic individual and social psychiatry. Souvenir Press, London
- Best P 2000 Theoretical diversity and clinical collaboration: reflections by a dance/movement therapist. The Arts in Psychotherapy 27(3):197–211
- Best P, Parker G 2001 Moving reflections: the social creation of identities in communication. In: Kossolapow L, Scoble S, Waller D (eds) Arts – therapies – communication: on the way to a communicative European arts therapy, vol 1. Lit Verlag, Munster, p 142–148
- Bion W R 1961 Experiences in groups. Tavistock/Routledge, London
- Bion W R 1964 Elements of psychoanalysis. Heinemann, London
- Bonny H 1994 Twenty-one years later: a GIM update. Music Therapy Perspectives 12(2):70–74
- Bowlby J 1969 Attachment and loss, vol I. Hogarth Press, London
- Bruscia K E 1988 A survey of treatment procedures in improvisational music therapy. Psychology of Music 16:10–24
- Bunt L 1994 Music therapy: an art beyond words. Routledge, London
- Butcher J N, Koss M P 1978 Research on brief and crisis oriented therapies. In: Bergin A, Gerfield S (eds) Handbook of psychotherapy and behavioural change. Wiley, New York
- Byrne P 1995 From the depths to the surface: art therapy as a discursive practice in the post-modern era. The Arts in Psychotherapy 22(3):235–239
- Case C 1990 Reflections and shadows: an exploration of the world of the rejected girl. In: Case C, Dalley T (eds) Working with children in art therapy. Tavistock/Routledge, London, p 131–160
- Case C 2000 'Our lady of the Queen', journeys around the maternal object. In: Gilroy A, McNeilly G (eds) The changing shape of art therapy: new developments in theory and practice. p 15–54
- Case C, Dalley T 1990 Working with children in art therapy. Tavistock/Routledge, London
- Cattanach A 1994a The developmental model of dramatherapy. In: Jennings S, Cattanach A, Mitchell S et al (eds) The handbook of dramatherapy. Routledge, London, p 28–40
- Cattanach A 1994b Dramatic play with children: the interface of DT and play therapy. In: Jennings S, Cattanach A, Mitchell S et al (eds) The handbook of dramatherapy. Routledge, London, p 133–144
- Chaiklin S, Schmais D 1986 The Chace approach to dance therapy. In: Lewis P (ed) Theoretical approaches in dance/movement therapy, vol 1. Kendall/Hunt, Iowa, p17–36.
- Chodorow J 1991 Dance therapy and depth psychology: the moving imagination. Routledge, London
- Clarkson P 1994 The nature and range of psychotherapy. In: Clarkson P, Pokorny M (eds) The handbook of psychotherapy. Routledge, London, p 3–27
- Courtney R 1974 Play, drama and thought. Drama Books, New York
- Dent-Brown K 2004 UK research register for DT. Online. Available: http://www.badth.org.uk/register.html 8 Oct 2004

- Department of Health (DoH) 2001 Treatment choice in psychological therapies and counselling: evidence based clinical practice guideline. Department of Health, London
- Dokter D 1994 Fragile board – arts therapies and clients with eating disorders. In: Dokter D (ed) Arts therapies and clients with eating disorders: fragile board. Jessica Kingsley, London, p 7–22
- Dokter D (ed) 1998 Arts therapies, refugees and migrants: reaching across borders. Jessica Kingsley, London
- Dubowski J 1990 Art versus language: separate development during childhood. In: Case C, Dalley T (eds) Working with children in art therapy. Tavistock/Routledge, London, p 7–22
- Duffy R A 1979 An analysis of aesthetic sensitivity and creativity with other variables in grades four, six, eight and ten. Journal of Educational Research 73(1):26–30
- Erikson E 1959 Identity and the life circle. International Universities Press, New York
- Foucault M 1967 Madness and civilisation: a history of insanity in the age of reason. Tavistock, London
- Foulkes S H 1964 Therapeutic group analysis. Allen and Unwin, London
- Freud S 1953 Three essays on the theory of sexuality. In: Strachey J (ed) The complete psychological works of Freud, vol 7. Holgarth, London
- Gardner H 1973 The arts and human development. Wiley, New York
- Garfield S L 1980 Psychotherapy: an eclectic approach. Wiley, New York
- Gergen K J 1985 The social constructionist movement in modern psychology. American Psychologist 40(3):266–275
- Gergen K J 1991 The saturated self. Basic Books, New York
- Gersie A 1996 (ed) Dramatic approaches to brief therapy. Jessica Kingsley, London
- Gilroy A 1989 On occasionally being able to paint. Inscape(Spring):2–9
- Gilroy A 1992 Research in art therapy. In: Waller D, Gilroy A (eds) Art therapy: a handbook. Open University Press, Buckingham, p 229–247
- Goodman N 1976 Languages of art. Hackett, Indianapolis
- Grentz S 1996 A primer on postmodernism. William B Eermans, Grand Rapids, MI
- Hadamard J 1954 The psychology of invention in the mathematical field. Dover Publications, London
- Haley J, Rocheport-Haley M 2003 The art of strategic therapy. Brunner/Routledge, New York
- Hargreaves J 1982 The development of aesthetic reactions to music. Psychology of Music (special issue):51–54
- Heal-Hughes M A 1995 Comparison of mother-infant interactions and the client-therapist pelationship in music therapy sessions. In: Wigram T, Saperston B, West R (eds) The art and science of music therapy: a handbook. Harwood Academic Publications, Switzerland, p 296–309
- Heathcote D 1991 Collected writings on education and drama. Northwestern University, Evanston, IL
- Hill A 1945 Art versus illness. George Allen and Unwin, London
- Hill A 1951 Painting out illness. Williams and Norgate, London
- Hogan S 2001 Healing arts: the history of art therapy. Jessica Kingsley, London
- Housen A 1983 The eye of the beholder: measuring aesthetic development. Unpublished EdD dissertation, Harvard Graduate School of Education
- Hughes R 1988 Transitional phenomena and the potential space in art therapy with mentally handicapped people. Inscape (summer):4–8
- Jennings S 1983 Models of practice in DT. Dramatherapy 7(1):3–6
- Jennings S 1990 Dramatherapy with families, groups and individuals. Jessica Kingsley, London
- Jennings S 1992 Reason in madness; therapeutic journeys through King Lear. In Jennings S (ed) Dramatherapy: theory and practice 2. Routledge, London, p 5–18
- Jennings S 1995 Dramatherapy for survival: some thoughts on transitions and choices for children and adolescents. In: Jennings S (ed) Dramatherapy with children and adolescents. Routledge, London, p 90–104
- Jennings S 1998 Introduction to dramatherapy: theatre and healing, Ariadne's Ball of Thread. Jessica Kingsley, London
- John D 1995 The therapeutic relationship in music therapy as a tool in the treatment of psychosis. In: Wigram T, Saperston B, West R (eds) The art and science of music therapy: a handbook. Harwood Academic Publications, Switzerland, p 157–166

- Johnson D R 1998 On the therapeutic action of creative arts therapies: the psychodynamic model. The Arts in Psychotherapy 25(2):85–99
- Johnson D R 2000 Developmental transformations: towards the body as presence. In: Lewis P, Johnson D R (eds) Current approaches in drama therapy. Charles C Thomas, Springfield IL, p 87–110
- Jones P 1996 Drama as therapy: theatre as living. Routledge, London
- Jung C G (ed.) 1990 Man and his symbols. Arkana, Penguin Group, London (first published by Aldus Books, 1964)
- Karkou V 1999 Art therapy in education: findings from a nation-wide survey in arts therapies. Inscape 4(2):62–70
- Karkou V 2003 UK research register for DMT. Online. Available: http://www.admt.org.uk/res_research.html 11 Dec 2004
- Karkou V in press Dance movement therapy in the community: group work with people with enduring mental health difficulties. In: Payne H (ed.) Dance, movement therapy: theory, practice and research. Routledge, London
- Karkou V, Sanderson P 1997 An exploratory study of the utilisation of creative arts therapies in treating substance dependence. The Journal of Contemporary Health 5(spring):56–61
- Karkou V, Sanderson P 2000 Dance movement therapy in UK education. Research in Dance Education 1(1):69–85
- Karkou V, Sanderson P 2001 Report: theories and assessment procedures used by dance movement therapists in the UK. The Arts in Psychotherapy 28:13-20
- Kellogg R 1969 Analysing children's art. Mayfield, Palo Alto, CA
- Kestenberg J 1975 Children and parents: psychoanalytic studies in development. Jason Aronson, New York
- Killick K, Greenwood H 1995 Research in art therapy with people who have psychotic illness. In: Gilroy A, Lee C (eds) Art and music: therapy and research. Routledge, London, p 101–116
- Klein M 1975 Collected works of Melanie Klein, vols I, II, III, IV. Hogarth Press and Institute of Psychoanalysis, London
- Laban R 1975 Modern educational dance. MacDonald and Evans, London
- Laing R D 1959 The divided self. Penguin Books, London
- Lawes C, Woodcock J 1995 Music therapy with people with severe learning difficulties who exhibit self-injurious behaviour. In: Wigram T, Saperston B, West R (eds) The art and science of music therapy: a handbook. Harwood Academic Publications, Switzerland, p 261–272
- Levinge A 1993 Permission to play: the search for self through music therapy; research with children presenting with communication difficulties. In: Payne H (ed) Handbook of inquiry in the arts therapies: one river, many currents. Jessica Kingsley, London
- Lewis R 2000 Recovery and individuation: two stage model in transpersonal drama therapy. In: Lewis P, Johnson D R (eds) Current approaches in drama therapy. Charles C Thomas, Springfield IL, p 260–287
- Liebmann M 1986 Art therapy for groups: a handbook of themes, games and exercises. Routledge, London
- Lowenfeld V 1957 Creative and mental growth, 3rd edn. MacMillan, New York
- Lyotard J F 1984 The postmodern condition. Manchester University Press, Manchester, UK
- McNab D, Edwards D 1988 Private AT. Inscape (summer):14–19
- McNeilly G 1983 Directive and non-directive approaches in art therapy. The Arts in Psychotherapy 10(4):211–219
- McNeilly G 2000 Failure in group analytic art therapy. In: Gilroy A, McNeilly G (eds) The changing shape of art therapy: new developments in theory and practice: Jessica Kingsley, London, p 143–171
- Mahler M, Pine F, Bergman A 1975 The psychological birth of the human infant. Basic Books, New York
- Malan D H 1976 The frontier of brief psychotherapy. New York, Plenum Press
- Mann J 1973 Time-limited psychotherapy. Harvard University Press, Cambridge, MA
- Maslow A H 1968 Towards a psychology of being, 2nd edn. D Van Nostrand, New York
- May R 1961 Existential psychology. Basic Books, New York
- Meekums B 2000 Creative group therapy for women survivors of child sexual abuse. Jessica Kingsley Publishers, London
- Meekums B 2002 Dance movement therapy. Sage, London
- Meichenbaum D 1977 Cognitive-behaviour modification: an integrative approach. Plenum Press, New York

- Meier W 1997 The teacher and the therapist. E-motion ADMT UK Quarterly IX(1):7–9
- Miller S D, Hubble M A, Duncan B L 1996 Handbook of solution-focused brief therapy. Jossey-Bass, San Francisco
- Moog H 1976 The musical experience of the pre-school child. Schott, London
- Moreno J, Brotons M, Hawley T et al 1990 International music therapy: a global perspective. Music Therapy Perspectives 8:41–46
- Mottram P 2000 Assessment and treatment in brief art therapy. In: Wigram T (ed) Assessment and evaluation in the arts therapies: art therapy, music therapy and dramatherapy. Harper House Publications, Radlet, p 9–19
- Mottram P 2001 1+1+1+. . . a model of art therapy for an assessment and treatment unit for adults with learning disability and mental health illness. In: Kossolapow L, Scoble S, Waller D (eds) Arts – therapies – communication: on the way to a communicative European arts therapy, vol 1. Lit Verlag, Munster, p 199–206
- Naumburg M 1966 Dynamically oriented art therapy: its principles and practices. Grune and Stratton, New York
- Nordorff P, Robbins C 1971 Therapy in music for handicapped children. Voctor Gollancz, London
- Nordorff P, Robbins C 1977 Creative music therapy. Harper & Row, New York
- North M 1972 Personality assessment through movement. Northcote House, Plymouth
- Odell-Miller H 2000 Music therapy and its relationship to psychoanalysis. In: Searle Y, Sterng I (eds) Where analysis meets the arts. Karnac, London
- Odell-Miller H, Westacott M, Hughes P 2001 An investigation into the effectiveness of the arts therapies by measuring symptomatic and significant life change for people between the ages of 16–65 with continuing mental health problems. Report on a research study jointly funded by Addenbrooke's NHS Trust and Anglia Polytechnic University, Arts Therapies Department, Fulbourn Hospital, Cambridge
- Odell-Miller H, Learmonth M, Pembrooke C 2003 The arts and arts therapists. Scoping Paper Commissioned by Nuffield Foundation
- Oldfield A 1995 Communicating through music: the balance between following and initiating. In: Wigram T, Saperston B, West R (eds) The art and science of music therapy: a handbook. Harwood Academic Publications, Switzerland, p 226–237
- Parsons M, Johnston H, Durham R 1978 Developmental stages in children's aesthetic responses. The Journal of Aesthetic Education 12(1):83–104
- Payne H 1990 Creative movement and dance in groupwork. Winslow, Oxon
- Payne H 1992 Shut in, shut out: dance movement therapy with children and adolescents. In: Payne H (ed) Dance movement therapy: theory and practice. Tavistock/Routledge, London, p 39–80
- Payne H 1994 Eating distress, women and integrative movement psychotherapy. In: Dokter D (ed) Arts therapies and clients with eating disorders: fragile board. Jessica Kingsley, London, p 208–225
- Pearson J (ed) 1996 Discovering the self through drama and movement: the Sesame approach. Jessica Kingsley, London
- Penfield K 1992 Individual movement psychotherapy: dance movement therapy in private practice. In: Payne H (ed) Dance movement therapy: theory and practice. Tavistock/Routledge, London, p 163–182
- Perls F, Hefferline R, Goodman P 1969 Gestalt therapy: excitement and growth in the human personality. Julian Press, New York
- Pflederer M R 1964 The response of children to musical tasks embodying Piaget's principle of conservation. Journal of Research in Music Education 12:251–268
- Piaget J 1972 The psychology of the child. Basic Books, New York
- Poincaré H 1982 Mathematical creation. In: Poincaré H (ed) The foundations of science: science and hypothesis, the value of science, science and method. University Press of America, Washington
- Priebe S, Röhricht F 2001 Specific body image pathology in acute schizophrenia. Psychiatry Research 101:289–301
- Priestley M 1995 Linking sound and symbol. In: Wigram T, Saperston B, West R (eds) The art and science of music therapy: a handbook. Harwood Academic Publishers, Switzerland
- Rabiger S 1990 Art therapy as a container. In: Case C, Dalley T (eds) Working with children in art therapy. Tavistock/Routledge, London, p 23–38

- Rees M 1998 Drawing on difference: art therapy with people who have learning difficulties. Routledge, London
- Rider M S 1981 The assessment of cognitive functioning level through musical perception. Journal of Music Therapy 18(3):110–119
- Rogers C 1951 Client-centered therapy: its current practise, implications and theory. Constable and Company Ltd, London
- Roth A, Fonagy P 1996 What works for whom? A critical review of psychotherapy research. The Guilford Press, New York
- Sandel S, Johnson D 1983 Structure and process of the nascent group: dance movement therapy with chronic patients. The Arts in Psychotherapy 10:131–140
- Sanderson P 1991 Factors influencing attitudes of secondary school pupils to aesthetic aspects of sport and dance. Unpublished PhD thesis, University of Manchester, UK
- Sanderson P, Karkou V 2000 Arts therapy in mainstream education: a case study. Research report, The University of Manchester, School of Education
- Sandler J, Dare C, Holder A et al 1970 Basic psychoanalytic concepts: 'acting out', British Journal of Psychiatry 117:329
- Schaverien J 2000 The triangular relationship and the aesthetic countertransference in analytic art psychotherapy. In: Gilroy A, McNeilly G (eds) The changing shape of art therapy: new developments in theory and practice. Jessica Kingsley, London and Philadelphia, p 55–83
- Scheiby B B 1999 Music as symbolic expression: analytical music therapy. In: Weiner D J (ed) Beyond talk therapy: using movement and expressive techniques in clinical practice. American Psychological Association, Washington DC
- Schmais C 1985 Healing processes in group dance/movement therapy. American Journal of Dance Therapy 8:17–36
- Sherborne V 1990 Developmental movement for children. Cambridge University Press, Cambridge
- Siegel E V 1984 Dance movement therapy: mirrors of ourselves. The psychoanalytic approach. Human Sciences Press, New York
- Silverstone L 1993 Art therapy: the person-centred way, art and the development of the person. Autonomy Books, London
- Sinason V 1992 Mental handicap and the human condition. Free Association Books, London
- Slade P 1954 Child drama. University Press, London
- Stanton-Jones K 1992 An introduction to dance movement therapy in psychiatry. Tavistock/Routledge, London and New York
- Stern D The interpersonal world of the infant: a view from psychoanalysis and developmental psychology. Basic Books, London
- Skinner B F 1953 Science and human behaviour. MacMillan, New York
- Sullivan H S 1955 The interpersonal theory of psychiatry. W W Norton, New York
- Swanwick K, Tillman J 1986 The sequence of musical development: a study of children's composition. British Journal of Music Education 3(3):305–339
- Thorne F C 1967 Integrative psychology. Clinical Publishing, Brandon, VT
- Tipple R 1992 Art therapy with people who have severe learning difficulties. In: Waller D, Gilroy A (eds) Art therapy: a handbook. Open University Publications, Buckingham
- Valente L, Fontana D 1993 Research into dramatherapy theory and practice: some implications for training. In: Payne H (ed) Handbook of inquiry in the arts therapies: one river, many currents. Jessica Kingsley, London, p 56–67
- Waller D 1991 Becoming a profession: the history of art therapy in Britain 1940–1982. Tavistock/Routledge, London
- Waller D 1992 Different things to different people: art therapy in Britain – a brief survey of its history and current development. The Arts in Psychotherapy 19:87–92
- Waller D 1993 Group interactive art therapy: its use in training and treatment. Tavistock/Routledge, London
- Waller D 2001 The methods of arts therapeutic communication. In: Kossolapow L, Scoble S, Waller D (eds) Arts – therapies – communication: On the way to a communicative European arts therapy, vol 1. Lit Verlag, Munster, p 117–120
- Waller D, Dalley T 1992 Art therapy: a theoretical perspective. In. Waller D, Gilroy A (eds) Art therapy: a handbook. Open University Press, Buckingham, p 3–24
- Walrond-Skinner S 1986 A dictionary of psychotherapy. Routledge and Kegan Paul, London
- Wheeler B 1987 Levels of therapy: the classification of music therapy goals. Music Therapy 6(2):39–49

- Whitehouse M 1979 C G Jung and dance-therapy: two major principles. In: Bernstein P L (ed) Eight theoretical approaches in dance/movement therapy, vol I. Kendall/Hunt, Iowa
- Whitelock J 1987 Dramatherapy in a psychiatric day centre. In: Jennings S (ed) Dramatherapy: theory and practice 1. Routledge, London, p 209–232
- Winnicott D W 1971 Playing and reality. Routledge, London
- Woddis J 1992 Art therapy: new problems, new solutions? In: Waller D, Gilroy A (eds) Art therapy: a handbook. Open University Press, Buckingham, p 25–48
- Wood C 1997 The history of art therapy and psychosis 1938–1995. In: Killick K, Schaverien J (eds) Art, psychotherapy and psychosis. Routledge, London, p 144–175
- Yalom I D 1970 The theory and practice of group psychotherapy. Basic Books, New York

Section 2
Arts Therapies as Separate Disciplines

Although arts therapies share common characteristics, influences and frameworks as described in Section 1, they also have unique traits that justify the presence of separate disciplines within the arts therapies field: art therapy (AT), music therapy (MT), dramatherapy (DT) and dance movement therapy (DMT). So far we have treated the field as one. At this point it is important to look at the different disciplines separately.

There are a number of reasons why arts therapies in the UK consist of four disciplines and deserve separate discussion (note: there are different developments in other parts of the world; for example in the USA 'expressive arts therapists' regard themselves as generic arts therapists). The difference in the artistic medium itself provides the first obvious distinction. For example, music therapists may include movement and dance when working with children, but the emphasis remains on music, and improvisational music in particular; some dance movement therapists will habitually use music or role playing, but preoccupation remains with the body and non-verbal movement; dramatherapists often revert to body work, art and music-making, but dramatic and theatrical processes remain the focus of attention. Similarly, the art therapist may pay attention to the physical body and relationships in space, but the major task within a session is to work with the process of the clients' image-making. The majority of arts therapists in the UK continue to be primarily drama, art, dance movement and music therapists.

Apart from the role of the specific art as a distinguishing factor amongst disciplines, separate historical developments and current practices perpetuate the subdivision of the arts therapies field into different professions. In order to understand each of these disciplines better, we will therefore look at these separate developments, discuss current professional achievements and offer definitions and important features of each of the subfields. We will also see their links with the overall therapeutic trends we have conceptualised over the course of our study and that we have discussed in Chapter 4, and we will describe some important practices that are unique to each of the separate fields. Case examples will offer snapshots of these practices and will provide more in-depth illustrations of what might take place within different arts therapies.

It should be noted that the practices we choose to describe within each arts therapies discipline are not neatly separated and do not readily fall under one or another of the overall therapeutic trends we have described. Since each separate arts therapies discipline claims internal cohesiveness and a separate professional identity, there is often an overlap amongst practices within each discipline and consequently a non-linear connection with arts therapies' broad therapeutic trends. Furthermore, the background, age and training of the therapist, and the needs of the client/s or the setting play an important role in the way most practices are shaped, as discussed in Chapter 4. The personality of the therapist might also play an important role. The approaches we describe are therefore just indicative of specific arts therapies disciplines and do not exhaust the wide range of existing practices.

From a cross-cultural perspective, Section 2 highlights what is different and unique in each discipline. Although at times our descriptions are again broad (e.g. we define the whole of MT, DT and so on), and at times we refer to other arts therapies disciplines, there is a strong emphasis upon descriptions of practices by arts therapists themselves. References are made to specific sessions, specific working environments and single clients or single groups. In comparison to Section 1, this section of the book finds us more closely aligned with relativism and emic perspectives.

Section Two • Arts Therapies as Separate Disciplines

Chapter 5

Music Therapy (MT)

Key issues:

- Music has been used for therapeutic purposes since, at least, the beginning of the last century. However, music therapy (MT) as a professional grouping was not established before 1958. It was the first of the arts therapies to reach this stage of development. Professional registration with the Health Professions Council is currently in place and has been since 1999.

- Music therapists work with a wide range of difficulties, although clients with learning and mental health difficulties form the two largest groups.

- Music therapists work primarily in the National Health Service (NHS) and education, but are developing their work in voluntary and private organisations.

- Within most British MT practices, improvisational music-making forms the basis for the relationship between the client and the therapist.

- MT draws less heavily upon related fields for validation of its practice than other arts therapies.

- Some major MT approaches found in the UK today are the interactive (or free improvisational), the creative and the analytical. Each of these approaches is outlined with reference to their pioneers, and illustrated further by means of case examples.

Introduction

Within the evolution of arts therapies, music therapy (MT) was one of the first disciplines to form a professional body. It is also an area that received early recognition and fairly wide acknowledgement, reflecting a similar acceptance and value attached to music as an art form in the west. In this chapter we will give an historical overview of the establishment of the discipline within the UK in the 20th century, and refer to early precursors of MT as well as its most recent professional development. With reference to research, we will also discuss theoretical influences and major approaches within the field. In order to unfold some current practices, examples of clinical work will also be included.

Brief MT history

From the beginning of the last century there have been testimonies to the use of music for therapeutic purposes. As we have already mentioned (see 'The Emergence of Arts Therapies in the 20th Century' in Ch. 1) there are accounts of medical professionals looking at the effects of music upon people's physiology. Generally, music was seen as a kind of 'sedative' and was used in a variety of experimental ways (Bunt 1994, Tyler 2000). Almost concurrently with the use of music within this medical framework, there are accounts of the use of music for recreational purposes within hospital environments. This latter type of music, i.e. music as a recreational activity, fitted well with an overall perception of the recreational value of music within British society before the Second World War.

Recorded music, performances, and hospital choirs and bands, were some of the uses made of music within hospitals (Ansdell 2002). In both cases, i.e. when music was used for experimental work or for entertainment, there were two main characteristics: (1) music was predominantly played *to* people; (2) music was perceived as having a benign social value.

After the Second World War, music became associated with boosting morale. Musicians were invited to play *to* and increasingly play *with* returning veterans who were physically and/or mentally scarred. However, it was not until 1958 that MT was established as a professional grouping. The first such group was the Society for Musical Therapy and Remedial Music (see Box 5.1), an organisation that eventually became the British Society for Music Therapy (BSMT). The BSMT is currently less of a professional body and more of a promotional body: a charity responsible for promoting the use and development of MT in the UK through organising conferences, workshops and meetings and through disseminating information, books and videos about MT (BSMT 2004a).

The founder of the original group, i.e. the Society for Music Therapy and Remedial Music, was Alvin (1975), one of the pioneers of MT in the UK. Her work has been particularly influential and, according to Tyler (2000), it has shaped MT as a modern profession. She was an established musician (a concert cellist and a teacher), emphasised improvisation, and worked primarily with children with learning difficulties and/or autism. The effect of Alvin's influence upon current MT practice is apparent: music therapists

Box 5.1: Significant dates in the development of MT in the UK (Ansdell et al 2002, BSMT 2004a, Bunt 1994, Tyler 2000)

Year	Development
1958	Alvin founds the Society for Music Therapy and Remedial Music, which eventually develops into the British Society for Music Therapy, a charity with aims to promote MT in public.
1968	Alvin develops the first training course at the Guildhall School of Music and Drama.
1974	Nordoff and Robbins teach at the Goldie Leigh Hospital in south London.
1976	The Association of Professional Music Therapists (APMT) is formed, which becomes the official professional body for MT.
1980	Discussion in the House of Commons regarding pay scales and career structures; assumption that MT and art therapy (AT) fall under occupational therapy (OT).
1982	The Department of Health and Social Security awards career and grading structure for MT and AT practitioners.
1999	Registration with the Health Professions Council alongside AT and dramatherapy (DT).

today are expected to demonstrate high levels of musicianship and strong improvisational skills. Following Alvin's example, many music therapists today work with children with learning difficulties and/or autism.

Another important contribution to the development of the MT field has been the pioneering work of Nordoff & Robbins (1971) (Box 5.1). Like Alvin, Nordoff was an accomplished musician (a pianist and composer), who developed his work within the remedial model predominating within the therapeutic care of children with learning difficulties of that time. Ansdell (2002) describes the Nordoff–Robbins work as deriving from the 'anthroposophical movement' and involving both intense private work and public performances. Precomposed music was also extensively used.

None of the early work of these pioneers was affiliated with any specific psychotherapeutic school of thought and this situation continued until the analytical MT work of Priestley (1975) and others in the 1960s and 1970s became more widely integrated within the developing mainstream MT practice. Storr (1993) claims that, in contrast to art therapy (AT), the development of MT towards acquiring psychological resonance was delayed due to the writings of Freud and Jung, who had a limited understanding of music and its therapeutic potential. Because of this delay, several music therapists in the USA turned to behavioural therapy and the direct observation and documentation of more external behaviours. According to Bunt (1994), this turn had been so radical that, until the 1970s, MT in the USA was considered to be a 'science of behaviour'.

American MT developments initially influenced MT practice in the UK. However, British music therapists embraced a wider range of psychotherapeutic schools of thought from the 1970s than just behavioural psychology. The Guildhall School of MT, for example, founded by Alvin (see Box 5.1), began to stress developmental and psychoanalytic concepts alongside selected behavioural ideas. The Nordoff–Robbins school, founded a few years later (Box 5.1), started introducing humanistic concepts and made frequent references to Maslow. Freudian and Jungian principles were particularly appreciated amongst followers of Priestley's analytical MT (Priestley 1995).

The foundation of the Association of Professional Music Therapists (APMT) in 1976 moved MT into a different stage of development. Despite initial internal frictions between supporters of one or another approach (Odell-Miller 2001), the Association managed to stick together and fight for professional recognition. In 1982 MT, alongside AT, got official recognition as a health profession alongside occupational therapy (OT), psychotherapy and speech therapy; recently (1999) MT, alongside AT and dramatherapy (DT), has become registered with the Health Professions Council.

Current MT professional development

There are currently more than seven training courses in the UK (see Appendix 2) and more than 500 music therapists registered with APMT. MT can be found in a variety of settings and with a range of clients. Table 5.1 presents these client groups as reported by the music therapists participating in our survey (comprehensive findings regarding client groups for all separate arts therapies disciplines can be found in Ch. 2) and highlights differences between this and other arts therapies disciplines.

MT practitioners work predominantly with children with learning difficulties – more than other arts therapists do – a trait closely linked with the early pioneering work of Alvin and Nordoff–Robbins. However, work in mental health has also expanded, especially as a result of Priestley's influence and consequent embrace of a number of psychotherapeutic influences. It is interesting that there are relatively few music therapists working with people with no apparent difficulties. A possible explanation is that the needs of people labelled 'normal neurotics' are seen as being catered for through musical workshops and musical events widely available in the public arena, and that do not necessarily require a trained music therapist as facilitator. If this explanation is indeed accurate, working with people with no apparent difficulties can be perceived as falling outside the remit of MT, a position that can raise heated debate amongst arts therapists.

MT has provided quantity and quality of research evidence for the positive effects of MT when working with a number of different vulnerable client groups. Wigram et al (2002), in their review of articles published in MT journals in the UK, USA and Scandinavia (*Nordic Journal of Music Therapy*) from 1998 to 2001, estimate that over 60 percent of these articles are research based. The majority of the research-based articles come from the USA and are of quantitative nature. Standley (1995) in her meta-analysis of studies completed in medical settings shows that the greatest positive effects are with clients with chronic migraines, respiratory problems, chronic pain or physical

Table 5.1: Main MT client groups and differences from other arts therapies

Type of difficulty	% for MT	% for other arts therapies	Chi-square (x^2) value	Degrees of freedom (df)	P-value (p)
Learning	50.0	15.6	64.27	1	0.000**
Emotional/behavioural	31.1	67.6	53.25	1	0.000**
Multiple	6.6	2.4	5.15	1	0.023*
Other	7.4	5.4	Not significant		
Physical/sensory/medical	3.3	3.3	Not significant		
No apparent	1.6	5.7	Not significant (3.47)	(1)	(0.062)
Total	100.0	100.0			

**Accepted at the 0.01 level of significance
*Accepted at the 0.05 level of significance

The table shows that learning difficulties were the most frequent types of difficulties faced by the clients of music therapists. The second largest group had emotional/behavioural difficulties, or in other words difficulties relating to mental health, while the third group had multiple difficulties. The 'other' category included, amongst other difficulties, communication difficulties and terminal illness.

Chi-square tests performed for the different client groups revealed a number of statistically significant differences between MT and other arts therapies. Music therapists tended to work more often with learning (p = 0.000) and multiple difficulties (p = 0.023) than other arts therapists, and less often with emotional/behavioural difficulties (p = 0.000). Similarly, music therapists were least likely to be working with clients with no apparent difficulties; however, the last finding was not statistically significant (p = 0.062).

impairment and greater effect when live music is presented by a trained music therapist than does recorded music. Given the improvisatory nature of British practice, randomised controlled trials (RCTs) with MT interventions that are closer to daily practice are more difficult to conduct and fewer in number. Still, there are several well-designed studies completed with clients with disabilities, autism, dementia, enduring mental health problems, the elderly, and cancer patients to mention just a few. Most of these studies show positive effects of MT interventions. References to these studies can be found in Payne (1993), Gilroy & Lee (1995), Aldridge (1996) and Wigram et al (2002). A number of studies have been completed as part of MPhil/PhD qualifications while others are independent projects supported by external funding. Further systematic reviews of studies, meta-analyses and RCTs are currently under completion and relevant CD-ROM and research databases are being developed.

As Table 5.2 shows, music therapists work primarily in the NHS and in education but are also expanding their work in voluntary and private organisations within the community.

Efforts by the APMT to establish work within the NHS and education are apparent within the early years of the profession (see the brief history section earlier in the chapter) and, recently, calls have been made for expanding towards community work (e.g. Ansdell 2002). However, despite the fact that there are several music therapists employed by voluntary and private organisations, social work is still an underdeveloped area of work for such practitioners. Similarly low is the incidence of music therapists working in private practice. Both of these features of MT are closely linked with the fact that music therapists tend to work with people who do have some difficulties rather than the 'normal neurotics'. It may also reflect limited attention paid to these areas of work by the MT professional association. Ansdell (2002) insists that future developments of this arts therapies discipline, may include the more 'public' sphere of social work and further expansion in community work, in addition to the strictly 'private' work undertaken in health and education services. We find this an interesting suggestion worthy of further consideration.

MT defined

According to the APMT:

> There are different approaches to the use of music in therapy . . . Fundamental to all approaches, however, is the development of a relationship between the client and therapist. Music-making forms the basis for communication in this relationship . . . (BSMT 2004b, p. 1)

We have already discussed changes of MT definitions over time (see Ch. 2). We have seen, for example, that earlier definitions of MT had closer affinity with humanistic thinking. The most recent official statement about the nature of MT, presented above, refers explicitly to the range of approaches followed by practising music therapists in the UK today. At the same time it identifies core characteristics of the field such as the significance of the client–therapist relationship and the role of music-making within this relationship. This description of MT also refers to an active involvement of client and therapist within the

Table 5.2: Main MT working environments and differences from other arts therapies

Working environment	% for MT	% for other arts therapies	Chi-square (x^2) value	Degrees of freedom (df)	P-value (p)
Health	48.7	48.4	Not significant		
Education	30.3	12.9	20.57	1	0.000**
Voluntary/private agency	10.1	13.3	Not significant		
Private practice	4.2	8.4	Not significant		
Other	4.2	2.6	Not significant		
Social service	2.5	14.4	12.71	1	0.000**
Total	100.0	100.0			

**Accepted at the 0.01 level of significance

Health services were the most frequently reported areas of work followed by education and voluntary/private organisations. Social services were areas of work where music therapists were least likely to be working.

When chi-square tests were performed for these different working environments, two statistically significant differences were found between music therapists and non-music therapists. In proportion, more music therapists were found working in education compared with other arts therapists, while fewer music therapists were found in social services/community and in private practice. These differences were accepted at the 0.01 level of significance.

session in the form of playing, singing and listening, and acknowledges the need for using a wide range of musical styles according to the client's needs. Improvisation is highlighted as a tool that is frequently used in the development of a specific client–therapist musical language.

According to Alvin (1978), there are a number of techniques used within MT practice. She claims that techniques range from those that encourage the client to be actively engaged in music-making (she calls these 'active' techniques) to those that have a more passive character, e.g. listening to music (the 'receptive' techniques). During 'active' improvisational techniques, clients are invited to play and respond with a number of percussion instruments such as bells, drums, xylophones, tambourines, cymbals and gamelan chimes as well as guitar, cello, violin or piano. Songs/vocalisations may also be used and at times verbalisations may be encouraged. Examples of 'receptive' techniques involve listening to the therapist or others making music, listening to prerecorded music or listening to one's own recorded music.

Bruscia (1988) in his study of improvisational MT internationally, claims that therapeutic processes also vary from those with clear session structures and those that are free flowing. In the former type, there is a move towards or away from a central event or activity within a session. During the latter, cycles are repeated or layered according to certain musical or emotional themes. While the first type is frequently found within group work, the latter is often a trait of one-to-one MT work.

Irrespective of the type of therapeutic process encouraged each time, the 'isoprinciple' (a term introduced by Altshuler in 1948) is an important characteristic of MT practice. According to Meyer (1999), the concept dates back as far as the time of Plato and is currently used almost universally by music therapists. According to this principle, music is chosen in a way that matches the mood of the clients. The match between music and mood is seen as reducing somatic and emotional inhibitions and as lowering cognitive states. This principle is particularly important at the beginning of the therapeutic process when therapists aim to achieve an initial rapport, client validation and trust.

Other more general therapeutic aims held by music therapists in the UK are listed within the BSMT (2004b) general account of MT: positive changes in behaviour, promotion of emotional well-being, increased sense of self-awareness and improvement of quality of life.

Main therapeutic trends within MT

MT, in comparison with other arts therapies, draws less heavily upon related fields in order to provide a theoretical justification of its practice. Differences between MT and other arts therapies disciplines presented in Table 5.3 highlight this tendency.

It appears that, although music therapists draw upon humanistic principles (and client-centred principles in particular), utilise active/directive techniques, value psychoanalytic/psychodynamic frameworks, and acknowledge the eclectic character of their work, they are relatively sceptical of such approaches in comparison to other arts therapists (all differences are accepted at the 0.01 level of significance).

Table 5.3: Main MT therapeutic trends and differences from other arts therapies

Therapeutic trends	Mean for MT[*]	Mean for other arts therapies[*]	t-test value	Degrees of freedom (df)	P-value (p)
Humanistic	3.79	3.92	– 2.71	578	0.007**
Eclectic/integrative	3.49	3.74	– 3.97	578	0.000**
Psychoanalytic/psychodynamic	3.18	3.39	– 4.47	171.53	0.000**
Developmental	3.17	3.22	Not significant		
Artistic/creative	3.10	3.14	Not significant		
Active/directive	2.97	3.10	– 2.64	578	0.009**

*The higher the score, the stronger the agreement with this group of statements (a five-point scale was used ranging from strongly agree = 5 to strongly disagree = 1)

**Accepted at the 0.01 level of significance

As the table shows, music therapists demonstrated the strongest agreement with the humanistic group of statements and least agreement with the active/directive group. Statistically significant differences existed between MT and other arts therapies in relation to the humanistic, the eclectic/integrative, the psychoanalytic/psychodynamic and the active/directive group of statements. In all cases music therapists agreed, to a lesser extent than their colleagues, with these groups of statements.

The uneasy relationship of MT with eclectic practices, for example, has been discussed in the MT literature. Pavlicevic (1997) is sceptical of the use of language that is borrowed entirely from related fields, mainly because it may create a 'package' that is 'a little too neat' and largely unquestioned. Meyer (1999), in her study of arts therapies in the USA, concludes that current MT practice leans towards discovering a unique language with which to describe itself. It appears that the British MT practitioners are involved in a similar pattern of development.

The interactive (or free improvisational) MT approach: starting with Juliette Alvin

We have already presented Alvin (1975, 1978) as one of the most important pioneers of MT in the UK. Alvin, as an accomplished musician, valued the role of music, highlighted improvisation as a major means of relating to clients and laid the foundations for future music therapists working with children with learning difficulties, as well as with other client groups. She also attempted to integrate a number of different theoretical perspectives in a 'theoretical harmony'. According to Tyler (2000), this synthesis consisted of integrating models such as the medical/physiological, recreational, educational, psychological and the musical. Alvin (1975) has made explicit references to some of these models. For example, adopting a physiological perspective, she claimed that the initial impact of music is often physical and sensuous, explaining that this is associated with musical tension and release, which matches human physical patterns of activity and rest. Alvin also discussed the effects of sound, in terms of frequency, intensity, tone colour, interval and duration, upon the body. She regarded the first three characteristics of sound: frequency, intensity and tone colour, as directly generating emotive responses, with interval and duration referring to intellectual processing.

In terms of psychological and psychotherapeutic theory, Alvin (1975) utilised a psychoanalytic viewpoint when claiming that she regarded music as able to bring out what was present in the individual. Alvin discussed music in terms of Freud's id, ego and superego, suggesting that at times, music can stir up or enable clients to express primitive instincts (*id*), strengthen the *ego* through release or control of emotions, or sublimate certain emotions through concentrating and satisfying high aesthetic and spiritual experiences (*superego*). At the same time she allowed space within MT for behavioural perspectives, using behavioural terms such as 'conditioning', explaining that:

> The function to which music is associated often helps to condition the listener to a certain mood, either receptive or adverse. This conditioning may happen suddenly or through a slow forming habit. (Alvin 1975, p. 80)

The result of this amalgamation of theoretical perspectives can be seen as easily falling under what we have termed the eclectic/integrative approach to arts therapies. Wigram et al (2002), referring to the Guildhall course that was founded by Alvin, describes it as a course with a strong eclectic character. The influence of its founder may explain why this could be the case, although many music therapists affiliated with this MT approach may disagree, arguing that different theoretical perspectives are incorporated in an integrated way, leading to an approach with distinctive MT characteristics (see Tyler [2000] above).

Alvin's (1975) contribution however, does not rest solely with her attempts to develop a new theoretical body that justified MT practice. As with most arts therapies pioneers, her approach has been first and foremost rooted in practice. As indicated earlier, Alvin (1975) valued improvisation as a central feature of the music therapist's role to such an extent that Bruscia (1988), in his survey of treatment procedures in improvisational MT, calls Alvin's approach 'free improvisational therapy'. Such an approach is 'free' because, according to Alvin (1975), there are no rules, structures or themes imposed by the therapist upon the client. Clients are encouraged to 'let go' on instruments and find their own way of sequencing and ordering the sounds. When working with groups a 'free atonal rhythmical improvisation' is encouraged. According to Alvin (1975), this technique aims to develop spontaneous expression and freedom, encourages the making of 'instant music' and does not require any specific musical ability on the part of the client. Despite Alvin's preoccupation with improvisational 'active' techniques (i.e. the client making music), within this approach 'receptive' techniques are also used (i.e. the client listening to music). For children within the autistic spectrum Bruscia (1988) summarises Alvin's (1978) approach in Table 5.4.

It appears that free improvisation does not stand on its own as a 'methodological panacea'. 'Active' techniques that favour free improvisation on the client's part, co-exist with 'receptive' techniques in which the client is less active. At times the therapist guides the client through an introduction to the therapist's instruments and music (first stage), through engaging in a musical dialogue and feeding back to the client a recording of the latter's music (second stage), or through offering themes for improvisation or facilitating specific musical, verbal or movement activities (third stage). Despite Alvin (1975, 1978) placing great value on free improvisation and consequently freedom of expression, freedom can be acquired only with a degree of structure. Amelia Oldfield's example of clinical work illustrates this point further.

Structure and freedom within an interactive MT approach for children with autism

Oldfield (1995) describes how freedom and structure can co-exist within a single approach. In the example presented in Table 5.5, the child is free to move in the room and explore instruments, while the therapist mirrors what the child is doing through singing and instrumental accompaniment (following the 'isoprinciple' described earlier as a way of the therapist matching the client's mood in music). However, this sense of freedom is framed with the therapist offering a starting and finishing activity (e.g. 'welcome' and 'goodbye' music/song). Like many other music therapists working with children with autism, Oldfield's (1995) sessions incorporate interventions of a directive and often repetitive nature (in this case at the beginning and end of the session) as well as interventions with a less directive nature (in this case in the middle of the session).

Table 5.4: Stages of therapy for children with autism – summary of Juliette Alvin's (1978) work by Bruscia (1988, p. 12) (Reproduced by permission of Sage Publications Ltd from K E Bruscia, A Survey of Treatment Procedures in Improvisational Music Therapy, Copyright © Society for Education, Music, and Psychology Research, 1988)

Needs of clients
[Children with autism]

Aims
[(1) Relating self to objects, (2) relating to self and therapist (3) relating self to others (each of these aims is targeted in each of the three stages of therapy)]

Stages of therapy
'Each stage is characterised by certain techniques, which can be either active or receptive. The therapist chooses the most appropriate technique according to the client's immediate needs and reactions, and any situational factors that may be relevant.

(1) In the first stage, "active" techniques are used to help the client to relate to instruments and to music and to develop sensorimotor awareness, perception and integration. Receptive techniques are used to introduce the client to the therapist's instrument and music. . . . Emphasis is given to deriving musical pleasure through the free use of instruments.

(2) In the second stage, "active" techniques serve to project the client's feelings onto the instrument and to develop some level of trust in the therapist. Examples include: improvised dialogues and duets, sharing instruments and territories and exploring the therapeutic components of each instrument. "Receptive" techniques aim at bringing the client an awareness of his/her own musical and personal problems and feelings. This can be done through various listening activities. Having the client listen to tapes of his/her own playing is particularly effective.

(3) In the third stage (which may not be necessary or appropriate for everyone), the client is transferred from individual therapy to a family or group setting. The musical activities and experiences developed with the therapist in previous stages now provide models for developing or improving relationships with significant others or peers. Group techniques include free improvisation, titled improvisation, listening, singing, discussion and movement activities.'

Authors' wording in [brackets]

Oldfield (1995) views structure and freedom, being directive or less directive, using active or receptive techniques and initiating or following, as one continuum that is determined by a number of different factors: the needs of the client, the aims of the therapy, the duration of the therapy, and the period of the therapy. Considering Bruscia's (1988) comment regarding structured or free-flowing sessions, we may also add to the above list: the type of therapy; working with groups is often more directive than when working with individuals.

Oldfield (1995), however, also raises potential dangers from very directive approaches: there might be less time for the therapist to simply listen to, and follow, the child. We may also add that within an extreme directive approach,

Table 5.5: Structure and freedom within an interactive MT approach with children with autism – Amelia Oldfield (1995, p. 231)

Description of session structure	Comments by the therapist and the authors
Needs of clients within specific setting: [Children within the autistic spectrum, family unit] '*Confused and isolated children.*'	'How directive I am will depend very much on the type of child I am seeing and the child's difficulties.' [The more damaged the *client*, the more directive the session may become]
Aims [Precise *aims*: such as to improve concentration, to help with physical aims (e.g. to sit better), to extend interest in communicating] [General *aims*: to improve quality of life]	[The more specific the *aims*, the more directive the approach] [The longer the *duration* of the therapy, the less directive the approach]
Structure of session 'When working with mainly non-verbal, isolated children who are either diagnosed as autistic or have a number of autistic tendencies . . . , I provide a *clear starting and ending point for the very first session and allow the child as much freedom as possible in between.* *I will help the child sit opposite to me for* the first few minutes and sing a greeting to the child, possibly accompanied by the guitar. If necessary, I will physically help the child to remain seated for a few seconds. I will end the session in the same way by singing goodbye and often accompanying myself with the bongo drums, which I will attempt to share with the child. In between, the child is free to roam around the room, exploring and discovering instruments on the way. I will support and encourage the child by mirroring the child's playing through song and instrumental accompaniment and at times identifying what we are doing by singing. For example: 'we are playing the piano together now' or 'I am playing the drum and John is marching'.'	'My rationale for this is that any child – particularly a confused and isolated child – is reassured by a framework surrounding an event.' [At the *beginning* of the therapy, the therapist is more directive than later on]

Authors' wording in [brackets]

the session may become rigid, the principle of freedom (valued by Alvin and many other arts therapists) may become extinct and the approach questionable in terms of whether it remains a form of therapy. We have already argued (see Ch. 4) that activity-based approaches that are not appropriately framed within a clear therapy rationale might better be described as forms of therapeutic arts or sensitive forms of musical education, in this case, therapeutic or educational music.

Moving away from the structure versus freedom debate, it is interesting to look at Oldfield's approach as a recent version of Alvin's approach. Theoretically for instance, Oldfield's (V Karkou, personal communication, 1993) approach incorporates components of a number of different theoretical frameworks, but avoids aligning with a single psychotherapeutic school of thought. For example, although she makes connections between her work and developmental models (e.g. she claims that her work often resembles a mother–baby interaction), she also adds that children with learning difficulties do not necessarily follow prescribed developmental patterns and as such she does not see her work as developmentally-based. Although psychoanalytic thinking may partly inform her work she avoids offering interpretations. Also, although her research work in particular is clearly informed by behavioural thinking (e.g. she looks at overt behaviour within experimental designs as evidence for the effectiveness of her practice with clients with learning difficulties [Oldfield & Adams 1995]), being directive is not a core characteristic of her clinical work (e.g. she incorporates directive and non-directive aims and techniques as described in the example above). Furthermore, she has a tendency to work in the here-and-now and from time to time to disclose her own personal feelings (e.g. she may say to a client, 'this made me feel sad' [V Karkou, personal communication, 1993]). Although these principles imply an underlying humanistic thinking, Oldfield (1995) does not acknowledge humanistic schools of thought as directly informing her MT approach. Instead, she prefers to refer to her work as 'interactive', a term that has been extensively used for MT practices that derive from Alvin's teaching.

An interactive MT approach with groups of cancer patients

Following a similar tradition to that of Oldfield, Bunt (1994) acknowledges the eclectic assumptions underpinning his work. He describes MT from a medical perspective where there is an emphasis upon the physiological effects of music on the body. He refers to the value of psychoanalytic thinking and the American tendency to view MT as a 'science of behaviour'. Finally he states his own bias toward 'an open-ended approach and a stress on active interaction' (Bunt 1994, p. 44). The example in Table 5.6 is taken from Bunt's diverse work and shows how an interactive MT approach can be applied to groups. This type of work is extensively evaluated and researched regarding the processes and effects of the MT input in the specific centre. The value of working collaboratively with counselling has been highlighted (Bunt 1994, Bunt & Marston-Wyld 1995), while evidence of links between MT and improved psychological and physiological states is provided (Bunt et al 2000, Bunt & Hoskyns 2002, Burns et al 2001). The specific client group discussed,

Table 5.6: An interactive MT approach with a group of cancer patients – Leslie Bunt (Example provided to V Karkou for 'Arts Therapies: from Theory to Practice' study [Karkou 2002, reproduced with permission])

Description of session structure	Comments by the therapist and the authors
Needs of a group within specific setting 'Cancer patients within the *Bristol Cancer Help Centre*. . . . Generally the group is about 10–12 people with usually a larger proportion of patients to supporters.'	'There is a very holistic emphasis to the work at the Bristol Cancer Help Centre with an integration of mind/body/spirit. The humanistic/ transpersonal underpinning of the music therapy approach fits within this holistic frame.'
Aims [There are *one-off group sessions* as part of the 1-week residential programme of the Centre] '. . . to explore the instruments in as free a way as possible. I try to help members of the group lose any inhibitions they may have in approaching the instruments. I expect that in most groups people will feel comfortable to make connections between the music they play and their emotions.'	'Each group is a unique experience.'
Structure of session 'The music session needs to be very self-contained with a clear beginning, middle and end. The patients and any supporters attending the group need to feel safe within the structure. The main approach is the use of *free improvisation* but there is some *listening* during some sessions depending on the nature of the needs of each group.	[Both *active* and *receptive* techniques are used]
My main interventions are therefore: free improvisation, relaxed listening techniques *(with or without guiding)*. Usually I need to be slightly more directive at the start of the group with less direction as members of the group feel more comfortable and lead themselves. The *issues arising from the music* lead to the next structure, e.g. if one piece creates feelings of sadness we may move on to explore these feelings more deeply in subsequent music.'	'My experiences as a trained practitioner in *Guided Imagery and Music* (GIM) informs any use of listening to music.' [see description of GIM in 'Other MT approaches' in this chapter] 'Opportunities for verbalisation are also part of the group.'

Authors' wording [in brackets]

that is people with life-threatening and/or terminal illness, is also very interesting, since this area of work is becoming increasingly relevant to arts therapies practice. Notice that on this occasion, Bunt, (L Bunt, unpublished interview, 2002) terms his approach as humanistic/transpersonal.

It is apparent from the clinical example presented in Table 5.6 that there are a number of differences in comparison to the Oldfield example in Table 5.5. The obvious differences are: the type of clients involved, the setting, and the duration of the therapy. These factors, along with distinctive personality traits and training backgrounds, contribute to differences in the way the same interactive MT approach is practised. Bunt (1994, 2002) acknowledges that his approach has a close resonance with humanistic and transpersonal psychology and includes 'Guided Imagery' techniques. Such perspectives are not explicitly mentioned by Oldfield (A Oldfield, personal communication, 1993).

Despite these differences, both practitioners share a belief in the value of free improvised music (active) as well as listening to music (receptive) and the presence of a clear structure that is perceived as inspiring safety. Finally, both agree on intervening in a more direct, or gradually less direct way either during one single session (L Bunt, unpublished interview, 2002) or within the time frame of the therapeutic contact as a whole (Oldfield 1995).

The creative MT approach: starting with Paul Nordoff and Clive Robbins

The creative MT approach is a type of work that is often associated with a 17-year collaboration between Paul Nordoff and Clive Robbins. This approach was developed almost in parallel with Alvin's contribution and was originally devised for clients with similar difficulties to those of Alvin's, i.e. children with learning difficulties (later on it is expanded to include adults). However, as we have already stated (see the brief history section earlier in the chapter), this approach is derived from a different tradition, the anthroposophical movement, and is grounded in the belief that 'everyone can respond to music – no matter how ill or disabled' (Nordoff–Robbins Centre 2004, p.1). There is also a belief in the associated idea that there is a 'musical child' in everyone and the role of the music therapist is to reach this child through musical improvisation. Music is therefore regarded as having unique qualities which when appropriately used (e.g. in therapy) 'can enhance communication and can help people to live more resourcefully and creatively' (Nordoff–Robbins Centre 2004, p.1). An emphasis on the therapeutic potential of music is particularly apparent in the first descriptions of Nordoff–Robbins' work (Nordoff & Robbins 1971, 1977) and continues to inform this approach to a great extent (Ansdell 2002, Nordoff–Robbins Centre 2004). Initially, the creative MT approach involved both private work and public performances (Ansdell 2002). Although the public character of the approach has been minimised over the years, creative MT is currently practised both individually as well as within groups. Ideally there are two therapists involved in either case, one playing the piano and the other one enabling clients to respond with improvisation. This two-therapist model reflects the tradition created by Nordoff and Robbins and their respective roles in the original version of this approach (Nordoff was often playing the piano, while Robbins was supporting the musical responses). According to Bruscia (1988), there are two main media within which clients in individual creative MT approaches may respond: vocalising/singing or initially playing a simple percussion instrument such as a drum or a cymbal, and gradually adding more instruments. In group work, clients are encouraged to sing, play a range of instruments and take part in 'musical dramas'. According to the same author (Bruscia 1988) an individual session can be broken down into three procedural phases: (1) meeting the client musically; (2) evoking musical responses; (3) developing musical skills, expressive freedom and inter-responsiveness (see Table 5.7).

Table 5.7: Stages for individual sessions – summary of Nordorff–Robbins' (1971, 1977) approach by Bruscia (1988, p.11)

Needs of clients
[Mainly children with learning difficulties but also adults]

Aims and Objectives
1. [To meet the child musically in order] '. . . to establish musical contact and rapport, to explore and gratify the client's musical tendencies and to develop a trusting, accepting relationship.'
2. [To evoke musical responses in order] '. . . to help the client develop a musical vocabulary, that will facilitate self-expression, and to create a musical context wherein client and therapist can build a working relationship.'
3. [To develop musical skills, expressive freedom and inter-responsiveness in order to modify or dispel pathological restrictions frequently encountered in this phase]

Stages of therapy
1. 'Meeting the child musically '. . . involves improvising music that matches the child's emotional state, while also accepting and enhancing its expression . . . Musical reflection is the most frequently used technique.
2. Evoking musical responses involves a variety of techniques . . . : presenting and demonstrating instruments, improvising music that stimulates or calls for a vocal or instrumental response, establishing musical turn-taking, helping the client phrase or shape his/her musical ideas or impulses, providing musical structures that support the client's improvising and make it more meaningful, and giving the improvisation musical form . . .
3. Developing musical skills may include establishing a basic beat, forming rhythm patterns or melodic motifs, or creating an instrumentation for a phrase.

Expressive freedom is developed by exploring the musical options and choices inherent in each musical skill . . .

In the process of discovering these expressive freedoms, the client also realises that there are many options for relating his/her music to that of the therapist . . . that the music can be 'inter-responsive' give-and-take with another person.'

Authors' wording in [brackets]

The three stages may occur spontaneously within one session. On other occasions they may develop over a number of sessions.

This approach comes closer to the artistic/creative approaches to arts therapies described in Section 1, where musical objectives and musical activities are perceived as sufficient for facilitating therapeutic change. Direct verbal references to people's psychological issues are avoided as are interpretations of the musical work. However, current practices of this very music-based approach are expanding in a way that they also incorporate a number of psychotherapeutic therapeutic principles. Expansion beyond an art-based practice is reflected in recent training content of the Nordoff–Robbins Centre (2003) and is apparent in the following example.

A creative MT approach with an adult with mental health difficulties

Ansdell, in his contribution to the study 'From Theory to Practice' (Karkou 2002), explains how his own approach, a MT practice with direct connections to the creative MT work of Nordoff and Robbins, draws primarily upon musical principles. His approach, however, also acknowledges the active/directive character of the work, humanistic (specifically Rogerian client-centred) underpinnings and the value of certain psychoanalytic principles, for instance the transferential/countertransferential relationship. He claims that there are theoretical contradictions in this work in that the therapist is directive by offering, for example, possibilities in music, but the therapy is client-led and so the client may reject possibilities or suggest alternatives. Other differences between Ansdell's (G Ansdell, unpublished interview, 2002) approach from the Nordoff–Robbins typical practice is that, as with most current creative MT practices, it also diverges from the original preoccupation of working mainly with clients with learning difficulties. The example presented in Table 5.8 involves an adult with mental health problems.

The similarities of Ansdell's work with the Nordoff–Robbins tradition are apparent. In the example in Table 5.8 there is a similar emphasis upon meeting the client musically and evoking a musical response. This becomes what Ansdell calls a 'musical conversation'. Music is the main emphasis of the work and is perceived as a tool for communication, a means of achieving creative potential and a way of expanding possibilities. The therapeutic aims are included within the musical aims. For example, encouraging someone to expand, change the rhythm and try new instruments is perceived as offering new possibilities in other areas of a person's life. The relational character of this approach is also highlighted. Linking the activity of making music with the client's difficulties, the person and the relationship, are some of what Ansdell (Karkou 2002) terms the 'meta-aims' of the work.

According to Ansdell (G Ansdell, unpublished interview, 2002), the music experience is a crucial characteristic of this work:

> There is a difference between being in the world musically and being in the world without music. It is almost as if a person enters the water for the first time; music creates a different environment. It is almost a surprise for the therapist to find out how a client will be in the world of music. The therapeutic change comes from engaging in the music.

Table 5.8: A creative MT approach with an adult with depression – Gary Ansdell (Example provided to V Karkou for 'Arts Therapies: from Theory to Practice' study [Karkou 2002, reproduced with permission])

Description of process	Comments by the therapist and the authors
Needs of client 'C. is a young woman with *depression and poor communication* who feels "unable to make a sound".'	Adult mental health
Aims 'Communication; creativity; motivation; freedom; enjoyment.'	'The therapeutic aims are included within the musical aims. By encouraging someone to expand, change the rhythm, try new instruments etc., you offer possibilities. Meta-aims: linking activity of making music with their illness, the person and the relationship.'
Beginning of MT process 'C. begins exploring the *sound of small instruments*. I play beside her . . . I *"tune into" her playing* – at first small gestures, tentative sounds.'	[Entering] ' "into" the world of spontaneous, creative music-making.' [*Meeting the client*]
Development of MT work and therapist's interventions [Gradually there is] 'louder and more expansive playing and singing – which finds an "answering activity" in my side of the *musical dialogue* with her. I am not just supportive, but co-creative with her. She says that she feels *permitted to explore* a less depressed, more active, more "noisy" side of herself. It's easier for her to play music with another person, than to speak. It's also "fun" – she enjoys being "playful" for a change. . . . MT makes C. feel better about herself.'	[*Musical conversation*] 'Instigating a "musical conversation".' 'Keep the conversation going.' [*Musical exploration*] 'I help the client explore the creative, communicative, relational possibilities of active music-making.'
Completion of MT work 'With C. the *agreed period* is 6 sessions; with other clients the process is open-ended.'	'The end mostly comes through mutual agreement, but like most artistic processes, the end is never certain. . . '

Authors' wording in [brackets]

With music-making being regarded as an important experience, Ansdell (G Ansdell, unpublished interview, 2002) adopts a phenomenological perspective and views music as:

- An experience of the body; it has an embodied quality.
- It has a time component; it takes place in time.
- It creates a 'virtual' space, a space defined by the sound.
- It encourages flow; flow of the body, emotions and thought.
- It offers form; musical phrases, rhythm, melody (this is very relevant to people with disorganised thoughts and emotions).
- One way or another it is connected to play even in its most serious expression (e.g. 'playing' music in a concert).

Similarities between the qualities of the music experience with experiences generated from some of the other artistic forms are apparent. For example there are obvious connections between music and dance in that the latter also offers an embodied and spatial experience; it takes place in time, encourages flow, and offers form. All artistic forms, when used within an arts therapies framework, may also take the form of play.

Analytical MT approaches: starting with Mary Priestley

The MT approaches described so far have drawn only marginally upon psychoanalytic/psychodynamic thinking. This section deals with a number of different MT practices that are more strongly informed by psychoanalytic/psychodynamic perspectives. The starting point for describing these approaches is the work of Priestley (1975, 1995). She was among the first music therapists to thoroughly compare MT theory with this dominant school of psychotherapy and develop a practice that brings together the two fields. Although Priestley's original MT training was with Alvin, influences from psychoanalytic/psychodynamic thinking are the characteristic features of her work, and are primarily influences from Freud, Jung, Klein and Adler (Priestley 1995). According to her, analytical MT is:

> . . . the analytically-informed symbolic use of improvised music by music therapist and client. It is used as a creative tool with which to explore the client's inner life so as to provide a way forward for growth and self-knowledge. (Priestley 1975, p. 3).

Despite the apparent influence of psychoanalysis upon this approach, Priestley (1975) claims that analytical MT can offer to individuals more than psychoanalysis, in that music enables feelings that are beneath the level of consciousness to be revealed with a greater force. Furthermore, through music these unconscious feelings become concrete and as such cannot be denied as easily as verbal expressions. She also regards the music as a 'sound matrix' that allows for containment of such feelings in a way that is not possible within classic psychoanalytic work.

Within this approach, the value of verbalisation is characteristically higher than in other MT approaches. Verbalisation may be an integral part of the beginning and end of a session or may take the form of an ongoing narrative next to music-based work. However, perhaps the most characteristic use of verbalisation is for stimulating the topic of music improvisations. 'Verbal titles' are offered to the client in order to develop musical improvisations that deal with 'central' work (i.e. confronting problems within the client's self or inner life) or with 'peripheral' work (i.e. confronting problems of everyday life and 'outer' life relationships).

Another characteristic of this approach is that the client is invited to sing, draw, paint, dance or engage in dramatic activities next to, or at the same time as, creating music. According to Scheiby (1999) these action-based components become one of the therapeutic factors for this approach next to the expressive and structural components of music, and the relationship between the client and the therapist.

Bruscia (1988) summarises Priesley's analytical session as a four-phase cycle (see Table 5.9). Once the cycle is completed, material emerging may trigger the whole process to get repeated again.

Table 5.9: The analytical MT phases – summary of Priestley's (1975) approach by Bruscia (1988, p. 13–14)

Needs of clients
[Mainly adults with emotional or interpersonal problems, but also couples and groups]

Aims
1. [Identify and entitle an issue for investigation
2. Define improvisational roles for the client and the therapist
3. Improvise the title
4. Discuss the improvisation experience afterwards]

Therapeutic phases
1. 'To identify an issue that needs investigation, the therapist may engage the client in a verbal discussion or an untitled musical improvisation, or simply observe the client's body language . . .
2. Defining what roles the client and therapist are to take in the improvisation depends upon several factors. These include: the therapeutic issues being explored, the role possibilities inherent in the title, the technique employed by the therapist, the client's need for direction or support, and the client's readiness for playing specific roles.
3. Improvising the title is aimed at putting the client in musical contact with his own feelings and letting the 'inner music' flow[1] . . . Depending on the purpose of the improvisation and the client's needs, the therapist may sit back and listen, or improvise along with the client . . . The improvisation is usually tape-recorded.
4. The final phase of the cycle is discussing the improvisation. The therapist usually begins by asking the client to verbalise his/her immediate reactions to the improvisatory experience . . . After processing immediate reactions and impression, the therapist may have the client listen to a tape of the improvisation for further analysis . . . The therapist may begin the entire cycle again by formulating another title to improvise. Or the therapist may ask the client to draw, paint or dance instead.'

[1]'Inner music' stands for the sounds of one's inner life.
Authors' wording in [brackets]

During the first phase of the therapeutic work, therapists pay special attention to discovering 'psychic blocks', i.e. finding out if clients' energy is blocked on a conscious or unconscious level. During the improvisatory phase therapists pay attention to clients' feelings through musical contact and also attend to their own feelings, a process that links closely with the psychoanalytic principles of transference and counter-transference. Also characteristic of this approach is the emphasis placed upon identifying areas of resistance, whether these areas are mainly musical or verbal.

In order to access unconscious material and work through this material, Priestley (1975) developed a number of techniques. The most commonly-used techniques found in current analytical MT practices are listed by Scheiby (1999) as follows: programmed or spontaneous regression, entering into somatic communication, free association, splitting, reality rehearsal, dream work, role playing, ritual acts, guided imagery, myths and holding. Some of these techniques make direct connection with Freudian psychoanalytic theory (e.g. spontaneous regression, free association, splitting, dream work); others seem to have a much more active/directive character and miscellaneous origin (e.g. programmed regression, role playing, ritual acts, guided imagery and use of myths). Influences from other psychotherapeutic practices (e.g. Jungian work) and other arts therapies (e.g. DT) are potentially present. Despite the overall analytical bias, this approach, once again, cannot be pinpointed specifically to one or two of the therapeutic approaches defined in Section 1 of this book. This is possibly the reason why in recent years it is also called 'exploratory MT' (Bruscia 1988), a title that may better reflect the wide-ranging influences incorporated in this approach.

Priestley's work, although particularly influential during the early days of MT as a modern profession, does not seem to be extensively used within current British MT practice; analytical MT deriving from Priestley's teaching is currently more popular in the USA (e.g. Scheiby 1999). However, her contribution to the field is apparent since it has opened the way for the development of a number of other psychoanalytically/psychodynamically-informed MT practices. The work of Sobey, Levinge and Odell-Miller cited below offers some examples of the ways in which this major school of thought is currently employed within British MT practice.

Psychoanalytically/psychodynamically-informed MT approaches with children

A psychoanalytically-informed MT approach with children aged 2.5 to 5 years with a diagnosis of autistic tendencies

There are a number of MT approaches that are deeply rooted within psychoanalytic thinking. One such example is provided by Sobey (K Sobey, unpublished interview, 2002). Her own training reflects her music and psychoanalytic bias; she originally trained at the Nordoff–Robbins course and acquired further training at the Tavistock Clinic. In her contribution to the study 'From Theory to Practice' (Karkou 2002), she clearly articulates her psychoanalytic bias, and presents the role of music within this work and the non-directive nature of her interventions. In relation to psychoanalytic thinking she believes that:

However, in Sobey's work, there is a clear emphasis upon the value of non-directive approaches in therapy and a strong psychoanalytic conceptualisation of the whole process (including whatever interventions may be made – see the case example in Table 5.10).

- *Differences.* Despite both Priestley and Sobey drawing heavily upon psychoanalytic/psychodynamic thinking, there are a number of differences. Firstly, Priestley's work is mainly with highly functioning adults, while Sobey predominantly works with children, some of whom may have severe difficulties such as autism. Secondly, Sobey's work does not include specific techniques developed within analytical MT such as musical role play, programmed regression and so on. Finally, Sobey retains a strong relational emphasis, a possible result of influences from the British object relations school of thought and her Tavistock training.

Psychoanalytically/psychodynamically-informed MT with children with learning and communication difficulties

Explicit references to the British schools of psychoanalytic/psychodynamic therapy (e.g. object relations theory), and Winnicott in particular, are made in the following example of the psychoanalytically/psychoadynamically-informed MT approach. Levinge (1993) regards the Winnicottian concepts of playing, transitional objects and holding, as issues directly translatable to MT practice. Playing becomes playing in music, which reveals the way in which the client perceives and relates to the world. The musical instruments, the music and sometimes the therapist become the transitional objects that enable the child to move from being merged with the original object (e.g. the mother) to a more independent state. Finally 'holding' (i.e. the process in which the mother/therapist reflects as a mirror the infant's emotional states) is created within MT. For 'holding' to take place, processes such as identification and adaptation take place beforehand. The therapist identifies with the child's music and may respond musically, adapting to the child's musical changes. Similarly, the child is enabled to identify and adapt to the therapist's music. Once both therapist

Table 5.11: Winnicott and MT for children with emotionally based communication difficulties – Alison Levinge ([a]Extracts from Levinge 1993, pp. 225–227; [b]material provided to V Karkou for 'Arts Therapies: from Theory to Practice' study [Karkou 2002, reproduced with permission])

Description of process with a specific case[a]	Comments on process by therapist and authors[b]
Needs of specific client [David was a lively, 3-year-old boy, described as having *language delay accompanied by behavioural difficulties*]	'Children with learning and communication difficulties based on a child development centre.'
Aims [David had difficulties separating from his mother] 'It was decided that mother and I would work together on helping David feel comfortable about being away from her.'	'To gain an understanding of what aspects of a child's internal psychological state of mind inhibits their development and to enable changes to occur in their capacity to relate.'
Beginning of MT work [The session started with David and *the therapist on their own in the room* but therapist felt that:] '. . . David seemed caught between his desire to explore and his desire for his mother. I decided to ask the mother to join us. With mother present in the room, David continued to explore the instruments, now playing a wider range of sounds. He moved quickly from one instrument to another, spending only a short time on each. David's musical expressions were more definite, but unsustained, often directed towards his mother.'	'A child might enter the MT environment and immediately begin to play. This play may consist of an exploratory period of examining the instruments, combined with improvised sounds. Depending upon the feeling at that initial moment, I may decide to accompany and support the child's sounds, movements or feelings.'
Development of MT work *'My role [as a therapist] was now very much in the background, sitting at the piano*. It seemed that my only way of safely *making contact* with David was through music. So I began making musical invitations on the piano. These took the form of short musical statements, which in some way *echoed or mirrored something of the quality or character of David's musical play*. Throughout these musical exchanges, mother made continuous comments, either praising, *encouraging or instructing David to be careful.*	'I will be involved in *finding out where I am placed*.' 'Initially my focus will be upon the development of the therapeutic relationship, which will involve such processes as: identification, adaptation and holding.'
Gradually David began to respond and his *musical explosions began to be directed towards me*. The music changed from being my invitations and affirmations of David's music, to David's imitations and responses to mine.	[1. *identification*] [2. *adaptation*] [In this example identification and adaptation were initially taking place between the child and his mother. Gradually there was a shift towards the therapist]

Continued

Table 5.11: Winnicott and MT for children with emotionally based communication difficulties – Alison Levinge – cont'd ([a]Extracts from Levinge 1993, p. 225–227; [b]material provided to V. Karkou for 'Arts Therapies: from Theory to Practice' study [Karkou 2002, reproduced with permission])

Description of process with a specific case[a]	Comments on process by therapist and authors[b]
We were creating *a language* together. We moved away from an uncomfortable place where relating and communicating seemed awkward and difficult to a place where we both felt safe enough to explore. As the session moved on, David allowed himself to be *fully held* in the music. He now came to join me at the piano. *Our music developed into a duet which led from dissonant, heavy chords into a waltz . . .* As we entered the waltz, David's whole body moved as if he was totally held in the music. I noticed that he had now become coordinated and more focused . . .	'These [processes] would occur primarily musically, through improvised music-making, but may include verbal comments on the process.' [3. *holding*] 'I will be involved in developing *a mutual space.* Winnicott named this place "the playground".'
However the original conflict re-emerged and David made an attempt to move away from the music and back to mother . . . David's tripping and falling were, I felt, *a rupture to our togetherness* and in the following sessions this emerged as a significant theme."	'As the relationship develops, I will expect to see expressions of the *issues affecting the child's development emerging* in more detail and with more intensity. Being a musical presence will eventually enable the child to rework their issues and develop a more healthy way of relating.'
Completion of MT work 'His inability to hold himself, both physically and emotionally, seemed to reflect part of David's experience of being with his mother. This was translated directly into our musical relationship. Without words it had been possible to recreate David's early experience of relating. *MT had been able to provide another opportunity for David to renegotiate this stage of development and hopefully to move on.*'	'The ending of my therapy is ideally arrived at through the *combination of the therapist and child's feelings* about the process. In the case of children, there are often external restrictions, such as moving schools, which may intervene.'

Authors' wording in [brackets]

and child feel sufficiently held within the music (i.e. feel heard by each other), exploration of difficult feelings becomes a possibility.

For Levinge (A Levinge, unpublished interview, 2002) the unconscious aspects of the client–therapist relationship are central areas of attention during her work (an emphasis common for most psychoanalytically-informed therapists). However, she also finds it important to take into consideration the whole environment; the therapist is part of this environment alongside the music and the musical instruments. This environment provides holding, handling and object-presenting, which allows children to respond playfully, visit and rework earlier developmental stages, and eventually create more functional relationships. Trusting that the environment (i.e. the therapist, the music and the musical instruments) is 'good enough' for children to reveal something about themselves, and to explore and deal with difficulties, is a key concept for Levinge's work and directly linked with the Winnicottian concepts of 'good enough' mothering.

A description of how the process may look when working with children with learning and/or communication difficulties is presented in Table 5.11. Extracts from published material (Levinge 1993) that refer to working with a specific child with language and behavioural problems are also included as an additional illustration of this work.

A psychoanalytically-informed MT approach with adults

The psychoanalytically-informed MT approach adopted by Odell-Miller (2000, 2002) does not have the same emphasis upon a single theoretician as the previous approach presented. Odell-Miller seems to be working with a different client group (i.e. adults with long-term mental health problems) and draws upon a wider pool of theoretical sources for achieving theoretical resonance (i.e. Freud, object relations theory, attachment theory, early mother–infant interaction theories such as those described by Daniel Stern). A lot of this work often takes place in groups and draws upon analytical group theorists (e.g. Bion, Foulkes) and interpersonal group theorists (e.g. Yalom). However, according to Odell-Miller, despite the presence of all these theoretical influences (most of which come from psychoanalytic thinking), the 'central driving force' remains the music. Through musical improvisation, unconscious processes are brought to clients' attention, while transference and counter-transference issues are worked through. Verbal interpretation also has a place within this approach as a means of giving meaning to the musical improvisations. Emphasis is placed upon both the internal world of the clients, as well as the linking of the internal world with the external and the day-to-day reality. A summary of the main MT assumptions of this work follows:

- Through the developing relationship (with the therapist and/or members of a group) change will occur which is reflected and brought about partly by the music itself, but also by the thinking and talking about the musical experience in between each improvisation.
- Music has an innate quality which is present before speech develops; therefore spontaneous non-verbal communication is accessible to most people.
- Music can be a way of taking hold of 'affect' or mood, and bringing about expression and change of these states within a containing holding environment where sometimes unacceptable feelings such as aggression can be expressed and 'channelled' in a creative acceptable way.

A detailed account of the way this approach is implemented in practice is presented in Table 5.12.

Odell-Miller's work has been extensively researched with research designs that are not always popular amongst psychoanalytically-informed arts therapists, e.g. RCTs. These studies offer hard evidence for the value and effectiveness of MT, and other arts therapies, with clients with mental health problems (Odell-Miller 1995, Odell-Miller et al 2001).

Other MT approaches

There are a number of other approaches to MT. The ones cited more often are: the 'guided imagery and music' (GIM) approach and the behavioural approach to MT. Both of these approaches come from the USA and as such their impact upon British practice is not necessarily that great. Nevertheless, references to such practices are still made within British texts. For example, Bunt (2002) talks about the use of his GIM training within his own work, while Wigram et al (2002) refers, amongst others, to behavioural MT. Pressures to operate within settings with a predominantly behavioural culture and the need to modify practices are also acknowledged (e.g. Sobey refers to expanding attention span through music as one of her colleagues' expectations from MT with the specific child described earlier [K Sobey, unpublished interview, 2002]).

GIM was founded by Helen Lindquist Bonny and involves imagery evoked during listening to music. It is described by its founder (Bonny 1994) as a humanistic and transpersonal model (notice that this is also how Bunt [L Bunt, unpublished interview, 2002] describes his own approach to MT) and is based on research on altered states of consciousness that was undertaken during the 1970s, and research on guided imagery influenced by Jung and Gestalt therapy. Clients are invited to enter into deep relaxation while the therapist chooses the music and guides them to shift their attention from the outer to their inner world, identify personal material, develop this material further, transform it and ideally re-integrate it (Wigram et al 2002). A more formalised reference to the GIM process involves the following stages: prelude, induction, music travel and postlude. The therapist is quite directive, especially during the first two stages of the work ('prelude' and 'induction'), while less so during the 'music travel' and the 'postlude' that follow. Despite the overall receptive musical techniques used within this approach, clients' own interpretations of their experiences are seen as authoritative (thus the humanistic affiliation), and the role of the music experience is regarded as central and transformative (thus, easily placed under the artistic/creative therapeutic underpinnings discussed in Section 1). According to Burns et al (2001), the relevance and value of this method for certain clients, such as cancer clients, are potentially high.

Behavioural MT is defined as an approach that uses music as a reinforcement or stimulus cue that aims to modify, improve or extinguish undesired physiological, motor, psychological, emotional, cognitive, perceptual or autonomic behaviours (Bruscia 1998, Wigram et al 2002). In general, symptoms are targeted at the whole personality and both active and receptive musical activities are involved with very specific goals (e.g. to improve motor skills with clients with Parkinson's disease, change a certain behaviour with clients

Table 5.12: Working with adults with mental health problems within a MT group – Helen Odell-Miller [Example provided to V Karkou for 'Arts Therapies: from Theory to Practice' study [Karkou 2002, reproduced with permission]]

Description of process with a specific client	Comments on process by therapist and authors
Needs of client 'This 55-year-old extremely *damaged*, but intelligent, lady was referred following her attendance at a movement therapy group at a day center . . . she had developed an interest in using *rhythm and music to express her feelings*. Her diagnosis on the referral form was given as possibly schizotypal personality disorder, with depression and an eating disorder. She needs to improve her self-image but also to increase her independence. She lives with her sister who is her main carer. She also needs an outlet for her emotions, and was described by others as having "pent up angry feelings". She needs a containing supportive place which will help her socially as well as provide a place for regular contact and interactions with others. She has a long history of problems, and still needs help with separation from her parents.' **Aims/expectations/assumptions** 'This lady . . . has multiple problems, and the expectation . . . is that the work will entail *close liaison with many other professionals* for it to be of any benefit . . .'	'The clients referred to MT have *continuing mental health* problems such as schizophrenia, bipolar, depression and or personality disorders.' '*Non-verbal* relating is crucial for this group of clients who have often found using words too direct or used them as a way of avoiding feelings.' 'MT with this patient group should always take account of the *multi-disciplinary teams*, and music therapists should liaise and maintain their role as a team member for the patient at all times . . . It is likely that the patient could use these multi-professional links to avoid change by "splitting", and this needs to be understood and managed by the music therapist in liaison with the other professionals, and the patient herself.'

'Therapy is often concerned with *trying to re-create a sense of life* for those who have lost it, literally for some and metaphorically for others.'
'*The musical relationship* with the therapist (and group members in a group) allows these [particular] aims to be realised.'

'Main carers need as much support as the patient and this will be a dynamic to be taken into account . . . in the care plan.'

'This group is *long established* with a core membership who are used to using music as almost another language.'
'The therapist would help the patient *integrate into the group* by listening and interacting with the group musical improvisations . . . ', [The group members also help integration and gradually the best means of the new patient using the group will emerge]

'This is not necessarily typical but given the fact that the person concerned is also musical and *used to play the piano* she was more quickly confident.'

'The patient began to *use the group to help her own mood* and to understand how her experiences in the music therapy group could help her in her life outside the group.'

Assumptions are that she will develop a high degree of *dependency* on the music therapy group, but that the process will be slow and gradual. Also that much of the work will be in *managing feelings*, in *developing a relationship* so that the person can regularly feel understood and listened to, but that with such a chronic history, change may be small.

It will be about managing and improving day-to-day living to make it more bearable for the patient and *main carers* (in this case her sister) . . .'

Beginning of MT work
'After a thorough assessment, the patient in this case was offered a place in a *weekly MT group*. . . .
The patient *engaged immediately* by trying out instruments, particularly the small drum (tambour) and by fitting in with other people's music and keeping a low profile . . . The patient experimented using movement as well which she found particularly useful in rhythm to the music being improvised, and she also started to realise she could use music to express her feelings at the time. The patient *integrated quickly* and made relationships musically and through talking to the other members, asking questions . . .'

Development of MT work
'. . . There were a few early sessions like the first one . . . She became more able to *assert her own music* without worrying all the time about what others thought.

Continued

Table 5.12: Working with adults with mental health problems within a MT group – Helen Odell-Miller [Example provided to V. Karkou for 'Arts Therapies: from Theory to Practice' study [Karkou 2002, reproduced with permission]]—cont'd

Description of process with a specific client	Comments on process by therapist and authors
'I used the piano a lot at this stage and gradually became *less and less directive* from the piano to a point where members began to make their own group music, the patient concerned daring to use the piano herself after the sixth session. After 6 months the patient's music became more demonstrative and also more flexible. She was putting on weight and seemed to think there might be a link in that she felt more able to relax and *"feed herself"* both *musically and literally*. She was also becoming more aware of the group's music and not only her own music. . . . whilst it is not an aim of the therapy, patients often develop a way of becoming more inventive and aware of the structure and form of the music itself, its aesthetic . . . and also its . . . more destructive qualities. For this lady this contrast was very relevant at different times. She became more able to experiment with spontaneously being in control and also not so "in control".	'The therapist helps to build up a musical language, with *less musical intervention by the therapist* as the new group membership becomes established.'
The therapist acknowledged this *by musical interventions*, which showed this has been heard, and also help the patient move on (by suggesting different rhythms for example). Equally in this [case], reflection, interpretation and understanding were crucial to help articulate the musical experience and its meaning for the patient in her life.'	The role of the music therapist is crucial in facilitating the patient's expression . . . This is sometimes understood in *symbolic terms* as a parental role. . . in some cases, my harmonic input from the piano can inhibit patients from being able to work through their own problems. However, there are times when the opposite is true and the basis for someone exploring a problem is that a musical dialogue with a supportive role taken by the therapist is necessary. Here, considerations of transference and counter-transference are essential.' 'The *therapist's main interventions* are . . . centred around musically supporting and helping the members develop their playing to bring out latent meaning and affect.' [As trust grows, members may discuss more freely, the effect on them of others' improvisations]

Completion of MT work

'For this lady, 9 months into her therapy we *discussed her attendance* as being for about 2 years. It was important to bear this in mind so that she had a feeling of working towards this, and the possibility of change. For this lady, at the end of the 2-year period, she managed to work on an ending musically and verbally.'

In discussion, she had made good relationships with members, which had been important to her, but she found the separation very difficult and it involved a lot of interaction between the therapist and other team members. In the last session *she led the group in an improvisation* from the piano which went through many sections (quite like sonata form), in which she interacted sensitively with each member and also had 'solos' for herself. She has since managed to move away from her sister and live on her own, taking a voluntary job in an old people's home for one afternoon a week. She is no longer under weight and whilst we cannot attribute this to the music therapy alone, together with all the input from the team and her family, she feels the various interventions have been significant.'

Authors' wording in [brackets]

'The *decision about ending* in this group is driven by the patient's whole care plan and in liaison with the multi-disciplinary team. As far as possible . . . patients make their own endings but helped by the therapists understanding of their own process . . . People leave at different times, so endings are used to understand events of comings and goings in relationships in the patients' lives.'

'Musically, usually when a patient leaves *there are improvisations* around that time that seem to express sadness and loss and also celebration (Odell-Miller 2002). The work might involve the making of a song or the working through of a piece of group music. Or an ending might be sudden.'

with learning disabilities, and so on). This approach is extensively researched in the USA using mainly experimental designs (e.g. Madsen et al 1968, Madsen & Madsen 1997, Standley 1991, Thaut 1985). Part of the same tradition is the vibroacoustic and vibrotactile therapy that focuses specifically on physical treatment and has been developed in the UK by Tony Wigram (Wigram 1996, Wigram & Dileo 1997). This approach to therapy involves specific vibroacoustic devices that enable clients to experience musical vibrations directly on their bodies (there are often speakers built into a chair where the client is sitting, through which low frequency tones are played in combination with appropriately relaxing music). Vibroacoustic therapy carries memories from the early medical/physiological interest in music and is not as popular in the UK as other approaches already described.

Finally, Bruscia (1988) refers to a number of other approaches to MT such as: the music and dance experimental therapy, the Orff model, the metaphoric MT, the integrative approach and the developmental. Although these approaches are well documented by Bruscia (1987, 1988, 1998), and some principles of these are present in current British practice, overall they remain fairly unpopular within the British MT context.

Summary

Music therapists were the first of the arts therapists to organise themselves into a professional group and develop training courses after the lengthy pioneering work of musicians and music teachers with special-needs populations. With the support of physicians and acceptance from the general public they have developed a practice that is based on music improvisation and have incorporated influences from humanistic psychology, psychoanalytic/psychodynamic thinking, and, up to a point, behaviourism, into a distinctive professional discipline. Memories from the pioneering work of Alvin, Nordoff–Robbins and Priestley can still be found within current practice. However, the scope of MT has expanded from working primarily with autism and learning disabilities to mental health populations, cancer care and dementia as well as a number of other client groups. A lot of the work undertaken with these clients has been extensively researched offering qualitative and quantitative evidence of the effectiveness and value of certain types of interventions. Extensive work has been completed in health services and education while further developments have recently begun in community MT. Examples of current practice that have been described and discussed in this chapter are interactive or free improvisational MT, creative MT, analytical MT and approaches strongly rooted within psychoanalytic/psychodynamic thinking. Other approaches primarily stemming from American practice are also briefly referred to, such as the 'guided imagery and music' (GIM) model and behavioural approaches to MT.

References

- Aldridge D 1996 Music therapy research and practice in medicine: from out of the silence. Jessica Kingsley, London
- Altshuler I M 1948 A psychiatrist's experiences with music as a therapeutic agent. In: Schullian D M, Schoen M (eds) Music and medicine. Henry Schumann, New York, p 226–281

- Alvin J 1975 Music therapy. John Clare Books, London
- Alvin J 1978 Music therapy for the autistic child. Oxford University Press, London
- Ansdell G 2002 Community music therapy and the winds of change: a discussion paper. Voices: a World Forum for Music Therapy 2(2):1–37. Online. Available: http://www.voices.no/mainissues/voices2(2)ansdell.html 26 Dec 2004
- Ansdell G, Bunt L, Hartley N 2002 Music therapy in the United Kingdom. Voices: a World Forum for Music Therapy. Online. Available: http://www.voices.no/country/monthuk_april2002.html 26 Dec 2004
- Bonny H 1994 Twenty-one years later: a GIM update. Music Therapy Perspectives 12(2):70–74
- British Society for Music Therapy (BSMT) 2004a The society. Online. Available: http://www.bsmt.org/the_society.htm 26 Dec 2004
- British Society for Music Therapy (BSMT) 2004b What is music therapy? Online. Available: http://www.apmt.org/mt_whatismt.htm 26 Dec 2004
- Bruscia K 1987 Improvisation models of music therapy. Charles C Thomas, Springfield IL
- Bruscia K E 1988 A survey of treatment procedures in improvisational music therapy. Psychology of Music 16:10–24
- Bruscia K E 1998 Defining music therapy, 2nd edn. Barcelona Publishers, Gilsum NH
- Bunt L 1994 Music therapy: an art beyond words. Routledge, London
- Bunt L 2002 Transformation, ovid and guided imagery and music (GIM). In: Bunt L, Hoskyns S (eds) The handbook of music therapy. Brunner-Routledge, East Sussex, p 290–307
- Bunt L, Hoskyns S 2002 The handbook of music therapy. Brunner-Routledge, Hove
- Bunt L, Marston-Wyld J 1995 Special feature: where words fail music takes over: a collaborative study by a music therapist and a counsellor in the context of cancer care. National Association for MT 13(1):46–50
- Bunt L, Burns S, Turton P 2000 Variations on a theme: the evolution of a music therapy research programme at the Bristol Cancer Help Centre. British Journal of Music Therapy 14(2):62–69
- Burns S J I, Harbuz M S, Huckerbridge F 2001 A pilot study into the therapeutic effects of music therapy at a cancer help center. Alternative Therapies 7(1):48–56
- Gilroy A, Lee C 1995 Art and music: therapy and research. Routledge, London
- Karkou V 2002 Arts therapies: from theory to practice. Unpublished report submitted to the funding body, University of Hertfordshire
- Levinge A 1993 Permission to play: the search for self through music therapy; research with children presenting with communication difficulties. In: Payne H (ed) Handbook of inquiry in the arts therapies: one river, many currents. Jessica Kingsley, London
- Madsen C K, Madsen C H 1997 Experimental research in music, 3rd edn. Contemporary Publishing Company, Raleigh NC
- Madsen C K, Cotter V, Madsen C H 1968 A behavioural approach to music therapy. Journal of Music Therapy 5(3):69–71
- Meyer G 1999 An exploratory study of the theory and technique of five expressive art therapy modalities. PhD dissertation, California School of Professional Psychology, Alameda
- Nordoff P, Robbins C 1971 Therapy in music for handicapped children. Victor Gollancz, London
- Nordoff P, Robbins C 1977 Creative music therapy. Harper and Row, New York
- Nordoff-Robbins Centre 2004 Training as qualified music therapist. Online. Available: http://www.nordoff-robbins.org.uk/html/training.html 26 Dec 2004
- Odell-Miller H 1995 Approaches to music therapy in psychiatry with specific emphasis upon a research project with the elderly mentally ill. In: Wigram T, Saperston B, West R (eds) The art and science of music therapy: a handbook. Harwood Academic Publications, Chur, p 83–111
- Odell-Miller H 2000 Music therapy and its relationship to psychoanalysis. In: Searle Y, Sterng I (eds) Where analysis meets the arts. Karnac, London
- Odell-Miller H 2001 Interview by Rachel Darnley-Smith. Historical perspectives interview series. British Journal of Music Therapy 15(1):8–13
- Odell-Miller H 2002 One man's journey and the importance of time in music therapy. In: Davies A, Richards E (eds) Music therapy and group work: sound company. Jessica Kingsley, London
- Odell-Miller H, Westacott M, Hughes P et al 2001 An investigation into the effectiveness of the arts therapies by measuring symptomatic and significant life change for people

between the ages of 16–65 with continuing mental health problems. Report on a research study jointly funded by Adderbrooke's NHS Trust and Anglia Polytechnic University, Arts Therapies Department, Fulbourn Hospital, Cambridge

* Oldfield A 1995 Communicating through music: the balance between following and initiating. In: Wigram T, Saperston B, West R (eds) The art and science of music therapy: a handbook. Harwood Academic Publications, Switzerland, p 226–237
* Oldfield A, Adams 1995 M The Effects of music therapy on a group of adults with profound learning difficulties. In: Gilroy A, Lee C (eds) Art and music: therapy and research. Routledge, London, p 164–182
* Pavlicevic M 1997 Music therapy in context: music, meaning and relationship. Jessica Kingsley, London
* Payne H (ed) 1993 Handbook of inquiry in the arts therapies: one river many currents. Jessica Kingsley, London
* Priestley M 1975 Music therapy in action. Constable and Company, London
* Priestley M 1995 Linking sound and symbol. In: Wigram T, Saperston B, West R (eds) The art and science of music therapy: a handbook. Harwood Academic Publishers, Chur, p 129–138
* Scheiby B B 1999 Music as symbolic expression: analytical music therapy. In: Weiner D J (ed) Beyond talk therapy: using movement and expressive techniques in clinical practice. American Psychological Association, Washington DC
* Standley J M 1991 The role of music in pacification/stimulation of premature students with low birth weights. Music Therapy Perspectives 9:19–25
* Standley J M 1995 Music as a therapeutic intervention in medical and dental treatment: research and clinical application. In: Wigram T, Saperston B, West R (eds) The art and science of music therapy: a handbook. Harwood Academic Publishers, Chur, p 3-22
* Storr A 1993 Forward. In: Heal M, Wigram T (eds) Music therapy in health and education. Jessica Kingsley, London
* Thaut M H 1985 The use of auditory rhythm and rhythmic speech to aid temporal muscular control in children with gross motor dysfunction. Journal of Music Therapy 22(3):129–145
* Tyler H 2000 The music therapy profession in modern Britain. In: Horden P (ed) Music as medicine: the history of music therapy since antiquity. Ashgate, Aldershot
* Wigram T 1996 The effect of vibroacoustic therapy on clinical and non-clinical populations. PhD psychological research thesis. St George's Medical School, University of London
* Wigram T, Dileo C (eds) 1997 Music, vibration and health. Jeffrey Books, New Jersey
* Wigram T, Saperston B, West R 1995 The art and science of music therapy: a handbook Harwood, Chur
* Wigram T, Pedersen I N, Bonde L O 2002 A comprehensive guide to music therapy: theory, clinical practice, research and training. Jessica Kingsley, London

Chapter 6

Art Therapy (AT)

Key issues:

- Art therapy (AT), also known as art psychotherapy, emerged as a modern profession after the Second World War. The British Association of Art Therapists (BAAT) was established in 1964 and is currently the largest arts therapies professional body. It gained professional recognition by the Health Professions Council in 1999, alongside drama- and music therapy.

- Research shows that emotional/behavioural difficulties constitute the major focus of AT practice, followed by learning difficulties.

- The main working environments are reported as the health services, then voluntary/private organisations and social services. Although the proportion of art therapists employed in educational settings remains relatively small, there are recent indications of renewed interest in this area of work.

- In AT a range of art materials is used and major emphasis is placed upon the client–therapist relationship.

- From research evidence it seems that in comparison with other arts therapies, AT places an increased significance upon psychoanalytic/psychodynamic principles.

- Approaches to AT found in the British context such as structured AT, client-centred, analytical art psychotherapy, object relations perspectives and group analytic AT are described and illustrated using case examples.

Introduction

Art therapy, or as it is also known, art psychotherapy, (AT) was the first of the arts therapies to form a professional association in the UK and, alongside music therapy (MT), to achieve professional recognition and conditions of work. Furthermore, the British Association of Art Therapists (BAAT) is currently the largest arts therapies professional body. In this chapter, historical and current developments will be discussed, AT will be defined, and current therapeutic trends and some AT approaches will be delineated.

Brief AT history

The multifaceted influences upon the emergence of AT are apparent in Waller's (1991) study of the profession in Britain (1940–1982) as well as other historical accounts of the development of AT as a modern profession (e.g. from Wood 1997, and Hogan 2001). For example, Waller (1991, 1992) suggests that AT has some roots in art education and especially the 'Child Art' trend that emanated from Cizek and the 19th century Vienna Secessions art movement. This movement affected art education in the UK and the USA and eventually developed into a child-centred approach to art teaching that had principles and techniques very conducive to the emergence of AT.

In parallel with the contribution of child-centred education during the first half of the century, psychoanalytic thinking also paid close attention to the visual arts as having psychological resonance. For example, Freud himself developed much of his theoretical work through studying literature and visual arts. With a number of artists, and surrealists in particular, also turning to Freud to find meaning in their imagery (Chilvers et al 1988, Hogan 2001, Malchiodi 1998), the link between psychoanalysis and visual art probably became stronger than with any other art form. Jung developed these links even further through his personal interest in art and his theoretical connections between image-making and the psyche. Similarly to Freud, he perceived art expression as accessing the unconscious mind. But unlike Freud, Jung did not see symbolic expression as a sign of unresolved issues but as a source for transformation and well-being.

Another important root of AT stemmed from collections of artwork produced by people with mental illness (Waller 1991). For example, the Swiss art collector Dubuffet and his 'Art Brut' collection of what is currently known as 'outsider art', received interest from a number of art students and psychiatrists. Art students for example, during their search for 'individual' modes of expression, saw 'psychiatric art' as an inspiration for their own work. Psychiatrists on the other hand, saw art as potentially advancing psychiatric diagnosis and/or supporting existing psychiatric treatments. After the Second World War in particular, interest from medical circles in the recreational and healing aspects of art began to increase. Occupational therapy (OT), in the form of creative crafts work emerged at this time, while a growing number of artists started getting employment within hospital environments.

According to Waller (1991), the emergence of AT as a modern profession in the UK began as a result of the above influences during and soon after the Second World War. Although it began at a similar time as American AT (with the American pioneers Naumburg [1966] and Kramer [1971]), British AT developed slightly differently, following a number of delays regarding professional identity and recognition. Overall, there are three periods that can be traced in British professional development. During the first period (from the 1940s up to the formation of the BAAT) certain individuals, either artists or psychiatrists/psychotherapists started recognising the therapeutic value of art-making but continued working independently. Waller (1991, 1992) refers to some important contributions made by artists during this period such as Adrian Hill and Edward Adamson. Both of them were originally trained as commercial artists, found employment in hospitals and are currently seen as important pioneers of AT in the UK. The Jungian-trained Irene Champernowne is another name associated with this period. Champernowne never described herself as an art therapist, but her contribution to the field and her active involvement with the first AT working party meetings was such (see Box 6.1) that today she is regarded as another important pioneer of AT next to Hill and Adamson. Waller (1991) also discusses the special attention paid to the visual arts by other psychotherapists such as Donald Winnicott, Marion Milner and Ralph Pickford, while Hogan (2001) adds contributions made by Kris and Pailthorpe.

The formation of BAAT in 1964 (Box 6.1) marked a second important period of AT development. During that time organised professional activity was launched that involved heated debates around AT identity and resulted in agreement on criteria for training and BAAT registration. The majority of the members of the Association of that time were artists with a teaching qualification. The client-centred emphasis of the studio work of Hill and Adamson became a popular way of working for art therapists to such an extent that Waller (1992) argues that AT of the period was not very different from a form of 'sensitive' art teaching. Gradually, practising art therapists became interested in humanistic thinking in general, as well as existentialism and the anti-psychiatry movement in particular (Wood 1997). There are some obvious reasons for this shift: (1) there was an increasing pressure from within the profession to acquire a psychotherapeutic justification for AT practices; (2) humanistic movements were on the increase during the 1960s and 1970s; (3) the original affiliation with art teaching, and client-centred teaching in particular, was conceptually very close to an overall humanistic rationale.

By the 1980s, AT had established training courses (some of which were founded in the previous period) and had achieved recognition within the National Health Service (NHS), first under an occupational therapy umbrella and a few years later, as a different profession alongside music therapy (MT) and other health professions (Box 6.1). Within the emphasis of the period to strengthen the professional basis of the profession, humanistic thinking was gradually abandoned for the more established and articulate

Box 6.1: Significant dates in the development of AT in the UK (BAAT 2004a, Hogan 2001, Waller 1991, 1992)

Year	Development
1940s–1950s	Series of working party meetings chaired by Hill, but also Champernowne and Adamson.
1964	BAAT is formed, which becomes the official professional body for AT.
1969	AT as an option within an Art Teacher's Diploma course, School of Art Education in Birmingham.
1970	Certificate in Remedial Art, St Albans School of Art; Adamson acts as its first consultant.
1974	AT as an option within the Art Teacher's course at Goldsmith's College of Art.
1980	Discussion in the House of Commons regarding pay scales and career structures; assumption that AT and MT fall under OT.
1982	The Department of Health and Social Security awards career and grading structure for AT and MT practitioners.
1999	Registration with the Health Professions Council alongside MT and dramatherapy (DT).

psychoanalytic/psychodynamic school of thought. As we will see in the following sections, further changes have taken place within the profession. Still, the alliance of AT with this psychotherapeutic school of thought remains strong up to this day as we will discuss later on.

Current AT professional development

The British Association of Art Therapists (BAAT) is currently the largest professional association amongst arts therapies with around 2000 full members (i.e. qualified art therapists). There are six training courses in AT based in England, Scotland and Northern Ireland (see Appendix 2). The minimum AT training required for BAAT and Health Professions Council (HPC) registration is 2 years full-time, a duration of training that, for many years, was longer than for most of the other arts therapies. Partly because of the longer training, but also due to relevant debates and distinctive traditions within AT, many practising art therapists prefer to call their practice art psychotherapy. As either art therapists or art psychotherapists, they all follow the same core training requirements and are obliged to meet the same professional standards.

Many art therapists work with individuals on a one-to-one basis, in addition to the currently expanding, AT group work. Tables 6.1 and 6.2 show that art therapists work with clients with mental health issues (otherwise termed as

Table 6.1: Main AT client groups and differences from other arts therapies

Type of difficulty	% for AT	% for other arts therapies	Chi-square (x²) value	Degrees of freedom (df)	P-value (p)
Emotional/behavioural	73.9	45.2	49.36	1	0.000**
Learning	11.1	35.2	47.10	1	0.000**
Other	5.8	5.7	Not significant		
Physical/sensory/medical	4.1	2.5	Not significant		
Multiple	2.7	3.9	Not significant		
No apparent	2.4	7.5	8.9	1	0.004**
Total	100.0	100.0			

**Accepted at the 0.01 level of significance

The table shows that emotional/behavioural difficulties (that is mental health issues) were, overwhelmingly, the most frequent types of difficulties faced by the clients of art therapists, with considerably fewer difficulties falling under the learning category. The third group of client difficulties was the 'other' category, most likely consisting of clients with a particular mental health diagnosis such as people with depression, schizophrenia or survivors of sexual abuse. Chi-square tests performed for the different client groups revealed a number of statistically significant differences between AT and other arts therapists. In proportion, there were fewer art therapists working with learning difficulties and fewer working with clients who did not present an apparent difficulty. All these differences were accepted at the 0.01 level of significance.

Table 6.2: Main AT working environments and differences from other arts therapies

Working environment	% for AT	% for other arts therapies	Chi-square (x^2) value	Degrees of freedom (df)	P-value (p)
Health	58.7	37.7	25.15	1	0.000**
Voluntary/private agency	14.0	11.2	Not significant		
Social service	11.6	12.3	Not significant		
Education	7.5	26.1	35.57	1	0.000**
Private practice	6.8	8.3	Not significant		
Other	1.4	4.4	4.63	1	0.031*
Total	100.0	100.0			

**Accepted at the 0.01 level of significance
*Accepted at the 0.05 level of significance

Health services were the most frequently reported areas of work followed by voluntary/private organisations and social services. Education, private practice and the other category (most likely to be Home Office establishments such as prisons or detention centres) were working environments that did not score as highly amongst art therapists.

When chi-square tests were performed for these different working environments, three statistically significant differences were found between art therapists and non-art therapists. In proportion, more art therapists were found working in health services compared with other arts therapists (p = 0.000), while smaller percentages of art therapists were found in education (p = 0.000) and in other settings (p = 0.031).

'emotional/behavioural difficulties') and within the NHS to a much larger extent than other arts therapies practitioners. These findings seem to reflect the pioneering work of Adamson and Champernowne with people with mental health issues during the first period of AT development, as well as the lengthy professional effort placed upon recognising AT within the NHS during the second and third periods.

Waller's (1991) study of the history of the AT profession discusses how the original alignment of BAAT with the National Union of Teachers (NUT) was subsequently perceived by some practising art therapists with increasing uneasiness due to the implication that AT was a type of teaching intervention. The alliance with the NUT was eventually dropped in favour of resolving intra-professional conflicts and pursuing a health services' recognition. Moving away from the teaching profession seems also to be reflected in the findings presented in Tables 6.1 and 6.2, where in comparison with other arts therapies, the proportion of art therapists working with either children with learning difficulties or educational settings is not as high. There is a fairly recent increase of publications relating to AT with clients with learning difficulties (e.g. Rees 1998) and AT in schools (Karkou 1999, Karkou & Glasman 2004, Sanderson & Karkou 2000). Publications of this kind and promotion of this area of work from the AT in education subgroup is expected to create a different picture of the profession in the near future.

In terms of research evidence available for the value of AT interventions, there are a number of completed studies that look at adult mental health, schizophrenia, eating disorders, addiction, abused children, autism and learning disabilities (Gilroy & Lee 1995, Payne 1993). Most of these studies are qualitative in nature and of a small scale. The few studies that have been completed in the UK with a randomised controlled trial (RCT) design refer to clients with severe mental health illness and dementia. Much more research activity with varied methodological emphasis is available in the American AT literature where research training is part of the basic training of the art therapists (Edwards 2004). However, Burleigh & Beutler (1997), in their critical analysis of AT and DT empirical studies, argue that further research work is required. Current changes in the British AT training are expected to offer stronger research skills to art therapists and support them towards generating stronger evidence for appropriate uses of AT with a range of client populations. Calls for collaborative research work with other professionals have also been made (e.g. Waller 2002), which if taken to heart, are expected to further increase research activity in the field.

AT defined

The nature of AT has changed over time, reflecting debates within the profession about its own identity. For example, we have already stated that during the 1980s AT became increasingly aligned with psychoanalytic/psychodynamic thinking. This was particularly apparent in the official definition of AT of 1989 (see Ch. 2), where psychoanalytic/psychodynamic language was used to define the field. Currently, BAAT (2004b, p. 1) describes AT as involving:

. . . the use of art materials for self-expression and reflection in the presence of a trained art therapist. . . The overall aim of its practitioners is to enable a client to effect change and growth on a personal level through the use of art materials in a safe and facilitating environment. The relationship between the therapist and the client is of a central importance . . .

Within this fairly broad description of AT, the psychoanalytic/psychodynamic language of the 1989 definition is dropped to make way for a wider diversity of practices. Furthermore, although references to the value of the client–therapist relationship remain, 'image making' is replaced with a reference to 'the use of art materials' in general. We see this as yet another indication of acknowledging diversity in current practice.

According to Schaverien (2000), a prolific AT writer and Jungian analyst, there are three types of AT practice: (1) art therapy, (2) art psychotherapy and (3) analytical art psychotherapy. These three forms of AT vary in terms of the emphasis they place upon the triangular relationship, i.e. the relationship between the client, the therapist and art making (see Ch. 3 for an introduction to the triangular relationship and the authors' understanding of its use within arts therapies practice in general). According to Schaverien (2000):

1. Art therapy places a strong emphasis upon the relationship of the client with the image on one hand and the therapist with the image on the other.
2. Art psychotherapy emphasises more the client–therapist relationship rather than the relationship of the two individuals with the image.
3. Analytical art psychotherapy has a dynamic quality in which all the corners of the triangle (i.e. the client, the therapist and the image) interplay equally with each other.

Within this theory, a valuable acknowledgement of different types of AT practice is made. 'Art therapy' is seen as a more art-based practice, while 'art psychotherapy' has a stronger psychotherapeutic bias. 'Analytical art psychotherapy' is presented as the most comprehensive way of working. Although Schaverien's (2000) suggested typology is clearly coloured by her own Jungian training, her contribution to the field is highly influential. Her contribution lies in making theoretical links between AT and psychotherapeutic thinking and discussing image-making processes that are unique to AT practice. For example, we find the five-stage image-making process she refers to (i.e. identification, familiarisation, acknowledgement, assimilation and disposal) as a particularly useful idea, which we will discuss in more depth later on. Another attempt to identify techniques and processes specific to AT comes from Mottram's (2002) research work on the skills and interventions used by art therapists in the UK. During this empirical study, broad categories of skills and interventions are identified: 'receptive', 'active' and 'interactive'. To a great extent, this categorisation resembles and expands on Alvin's (1978) categories of techniques used for her interactive MT approach; Alvin (1978) talks about 'active' and 'receptive' types. Mottram (2002) also talks about different skills and interventions required to facilitate an image, to view image-making and to work with completed images:

1. 'Art-based', 'inter-personal' and 'intra-personal' skills and interventions that are essential for facilitating the making of an image.

2. When viewing image-making, art therapists are engaged in either 'looking at the image or process' in a phenomenological way (i.e. attention is placed on the formal qualities of the image) or 'looking into an image interpretively'. Mottram (2002) calls these either 'outsight' or 'insight' skills.

3. Finally, when the image is completed, art therapists either try to establish a specific meaning for the client or encourage an open-ended exploration. She names these 'meaning' or 'mystery'.

Overall, AT practice in the UK places a preference upon 'non-directive' techniques. Still, there are some British publications that describe themes, techniques, activities and games of a fairly directive nature (e.g. Campbell 1993, Liebmann 1986, Silverstone 1993). Examples of both 'directive' and 'non-directive' approaches to AT will be presented later on in this chapter.

Main therapeutic trends within AT

Despite BAAT's (2004b) attempts to acknowledge a diversity of practices within the current AT practice, findings from our study (see Table 6.3) suggest that, in comparison with other arts therapies, art therapists place a particular emphasis upon psychoanalytic/psychodynamic theoretical underpinnings (p = 0.000). The history of AT may account for this finding. Strong alliance with psychoanalytic/psychodynamic thinking has been a feature of AT practice during the 1980s and 1990s to a greater extent than for any of the other arts therapies. This alliance has been supported by the long-standing interest of psychiatric/psychoanalytic circles within the visual arts and the equally strong interest of artistic circles in psychoanalytic thinking (see the brief history of the profession at the beginning of the chapter).

AT is also different from other arts therapies in relation to the artistic/creative aspects. Despite the fact that BAAT (2004b) acknowledges a central role for art-making within AT practice, findings from our study suggest that, in comparison with other arts therapies, artistic/creative principles feature in a less prominent place within AT (p = 0.007). The pioneering work of Hill and Adamson, who emphasised the artistic side of AT practice, appears at the moment to be, somehow, less popular. An important reason for this may be the strong belief amongst contemporary art therapists that art, on its own, offers a limited way of achieving a theoretical justification for AT practice. The rather weak theoretical articulation of the work of the art-based pioneers of AT may offer an additional explanation for this result as we will see in the next section.

The artistic AT approach: starting with Adrian Hill and Edward Adamson

Adrian Hill (1945, 1951) is one of the pioneers of AT in the UK and the person who first coined the term 'art therapy' in this country. Hill was originally an art lecturer with a 'commercial art' background. According to Waller (1991), his involvement with what eventually became AT was accidental. As a patient in the King Edward VII sanatorium in Sussex, after contracting TB,

Table 6.3: Main AT therapeutic trends and differences from other arts therapies

Therapeutic trends (p)	Mean for AT[1]	Mean for other arts therapies*	t-test value	Degrees of freedom (df)	P-value
Humanistic	3.86	3.93	Not significant	578	0.062
Eclectic/integrative	3.70	3.67	Not significant		
Psychoanalytic/psychodynamic	3.45	3.24	5.92	561.44	0.000**
Developmental	3.21	3.22	Not significant		
Active/directive	3.10	3.05	Not significant		
Artistic/creative	3.07	3.20	−2.73	577	0.007**

[1]The higher the score, the stronger the agreement with this group of statements (a five-point scale was used ranging from strongly agree = 5 to strongly disagree = 1)

**Accepted at the 0.01 level of significance

As the table shows, art therapists demonstrated the strongest agreement with the humanistic group of statements and least agreement with the artistic/creative group. Statistically significant differences existed between AT and other arts therapies in relation to the psychoanalytic/psychodynamic and the artistic/creative group of statements. AT respondents presented stronger agreement with the former and less agreement with the latter in comparison with other arts therapies participants. The table also shows some differences between AT and other arts therapies in relation to the humanistic group of statements (AT scored lower on this group of statements). However, this difference was not statistically significant.

he started using art-making as a means of recovery, initially for himself, and later on, with the support of medical staff, for other patients in the sanatorium. Hogan (2001) describes Hill's work as follows:

- He would introduce an initial theme such as 'a view from the window' in order to help clients start.
- He would then suggest rough sketches to plan the drawing or painting.
- If this seemed too daunting, he would recommend doodling.

Hogan (2000) claims that Hill's work often resembled the emerging profession of OT, a form of OT via art. Although he encouraged expression of difficulties in a pictorial form, he also valued the idea of using art as a form of deflection of anxieties and distress in order to establish a 'more hopeful mental attitude' (Hill 1945, p. 33). Deflection meant encouraging clients to create pictures that were opposite in content and style to the actual distressing experience. Using art as deflection is perceived by contemporary art therapists as significantly different from working through issues via the art and therefore, different from therapy.

Waller (1991) is particularly critical of Hill's work on this account. She also claims that Hill's work was strongly linked with the post-imperialistic ideas of his time where popularising the arts and 'high art', in particular, was prevalent and was seen as having an unquestionable benefit for the 'culturally deprived' and 'disadvantaged'. Consequently, Hill saw art as having an inherent capacity to restore health as long as an 'appropriate' type was encouraged. In pursuit of an 'appropriate type', he was not afraid of expressing clear preferences regarding clients' artistic content and style.

Hill never developed a very articulate theory of his understanding of AT. However, his vision and endless campaigning for an emerging profession made a substantial contribution to the field. His important role in the formation of the British Association of Art Therapists (BAAT) has already been mentioned (see the brief history section earlier in the chapter). Furthermore, his campaigning made the term AT increasingly known amongst health professionals, brought pictures into hospitals (up to then there was very limited artistic input on hospital walls) and, in cooperation with the Red Cross, introduced a number of art classes within hospital environments.

Edward Adamson (1970, 1984), another important pioneer of AT in the UK, had a similar 'commercial' art background to Hill. Soon after the Second World War and after he worked briefly at the TB sanatorium with Hill, he was employed at the Netherne Psychiatric hospital, in order to assist with psychiatric-led experiments that looked at image-making for diagnostic purposes. According to historical accounts of this period (e.g. Byrne 1996, Hogan 2000, Waller 1991), within this environment, Adamson was given a very clear brief from the medical team of the hospital (i.e. Dax and Reitman) to avoid communicating with patients regarding their creative efforts. The only active input this brief allowed Adamson to have was to offer very basic instructions on how to use standardised materials provided for each patient (e.g. certain colours, two brushes, one size paper, a specific pallet) if such instruction was requested by them. The aim of this brief was to protect the images created from being 'spoiled' from a facilitator's interventions/interpretations. Waller (1991) claims that Reitman was particularly sceptical about Freudian and Jungian interpretations shared with patients, believing that such interpretations, when initiated from the therapist, have an impact upon subsequent images created; patients would take on board such interpretations and create images with Freudian or Jungian symbolism. More interpretations from the therapist would lead to further 'training' of the patient in psychoanalytic thinking and eventually images would be created that would fit the preconceived theory of the therapist rather than to serve any of the 'real' needs of the client.

The brief Adamson received suggested that images created in the studio were passed on to the medical team for them to gain more insight about the patients' state of mind. The brief also suggested that Adamson's presence in the studio had to be particularly passive. Although he was later given more freedom to intervene in client's art work, initial restrictions to his work created the blueprint for his subsequent approach to AT. Adamson (1984, p. 3)) describes his work as follows:

> In the studio, I considered it my role to facilitate, rather than direct. I never suggested what anyone ought to paint, because it seemed essential that the idea should be entirely theirs. If someone wished to discuss a possible topic for a painting, I would merely try to explore what he wanted to do. Invariably, when we had finished talking, he would go away and paint something entirely different. I never criticised, and I never praised the paintings. I just welcomed them. I certainly never tried to interpret them. I did pass them on to the individual's doctor, whom I hoped would use them to get a little closer to his patient.

The doctors themselves particularly valued Adamson's presence during art-making. For example, according to Waller (1991), Dax found that patients' attendance at the studios would decline when Adamson was not around; similarly their work would be 'poor' with 'little psychiatric value'.

Waller (1991) claims that Adamson's approach was very similar to the prevailing approach to art education of that time, where intervening in children's art was seen as detrimental to truly child-centred artistic development. Hogan (2000) on the other hand claims that Adamson's approach was essentially Jungian in that he believed, alongside other Jungian art therapists, that art is healing. However, Adamson himself made no explicit references to either child-centred education or Jung. His approach, an open-studio group approach to AT, became the first form of AT group work and is still practised in a number of settings and with a number of different client groups (e.g. Case & Dalley 1992, Deco 1998).

The fact that both Hill and Adamson believed in the healing power of art-making in itself and perceived themselves primarily as artists, qualify them as the first and most important names associated with an artistic bias to AT practice. Furthermore, both of them were heavily involved in exhibitions of artwork made by patients, an area of work that got increasingly abandoned in later days of the AT profession. Unlike Hill however, Adamson's work is currently perceived as a non-interventionist approach to AT which strongly opposed interpretations from the therapist (Hogan 2000).

Today, when the artistic components of AT are highlighted, AT practitioners tend to frame their work within theoretical perspectives borrowed from psychotherapy. Very few examples of artistic/creative models have been found in current AT literature that highlight the artistic/creative side as providing a theoretical framework. One such example comes from the USA: McNiff's (1992) book entitled *Art as Medicine*. Another is the British model devised by Mottram's (2000, 2001) for a brief AT intervention within an assessment and treatment unit for adults with a learning disability and mental illness. This model places a central role to the image and highlights creativity theory as the main conceptual framework (see Wallas' ideas of the four stages of the creative process [Arieti 1976] already discussed in Ch. 4). However, Mottram (2000, 2001) also makes explicit references to certain principles borrowed from Gestalt therapy, brief therapy and the conversational model of psychotherapy. Despite the artistic/creative emphasis of this model, the input from psychotherapeutic thinking to the conceptualisation of AT practice is apparent.

Practices that emphasise the artistic components of AT are also presented by Marian Liebmann and refer to structured or thematic AT groups. This type of work seems to echo Hill's somehow directive approach to AT, as we will see in the following section.

A structured AT group with ex-offenders

In the 1986 publication of *Art Therapy for Groups*, Marian Liebmann presented a compilation of games, themes and exercises, and described a number of practices taking place in the UK with different client groups and in different settings (Liebmann 1986). This publication was the result of Liebmann's (1979) empirical study and involved contributions from more than 50 art therapists practising in the UK. Most of the examples of practice included in this work were primarily about structured/theme-centred AT groups, highlighting the value of the art (see Hill's perspective discussed earlier), and were loosely connected with humanistic thinking (e.g. Yalom is mentioned in the introduction of Liebmann's 1986 book).

One such example is presented in Table 6.4. It comes from Liebmann's own work with ex-offenders and takes place at a day centre. This example, being part of a 'resource book for AT groups' does not necessarily give sufficient explanations of therapeutic choices and/or lengthy descriptions of therapeutic processes. For example, it remains unclear why this game was chosen for this particular session, how the activity selected became less threatening for vulnerable clients and non-abusive for the 'unpopular' member.

Due to this initial limited theoretical justification and the, at times, strongly directive nature of practices described, when Leibmann's publications came out (1979, 1986), they gave rise to a heated debate within the field surrounding 'directive' versus 'non-directive' approaches to AT (for further discussion of this topic regarding arts therapies, see 'The Active/Directive Trend' in Ch. 4). This debate is well recorded in the AT literature (e.g. Case & Dalley 1992, Skaife & Huet 1998, Waller 1993). Briefly, we can say here that the opponents of directive approaches to AT regarded structured AT groups as activity-based practices that resembled OT and therefore had limited value as an AT approach (McNeilly 1983, 1987, Molloy 1988). They saw the introduction of themes as addressing the therapist's rather than the client's anxieties and as such, as potentially threatening for the client. On the

Table 6.4: A structured AT group with ex-offenders – Marian Liebmann (1986, pp. 77–78) [Reproduced with permission]

Description of session	Comments by the therapist and the authors
Needs of clients in specific setting [Clients were ex-offenders with social and personal problems attending a *day centre* on a voluntary basis. One of the activities they could choose from in the Centre was to attend an 'art group']	[Other activities included in the centre were woodwork, community service projects, discussion groups, video role plays, literacy and numeracy tuition]
Aims/expectations/assumptions [Clients and members of staff agreed to work on *interpersonal communication* in a 4-week series of sessions]	[The type of work to be focused on was agreed in negotiation between clients and members of staff]
Use of activity [There were six clients attending the session, aged 17–32 years, and three members of staff. A game was *introduced by the therapist* called the 'Metaphorical Portraits' game as follows:] 'I outlined the idea: we would all try to draw portraits of all the other members of the group, not as they looked but in shapes, colours and lines to suggest something about their personality.' One of the women was *very unpopular* with other members generally, and knew it; she was also overweight and self-conscious about this. We took about 30 minutes to complete our drawings, using oil pastel crayons, and I joined in as a member of the group. Then I suggested that we played a game with the resulting portraits. I held one of mine up and asked the group to guess who it was meant to be. When the group had guessed, I gave it to that person as a gift, and she/he in	[*Value of selected activity:* the therapist claims that the game can be used in many variations and in many situations. Also that:] It enables people to communicate how they see others in an indirect and playful way; and also to reflect on their part in choosing a particular metaphor. [*Concerns:* Caution is raised regarding the possibility that some clients might find this activity too threatening or that the activity could be used to get at members of the group who are not popular]

turn held up a portrait of someone else. We continued until each person had a pile of gifts of portraits drawn by others.

There were some predictable [images created], e.g. I received a paintbrush, and also a series of brown wavy lines (my hair), but there were also some surprises. My co-leader was startled to find that one member drew him as a black cloud, and was worried about him.

[The] *unpopular member* received several ["gifts"] such as flowers . . .'

[The gifts received by the unpopular member] 'suggested that *others could see past her difficulties* and appreciate her inner sensitivity.'

'The session had been revealing, but in a *gentle way*, so as not to be hurtful.'

[There was *hilarity and warmth* in the group]

Authors' wording in [brackets]

other hand, the supporters of theme-centred work argued that themes could get people started, especially those who found it difficult to begin with AT, could give a clear idea of what AT was about, could offer structure to groups that were very insecure and would not operate otherwise, could weld the group together, and could challenge some groups that were 'stuck' (Liebmann 1986, Thornton 1985). They also saw them as particularly relevant to short-term work because key issues could be addressed more quickly. Finally, they criticised the supporters of the opposite view as placing a questionable value on the artistic elements of AT practice.

In the middle of the debate, Greenwood & Layton (1987) described an approach to community-based AT practice with people with severe mental health problems. Their approach seemed to fall in between a highly directive or highly non-directive AT practice. In this work, the therapists would introduce flexible themes for optional use emerging from an initial group discussion, while they would also take on board group dynamics and boundaries. Greenwood & Layton's (1987) approach had strong similarities with a number of group practices found in other arts therapies (see for example, interactive and analytical approaches to MT [Ch. 5] and most approaches to DT and dance movement therapy [DMT] [Chs 7 and 8 respectively]).

Despite the fact that the directive/non-directive debate created strong polarisation, it has given rise to an acknowledgement of different types of work within AT and an understanding that different degrees of structure and boundaries can be useful for different clients and/or client groups. Theme-centred AT groups are now featured in AT handbooks and are regarded as potentially appropriate for short-term interventions and/or for vulnerable clients such as clients with disabilities, children with hyperactivity, certain adolescent groups, clients with severe psychopathology, and/or long-stay psychiatric clients (Case & Dalley 1992).

Humanistic AT approaches

Wood (1997), in her history of AT and psychosis, identifies that in the early writings of art therapists there is a repeated reference to respect, a willingness to see beyond labelling and stigma, and an emphasis upon treating people as individuals no matter how disturbing their condition might be. These principles bore the seeds for humanistic perspectives to find a fruitful ground within the emerging AT practice. Indeed during the 1960s and 1970s, when humanistic schools of thought became widespread, a number of art therapists found themselves aligned with such ideas. Amongst others, Wood (1997) mentions the works of Ervin Goffman and RD Laing as particularly relevant for art therapists working with clients with psychosis. The movement, which became more widely known as the anti-psychiatry movement, offered art therapists a way of regarding mental health institutions and opened up possibilities for attempting to understand people diagnosed as psychotic. Laing's (1959) ideas for example, of psychotic despair as involving issues of 'engulfment', 'implosion' and 'petrification' are regarded by Wood (1997) as a helpful step towards understanding her own clients. Principles of care and respect were highlighted during this time and a search for understanding clients' experiences through image-making enabled a number of art therapists practising, mainly within the public sector, to form deep and helpful therapeutic relationships. However, unlike other arts therapies disciplines, a recording of specific ways in which AT practice took place is not available. Wood (1997) herself also notices that despite the fact that many art therapists were influenced by humanistic principles, she found no written evidence of detailed examples of practice from that period.

Accounts of British AT practices that are informed by humanistic thinking (i.e. client-centred, Gestalt, existential, transpersonal) remain sparse. The only published book in the UK with such an orientation is by Silverstone (1993), an art therapist and client-centred counsellor. Silverstone's (1993) publication makes direct references to Rogerian person-centred therapy and describes a number of exercises that can be used within an AT situation. However, her writing is framed within a counselling training context (she describes the content of this training over a period of a year) and as such it is not clear how her approach would be applied within an AT clinical situation.

The humanistic approach to AT practice can be better understood through the following work of Derryn Thomas, an art therapist who is also trained as a client-centred counsellor.

A client-centred approach to AT with children in foster care

Derryn Thomas (D Thomas, unpublished interview, 2002) describes her AT work as clearly informed by Rogerian thinking and thus as clearly working within a model of health rather than focusing on pathology. The aim is to enable people to reach their potential; in other words to become fully functioning. The core conditions outlined by Rogers (1951) as essential and sufficient for therapeutic change, are highlighted in Thomas' work and apparent in the case example presented in Table 6.5. Valuing the Rogerian core concepts means having:

- *psychological contact*: the therapist is checking whether client and therapist are open to each other and subject to mutual influence
- *congruence*: therapists attempt to be real, genuine and authentic. Thomas (D Thomas, unpublished interview, 2002) notes that if therapists present themselves in mysterious ways, clients have difficulties accessing the therapist
- *unconditional positive regard*: therapists accept people unconditionally, even if their behaviours are not accepted
- *empathy*: therapists are engaged in the process of knowing their clients deeply, echoing their feelings and experiences without being judgmental or evaluative.

In Thomas' case, these basic Rogerian principles are met through not only the presence of the therapist but also of the art. For example, Thomas talks about 'self-empathy', a term she uses to refer to trusting that the relationship of the client with art-making has value in itself. This idea, although discussed within a client-centred framework, is strikingly similar to the belief shared by pioneers of AT such as Hill and Adamson in the healing power of art. It is therefore not surprising that Thomas acknowledges that in relation to the triangular relationship (see discussion of the triangular relationship in a number of places in this book, for example Schaverien's [2000] typology of AT practices in the 'AT Defined' section earlier in this chapter), she finds in her work that there is a stronger emphasis upon the client–art relationship; a similar emphasis upon the client–art relationship has been given by the above-mentioned pioneers of AT.

We believe that in Thomas' work the therapeutic relationship is also closely linked with what we have termed in Chapter 3 of this book as the 'active' relationship, a therapeutic relationship that closely resembles the 'real' relationship advocated by humanistic psychotherapists. However, within this active relationship, Thomas avoids offering direction. She terms her work as a non-directive client-centred AT with verbal and artistic communication being led by the client. In this respect, she remains in line with Rogerian principles of non-directiveness and diverges from other, more directive, approaches to AT (see earlier examples), and other humanistically-informed arts therapists (see 'other approaches to AT' section, this chapter). Her non-directive emphasis makes her approach also significantly different from Silverstone's (1993) directive client-centred approach to AT as Table 6.5 illustrates.

Other humanistic approaches to AT originate mainly from an American context and will be briefly discussed in the last section of this chapter.

The psychoanalytic/psychodynamic AT approaches: starting with Irene Champernowne

Irene Champernowne is the third important person we have mentioned in association with the emergence of AT in the UK. Her contribution, however, is very different from the other AT pioneers, e.g. Hill and Adamson, in that she had a strong psychotherapeutic orientation. As we have already stated, Irene Champernowne did not consider herself to be an art therapist, but remained a psychotherapist with an interest in art. She is often regarded as the equivalent to Naumburg (1966) in the USA; they have both been pioneering figures in their respective countries and have introduced analytical thinking within AT. However, unlike Naumburg who was primarily Freudian, Champernowne was a Jungian analyst. Thus, her contribution to AT remained different from her American colleague.

Most of Champernowne's work took place at the Whithymead Centre for Remedial Education through Psychotherapy and the Arts, a private centre she ran with her husband in Devon. Waller (1991) and Hogan (2001) describe the Whithymead Centre as a form of therapeutic community which valued Jungian principles throughout: therapy staff had to undergo in-depth Jungian analysis as a prerequisite for employment; visiting professionals and artists attended the centre on a more short-term basis in order to acquire analytical support and further insight into Jungian thinking. Patients would stay there for up to 3 years, sometimes longer, and there was a stream of patients who would come for short-term stays; all of them would be engaged in analytical work. In some cases, patients who underwent lengthy analysis would become members of staff. Moreover, as Hogan (2001) records, visitors to the

Table 6.5: A client-centred AT approach with children in care – Derryn Thomas [Example provided to V Karkou for 'Arts Therapies: from Theory to Practice' study [Karkou 2002, reproduced with permission]]

Description of AT process	Comments by the therapist and the authors
Needs of children 'Female *child* (8 years of age) in foster care; some contact with mother, none with father.'	[*Referrals* are made from social services and/or foster care association. Referrals are fairly formal for children. Background information is acquired]
Aims/expectations/assumptions 'Child has not been provided consistently with core conditions (has moved from foster carers several times).'	'I expect that the clients will come to terms with difficulties and become more *"fully functioning"*. In order to become "fully functioning" creativity plays an important role.'
Beginning of AT process *I introduce myself and the room and the materials.* I explain that we will be working for 50 minutes each week. I inform child that they can choose what they want to do. *I allow child time to adjust to this freedom.*	[*Establishing psychological contact*]
'I *respond empathetically* to questions and feelings of "not knowing what to do".'	[*Empathy*]
Development of AT process 'I respond to the child and *will answer questions* about myself in a way that I believe is helpful to the child. I do not *disclose* unnecessary information.'	[*Congruence*] [The therapist discloses information about herself but such disclosures are made in an '*economic*' way. Information is given after request.]

Continued

Table 6.5: A client-centred AT approach with children in care – Derryn Thomas [Example provided to V. Karkou for 'Arts Therapies: from Theory to Practice' study [Karkou 2002, reproduced with permission]—cont'd

Description of AT process	Comments by the therapist and the authors
I will allow the child to give me instructions in regard to their play. *I will become their 'apprentice'* in terms of playing or art work. For example if the child asks me to paint with them I will ask them what colour, what brush strokes, etc.	[*Lack of direction from the therapist:* the client is seen as the expert, while the therapist is an 'apprentice']
In time I will reflect on the work with the child and check out its particular meaning. If the child responds positively to this verbal interaction I will continue in a very tentative way. If the child does not respond and is not ready for verbal intervention or able to understand metaphorical meaning I would not persist and *trust that the artwork had value in itself. . .*	'Self-empathy'
Completion of AT process	
'I [check] whether psychological contact is in place.'	
'The child can choose to finish.'	
'Therapist with carers, social services and agency evaluate if the child is *functioning more fully* as a result of therapy.'	'The work is *regularly reviewed* by social services and agency (12-weekly meetings).'

Authors' wording in [brackets]

Whithymead Centre (amongst them Storr and Michael Edward) would report that during their initial visits, they could see no obvious distinctions between patients and members of staff. People were identified as residents (patients and staff who lived in the Centre) and non-residents (people who were not living in the Centre). The lack of clear separation between patients and staff members was similar to the Zurich Psychological Club, a place where Jungian developments were taking place at the time. In the Zurich Club, people in analysis were able to attend the Club as a step towards becoming analysts themselves.

AT and the arts in general had a central role in the function of the Whithymead Centre; visual artists, musicians and dancers were employed to assist with the therapeutic programme. This high regard of the arts was in line with Jungian understanding of the arts as a means of offering possibilities for fluidity, change and growth. Champernowne regarded the arts (not only visual arts but also poetry, dance, mime and music) as a way for patients to discover themselves, a way of allowing the unconscious to 'speak'. Art-making was seen as having a compensatory function in that the unconscious, or in Jungian terminology the 'shadow self', was enabled to be expressed. Art-making had therefore a similar function to the one of dreams and symbolism and was seen as deriving from the unconscious mind.

'Active imagination', a central technique in Jungian analysis, was at the centre of art-making at the Whithymead Centre. Active imagination was seen as a way of 'dreaming with the eyes open'. During this process, patients were encouraged to concentrate on a specific mood or event and follow the subsequent fantasies arising from this starting point (see similar applications of this principle to 'authentic movement' by Mary Whitehouse [Ch. 8] and its relevance to the Sesame approach [Ch. 7]). Champernowne herself would encourage patients within a psychotherapeutic situation to go away and enlarge a certain issue by making a picture (or any other artistic product); thus concentrating and amplifying the starting point of interest. She has also been reported as encouraging her patients to 'take parts of it and dream the dream onwards on paper . . .' (Hogan 2001, p. 239).

In order for patients to become able to 'dream with their eyes open', and therefore access deep parts of themselves, staff members would avoid interfering with the process. Patients were encouraged to engage in the artistic process in a 'natural' way, i.e. in the time and way they wanted to. But, although the unconscious was admired and respected (thus the natural engagement with the artistic process), it was also feared. Art therapists working in the painting and pottery studios were therefore often there to play a regulatory role; at times they would also be intervening in order to stop patients from becoming overwhelmed (e.g. by asking them to change artistic medium). The role was one of a 'midwife', a role that enabled the 'birth' and 'rebirth' of the patients via the arts. Interventions varied depending on their training and understanding of Jungian analysis. The least trained artists/art therapists would retain an attitude of positive encouragement towards the patients' work. The more trained the practitioners, the more they would engage in further interventions about the meaning of the artwork, e.g. in relation to the Jungian theory of function types (i.e. sensation, feeling, thinking, intuition). Overall, a lot of interpretation in the presence of the patients was discouraged as it created over-intellectualisation, and thus hindered unconscious work.

Despite this central role of AT within the Whithymead Centre, analysts remained the ones who were seen as having further insight into the unconscious by virtue of experience and training. This is very similar to Adamson's case described before and characteristic of this early period of the arts therapies development. Alongside community staff meetings in which all members of staff were involved (including artists/art therapists), analysts held separate meetings in which there were in-depth discussions of certain patients. Hogan (2001) claims that the overall running of the Centre resembled the Jungian perception of the self. The meetings held by analysts involved discussions about deeper parts of the unconscious life of the Centre that all attendants of the Centre did not have access to, in the same way as there was limited access to the deeper parts of the unconscious self. According to Waller (1992), the Centre kept a clearly hierarchical order with Irene Champernowne being ultimately in control, a powerful mother figure, through whom all final decisions were made.

The Whithymead Centre eventually closed in the late 1960s due to financial reasons. Some of the artists/art therapists mentioned by Hogan (2001) as residents at the Centre were: Jo Guy, Norah Godfrey, Peter Lyle, Richard Fritzsche, Elizabeth Colyer, and Rupert Cracknell. Michael Edwards was another person who visited and stayed at the Centre. Later on he became one of the leading figures in the efforts of BAAT for professionalisation and the founder of one of the first training programmes in AT in Birmingham. Given the absence of formal training in AT at the time, the service the Whithymead Centre offered to the AT field is immense. It informally trained artists to view their work with clients through a psychotherapeutic perspective. However, despite its merits, the Centre retained the distinction between analytical and artistic work, at least insofar as the ultimate responsibility for the psychological well-being of the patients was concerned.

Within contemporary AT practice the psychological responsibility is held with the art therapist, especially since training courses in AT developed and psychotherapeutic thinking became an integral part of the practice. Moreover, AT with a Jungian perspective is now seen as just one approach to AT, next to psychoanalytic/psychodynamic practices that are informed by object-relations theory and group analytical work (see examples of this work in later sections of this chapter). Due to the important contribution of Champernowne in the early days of the emergence of AT, however, Jungian thinking remains a strong influence upon AT for a number of contemporary art therapists. One such example is described in the following section.

An analytical art psychotherapy approach with adults

Joy Schaverien's work is a good example of contemporary AT practice that shares a similar philosophy to Champernowne, i.e. Schaverien is also a trained Jungian analyst. At the same time, Schaverien's work is different from Champernowne's contribution, primarily because AT is not seen as an adjunctive practice to verbal analysis, but as a practice that stands on its own. A number of other differences also exist that can be explained as a result of

AT developing its own theoretical and clinical basis independently from verbal psychotherapy.

We have already acknowledged Schaverien's (2000) contribution in relation to identifying different types of AT practice (see the section on 'AT Defined' earlier in the chapter). Her most important contribution, however, lies in her attempts to conceptualise artistic processes that take place during AT practice (Schaverien 1987, 1991, 1994, 1995, 2000). For example, she often talks about different types of images created during AT sessions; images that are: (1) 'diagrammatic', that is images that can also be conveyed in many different ways, other than the visual medium, and (2) 'embodied' images, i.e. images that convey a state of being that cannot be represented in a mode other than a graphic representation. This latter type of image requires full engagement of the client in the process of art-making (Schaverien 2000). We understand this distinction as one between a linear/concrete expression of an issue ('diagrammatic' images) versus an expression of material with multiple layers of meaning that we have termed as symbols ('embodied' images). In Chapter 3 we borrowed language from semiotics to refer to the former type of artistic expression as 'iconic', while we discussed the latter as 'symbolic'.

Another important concept that is attributed to Schaverien (1987) is the idea of 'scapegoat transference'. Schaverien (1987) regards this as an additional type of transference that takes place during AT alongside the real relationship, the therapeutic alliance and the common psychotherapeutic transference. The scapegoat transference is the transference of the client's material onto the visual product. According to Mann (1989) it strongly resembles the Kleinian concept of 'projective identification' (i.e. the projection of parts of the self onto others and subsequent identification with these parts now located externally). Despite the similarity of scapegoat transference with projective identification, the significance of Schaverien's contribution to AT lies in the fact that scapegoat transference refers specifically to image-making processes. In her 2000 publication Schaverien delineated the following processes as relevant to the scapegoat transference:

1. *Identification*: the client is unconsciously identifying with the picture he or she is creating. We have already described this relationship as one in which the client is the artist (see Ch. 3). Schaverien (2000) goes even further to suggest that there is an undifferentiated state between the client as an artist and the image, while the therapist is a witness offering containment. This process is mainly non-verbal.

2. *Familiarisation*: the client begins to differentiate from the image and becomes a spectator of his or her work. Stronger conscious processes are possibly involved while the client moves further away from the picture and observes, but the relationship remains primarily one of him or her and the image. The therapist is not called upon to intervene. This process is again non-verbal.

3. *Acknowledgement*: The artist/client acquires a much more conscious attitude towards the image and calls upon the therapist to act as an active spectator with whom the image can be discussed. At this point, the therapist may also offer any relevant interpretations. This process is primarily verbal and resembles what we have broadly termed in

Chapter 3, the 'projected' relationship, i.e. a relationship between the client and the therapist that that takes place via the arts. In our conceptualisation of this process, both verbal and non-verbal activity might take place.

4. *Assimilation*: the client returns to viewing the original image but with renewed understanding. This is a result of integrating the previous discussion ('acknowledgement'). It is primarily a non-verbal process.

5. *Disposal*: the client–therapist relationship is activated during attempts to consciously dispose of the object/picture and unconsciously to resolve the client–therapist transference. The physical disposal of the image requires prior assimilation of the image and involves action. Given the need to also resolve the client–therapist transference, the client–therapist relationship becomes of paramount importance. Because of the emphasis upon the client–therapist relationship, this process has similarities with verbal psychotherapy (see Ch. 3).

Schaverien (2000) discusses these processes within the three different types of AT she has identified, i.e. art therapy, art psychotherapy and analytical art psychotherapy, and claims that they are manifested in different ways in each AT type. Table 6.6 presents an example of how these processes can become activated within an analytical art psychotherapy context, the type of AT that Schaverien prescribes to.

The influence of Schaverien's understanding of artistic processes upon the AT practice is very strong. AT practitioners may often refer to her work and the concepts she has identified even if these practitioners neither acknowledge a Jungian perspective in their work, nor refer to their practice as a form of analytical art psychotherapy. However, it is worth pointing out that Schaverien's work is developed mainly as a result of working in mental health and, to a large extent, in a private practice context. Her work can therefore be seen as more relevant to adults who are fairly highly functioning and able to engage in a therapeutic process for a lengthy period of time. For example, the client presented in Table 6.6 undertook therapy for a period of over 4 years. In most working environments today, engaging in such a lengthy treatment is not realistic anymore.

An object relations approach to AT with a rejected child

Caroline Case is another example of an art therapist and child psychotherapist with a clear psychoanalytic/psychodynamic orientation in her work. In contrast to the Jungian perspective of Schaverien discussed before, Case draws primarily upon object relations theory and the work of Bion (1964), Klein (1975) and Winnicott (1971) in particular. She favours concepts such as the use of 'objects' (i.e. inner representations of a real or phantasised person or aspects of a person that either satisfies or frustrates individual needs), and the relevance of defences such as splitting, projection and introjection. She also values the Winnicottian idea of the 'good enough' mother. The role of the art therapist, similar to the role of the analyst, is to offer 'good enough' mothering that is a reparative experience to the client who has had an inefficient or absent experience of early 'holding' (Winnicott 1971) or

Table 6.6: The scapegoat transference within analytical art psychotherapy with an adult with suicidal feelings – Joy Schaverien (2000, pp. 73–80)

Description of process	Comments by the therapist and the authors
Needs of client [Female *adult*, called Lisa, with suicidal impulses. Feelings of loneliness, isolation and abandonment]	[Adults seen in private practice for a long period of time. In this case the client undergoes more than 4 years of therapy]
Aims/expectations/assumptions [Lisa needed to recognise her anger and deal with her suicidal impulses]	[The expectation is that clients will go through the processes of identification, familiarisation, acknowledgement, assimilation and disposal of the image and become able to acquire a different way of dealing with painful feelings]
Beginning of AT process [A few months after having started with AT and after going through a difficult time when she felt she was not able to continue living, Lisa *drew a picture in which a figure was lying on the ground surrounded by blood*. The picture was not drawn in the presence of the therapist but Lisa brought it to the first session soon after she made it]	'The picture became a *scapegoat* in that it embodied the current feeling state.' [The picture is seen as a rehearsal of the suicide act and an expression of anger turned inwards]
Development of AT process When Lisa made her picture it seemed that she *was probably totally engaged in it*. She [probably] stood back and regarded it . . . Graphically conveyed, she was now able to view both the act and its potential consequence.	[1. *Identification*] 'At that time there would be no separation between herself and the created image.' [2. *Familiarisation*] 'It seemed there was some release in the intensity of the feelings as she became familiar with it . . . The impulse was now held outside of herself within the picture. The image was sufficient to contain the situation until her session the next day.'

Continued

Table 6.6: The scapegoat transference within analytical art psychotherapy with an adult with suicidal feelings – Joy Schaverien (2000, p. 73–80)—cont'd

Description of process	Comments by the therapist and the authors
[Lisa brought the picture to the session and *discussed it with the therapist.* By doing this however, additional concerns were evoked. She] *was worried about how the picture would be received* – was it good enough? An additional concern was, would [the therapist] believe and take her seriously?	[*3. Acknowledgement*] [*transference*] 'She would often stand outside herself and view her emotions in a critical and disbelieving manner. Thus her concern about whether the work was 'good enough' was also a concern about whether she would be acceptable when she revealed the extent of her distress.
[The picture she drew] was not pleasing to Lisa but it did impress on her the reality of the potential outcome of the impulse; *she could stand outside and view herself lying on the floor bleeding.*	[*differentiation from the image*]
Gradually a transformation in her state began to take place and this [was revealed in subsequent] pictures made at disparate intervals during the process of therapy. [The most important theme presented and described in these pictures was anger. *In one of them, which was also titled anger, Lisa talked about how the picture represented an explosion of her feelings*].	[*4. Assimilation*] 'She was previously unconscious of the connection between her anger and her suicidal feelings. However, through the manifestation of it in such pictures and through interpretations, this gradually began to become conscious.'
Completion of AT process 'Lisa valued her pictures and *took them with her when she concluded her treatment.* This was fully discussed, and thus it seemed that the elements which she initially held in the pictures had become integrated. Lisa could recognise her anger and no longer had the impulse to cut herself when she experienced painful feelings.'	[*5. Disposal*] [Disposal can take place in a number of different ways, the therapist may keep them, the client may keep them, client and therapist may agree on a different course of action]

Authors' wording in [brackets]

'containment' (Bion 1964). During the process of containment, for example, the parts of the client's self projected onto the therapist are mediated back to the client in a more digestible form. In an AT context, however, art therapists argue that it is not just the therapist who offers holding/containment but also the image created by the client and the AT room (e.g. Dalley 2000, Killick 2000) (further discussion of this process for arts therapies as a whole can be found in the 'The Psychoanalytic/Psychodynamic Trend' section in Ch. 4). The scapegoat transference discussed earlier (Schaverien 2000) is one example of the image acting as a holding/containing device. Expanding on this idea, Case (2000) discusses the relevance of one more type of transference that can take place within AT sessions, that of 'refractive transference'. Refractive transference is a split transference onto the therapist and the image as well as onto objects in the AT room. It can be experienced with clients who can be described in Kleinian (1975) terminology as being in the paranoid-schizoid position, i.e. people with a very damaged psychic state, or as Case (2000) terms it a 'liquid' psychic state. According to Case (2000), refractive transference takes place beyond the limits of the triangular relationship. In that respect, it can be seen as a theoretical expansion of Schaverien's notion of the scapegoat transference that refers primarily to the transference of client's material to the image (in the presence of the therapist) to also include transferences that take place to the room itself.

Typically of most arts therapists, and even more so of art therapists with an object relations orientation, Case (1990) also refers to Winnicott's (1971) notion of the transitional object and transitional space (or playground) as equivalent to the art-making process and the AT room respectively. She incorporates in her AT work Winnicott's understanding of child development: the therapeutic process may involve regression to an early developmental state such as merging and a shift from a merged state to a differentiated state. In the merged state, the child/client needs empathetic responses from the mother/therapist; the therapist takes up the role of creating meaning on the child/client's behalf. As the therapy progresses and depending on the child's/client's pace, further objectivity is acquired and separation is facilitated.

Some of the above ideas can be traced in the AT example presented in Table 6.7.

Object relations theory seems to predominate in the AT literature. For example, most of the key AT texts in the UK refer to practices that are closely aligned to this perspective (Case & Dalley 1992, Gilroy & McNeilly 2000, Waller & Gilroy 1992). Where groups are concerned, group analytic AT is often chosen, as illustrated in the following section.

Group analytic AT with adults with mental health issues

The person closely linked with group analytic AT is Gerry McNeilly (1983, 1987, 1989, 2000), an art therapist and group analyst. As we have already mentioned, McNeilly was heavily involved in the directive versus non-directive debate in the field during the 1980s. Given his group analytic training, he was one of the strong supporters of the non-directive 'camp', of group AT. Although in his more recent writings there has been an acknowledgement of the need to modify purist perspectives according to the needs of the clients, he remains

Table 6.7: An example of working with a child in AT with an object relations perspective – Caroline Case (1990, pp. 131–160) [Reproduced with permission]

Description of process	Comments by the therapist and the authors
Needs of client [Female *child* aged 9 years, called Ruth, having experiences of rejection, abandonment and ambivalence. She has been in and out of care. She looked small for her age, spoke with a superficially 'adult speech' and had taken the role of the mother to her siblings and a companion to her mother]	[The *setting* was an assessment centre supported by the social services department]
Assumptions [Ruth needed to work through her sense of loss, depression and merger towards separation]	[Children who have experienced rejection] '. . . need to experience what they have never fully had before separation can be negotiated.' [Rejected girls may attempt to merge with the female therapist, while rejected boys often re-enforce differences]
Beginning of AT process 'During the first weeks of AT Ruth made tentative explorations in the sessions, remaining almost hidden from sight in the group of children attending together. She chose to play with the doll's house, a perpetual re-arranging of furniture and making of beds, a *"being lost in housework"*.' 'Her first statement on paper was a pattern with a *heart at the centre*.'	[This] 're-flected her "mother's helper" role in the family and a need to put the "house of the self" in order.' [Vulnerability is shown and there is a cry to the therapist, but at the same time the drawing is stereotyped and therefore the child can easily deny its importance]
Development of AT process [In a group drawing involving liquid, powder, and finger paint Ruth started playing with *getting dirty with paint*. She gradually became completely covered in paint. At the end of the session she claimed that this was the best time of her life and that she would like to make a *mess* again.	[*Regression to earlier developmental position*] [*Fragmentation/splitting*] 'Torn fragments [were] scattered around the room. [This] had had a partly joyful feel of an [internal] breaking down to make ready for a new formulation.'

In following sessions and after Ruth requesting specifically to become messy she attended *one-to-one sessions* in which messiness was explored with paint, on her face, on her body (she was wearing a swimsuit), sliding on a paper paint floor, *covering the therapist's hands in paint and so on*. After each messy session there was a cleaning ritual.

[*Containment*]
'The role of the therapist is to contain a structure around the movement made, trying to support emerging forms and to reflect on the process that is happening.'
[*Merging*: The therapist's separateness and boundaries were briefly denied]

Messy sessions were interchanged with clean sessions and individual with group sessions. Using stories, sandplay and painting, *archaic images of Cyclops, the 'Dark Lady' and the 'Queen of Hearts' were revealed and explored*.]

[*Good and Bad objects* Some 'archaic' images can tolerate creativity, rage, anger and destruction]

Completion of AT process
[Earlier themes were revisited towards the end of the process and expressed as follows:]

'She used an enormous amount of *glue* . . . Pictures were attempted with ready-made sticky shapes, chaotically arranged on the paper, interspersed with flat, black paintings, completely featureless. There was a sense of formlessness, just sticking shapes together anywhere, often accompanied by worries about and for her mother. . . . Ruth was often literally sticking to my side.

[*Sticking* Activities gave a sense of] 'being stuck in depression and of putting a skin over fragmented pieces.'

[She made] requests and then ordered commands for us to *paint paintings together* ... We had to paint exactly the same shapes ... and each had to have the same number and colour. Then a piece of tape was

[*Merging*]
'There was a denial of our difference, a wish to return to a symbiotic relationship . . . [Her need to merge] was expressed in a symbolic way, not

attached to the top and the bottom of the picture. At the top, "By Ruth",
by regression to behaviour like a younger child.'
 and at the bottom, "By Caroline Case".

Table 6.7: An example of working with a child in AT with an object relations perspective – Caroline Case (1990, p. 131–160) (Reproduced with permission)—cont'd

Description of process	Comments by the therapist and the authors
[After Christmas] Ruth began showing me how they had made cards	
[*Good and Bad*]	
with angels on in the classroom and from this there developed several	'[This image] seemed a more punishing expression of
painting of *Yellow Angels and Red Devils*. These too were interspersed	"goodness" and "badness".'
with black, shapeless paintings and were sad, whiny, depressed sessions.'	
'. . . Ruth asked me to paint with her but this time to do *separate paintings*	
[*Separation*]	
and she would choose the subjects.'	'.
. . there was a sense of separate identities, but shared experience, a	
statement of difference and the coming parting.'	
[In the *last session* Ruth made:	
Evaluation of process	
An unfinished painting of a landscape.	
[The last session reflected the position the child had arrived at:	
A house out of cardboard boxes to take with her with a clear structure,	
There was still work that needed to be done (unfinished painting), but she	
ready for things to be added in.	
took a structure with her that she could add things to (house). The	
A chalked baby-looking figure of a person with hooves, heart and belly	
chalked figure:] '. . . did represent that this "bad" baby had had	
button that had the same colour of eyes as her own]	
recognition and acceptance in art therapy. We had been able to explore	
the messy side with the exposed vulnerable heart at the centre.'	

Authors' wording in [brackets]

strongly influenced by Foulkes, the person regarded as the father of group analysis. According to Foulkes (1964) the individual is a 'nodal' point within a network of communication. Within a group situation, communication can be understood fully by taking on board the whole web of communication and relationships within the group (i.e. the group 'matrix'). There are four levels of communication that can take place simultaneously within a group: (1) current reality, (2) individual transferences, (3) intrapsychic processes (or object relations level) and (4) universal/transpersonal processes. The therapist's role is to support a significant involvement of group members with each other, despite upsets and difficulties, and enable the group members to bring all the different levels of communication into conscious awareness. However, the therapist's responsibility for change is shared with the group; analysis of the group takes place by or through the group, including the facilitator. As a result of this, the group becomes able to treat itself.

McNeilly (1989) values the above principles as being fundamental to group work and has attempted to apply them to his group analytic AT approach. Given that AT is different from verbal psychotherapy (i.e. with the fundamental difference being in the presence or absence of image-making), he discusses the relevance of at least five types of images that can be found in AT groups and that can be understood from a group analytic perspective. For example:

- *The blank page*: it can occur at the beginning of the group process, although not only then, and can communicate powerful messages. For example, it may show a wish to let go and become engaged with drawing/painting and at the same time a fear in doing so. It might be associated with the facilitator's expectations of offering the client psychological 'food' and/or treatment by directing the process of the therapy. This is similar to Bion's (1961) discussion of the basic assumption of dependency. It may be an indication of emptiness and/or hidden rage.
- *The written word*: it occurs more often in the beginning of the group and diminishes as people become more comfortable with image-making. McNeilly (1989) sees the written word as having a complex dynamic that can often be associated with the need for control. While images can enable people to get in touch with more primitive parts of themselves, words leave limited space for exploration of different meanings and/or feedback from other group members.
- *The shocking image*: this can be an expression of the object relations level of communication (i.e. the intrapersonal level) in which there might be a conscious attempt to shock the group and an unconscious attempt to attack the external objects. It might also be an expression of the group fears and fantasies as a whole. Tolerance and understanding of the meaning of this image may lead to the process of containment as defined by Bion (1964) and discussed in the previous section.
- *The recurring image*: this might be an image with an emotional content that is repeated in order to resolve an associated 'prototype experience'. It might also be a recurring image with little 'affect' content that is used as a defence in order to avoid change. It can take place at both an individual and group level and can create complex dynamics, e.g. when one individual is involved in the same image-making process, it can trigger

other group members to attempt to change this in an unconscious wish to make changes in the parts of themselves that have been projected onto this person and/or the image.

- *Copied pictures*: these can stand for similar images emerging from two or three different group members simultaneously without apparently copying each other and can be a form of resonance. It can also be a direct copy of somebody else's image that is presented as one's own image. This resembles Bion's (1961) basic assumption of pairing that enables weaker group members to be in the group by attaching themselves to other group members who they perceive as somehow strong. Copying might also protect from what Bion (1961) has described as the 'fight or flight' response. On an individual level it might signify emptiness; on a group level it might be encouraged as an unconscious wish to create a saviour.

In terms of clinical methodology, McNeilly's sessions are divided into two parts: during the first half, clients are expected to draw/paint, and during the second half discussion takes place in an analytic manner. This means that the therapist refuses to take responsibility for the dependency wishes of the group, believing that this would hinder group members from achieving understanding for themselves and mobilising their own self-healing capacities. The therapist also avoids saying anything that other members of the group could not have said. When the therapist makes interpretations, the whole group is addressed. An example of what this approach looks like in practice is presented in Table 6.8.

Despite the criticism of this approach that image-making is seen as of limited value and that applicability to certain client groups is questionable (see 'A Structured AT Group with Ex-offenders' earlier in the chapter for further discussion of the pros and cons of this work), McNeilly's group analytic AT is particularly useful for its emphasis upon the group as a whole and the need for the art therapist to be sufficiently trained in order to be able to facilitate such groups. Furthermore, it has opened the way for other group approaches to AT to emerge such as Waller's (1993) interactive model which is described briefly in the following section.

Other approaches to AT

Closely linked with McNeilly's group analytic AT is the group interactive AT approach introduced by Waller (1993). Like McNeilly, Waller (1993) acknowledges and values group analytic thinking and Foulkes' contribution to group psychotherapy. However, her approach also includes principles from other group psychotherapy models, the most important of which is the interactive/interpersonal perspective developed by Sullivan and Yalom. The main theoretical principles that differentiate interpersonal thinking from group analysis, and that are discussed by Aveline & Dryden (1988) and referred to by Waller (1993), are:

1. Human actions are not predetermined; freedom is part of the human condition.
2. The corollary of this is the importance of choice in human life and

Table 6.8: An example of a group analytical AT session – Gerry McNeilly (2000, pp. 163–165) [Adapted with permission from G McNeilly 'Failures in Group Analytic Art Therapy: New Developments in Theory and Practice'. London, Jessica Kingsley Publishers. Copyright © Jessica Kingsley Publishers]

Description of session	Comments by the therapist and the authors
Needs of client [There were *two male therapists and four female core members* with emotional and relationship difficulties, some of whom had specific clinical diagnoses such as depression, neurosis and eating disorders. The session described occurred 14 months into the group]	[The group members were *selected* after stringent assessment with each person individually. Therapist and client established that group AT was the most relevant form of therapy over other forms. All selected individuals received a written list of group guidelines]
Aim [The aim was to facilitate neurotic symptoms to become transformed into a shared experience and encourage group members to achieve greater understanding of the group processes]	[The task of the group was *analysis* of the group by the group]
First part of session: image making [*Images* created in the first part of the session were:] 1. Sam: a picture of . . . two clowns' faces 2. Alison: painting of numerous feet 3. Mel: painting herself both free and in a cupboard 4. May: two paintings, one an undefined abstract and the other a circle.	[There was *no warm-up* section as in most other AT or arts therapies sessions. Clients were invited to draw/paint straight away for the first half of the session]

Continued

Table 6.8: An example of a group analytical AT session – Gerry McNeilly (2000, pp. 163-165) [Adapted with permission from G McNeilly 'Failures in Group Analytic Art Therapy: New Developments in Theory and Practice. London, Jessica Kingsley Publishers. Copyright © Jessica Kingsley Publishers]—cont'd

Description of session	Comments by the therapist and the authors
Second part of session: discussion	
'. . . Sam . . . took the initiative and . . . moved from speaking of her holiday to the struggles about coming back. . . . She pointed out that the clown faces in her picture were representative of herself and how she had swings of feeling up and down or happy and sad. . . . She went on to speak of how she felt as if she was brought back down to earth through being back from holidays, in that when she was away things were so much more free and she could be more herself. Now that she was back she was either *someone's mother or wife or indeed some other piece of property. As she spoke she kept moving from serious statements to superficial laughing.*	[The therapist regards this as a *dependency demand that reflects not only Sam's needs but also the group's needs as a whole*] 'This seemed to be *an enactment of the clown imagery in her picture.*'
Alison went on to speak of her picture of feet as representing *either being walked on by others or how she had walked over others herself.* She initially spoke of her son leaving home and how she felt walked on by him. There was some dialogue about his illness [he had had a stroke] and how he did not look after himself. . . . There were mixed feelings of anger and relief, alongside a continuing concern for her son's health. *It was interesting that she spoke of him not learning the lesson of his stroke, . . . and how this had left him with a physical disability.*	[The therapist associates this image with *feelings of resentment and anger that are seen as relevant to the group as a whole*] [While Alison was talking about her son the therapist noticed that Alison's problems were also physically related; although she had circulation problems she did not consider the consequences of her smoking. However, the *therapist avoided sharing his observations with the group, waiting for the group members to do it themselves*]

This led to further discussion about how people did things, even when they knew that it was either wrong or would do them damage in the end . . . Mel [talked] about how she did not allow herself to say things, even though she disagreed with what was happening, and how this was reflected in many parts of her life; she either *restricted herself or felt restricted by others*. She linked this directly to her early childhood . . . [and] made a direct reference to her picture of either being free or being locked in a cupboard. There followed a lot of questioning about Mel's childhood, which developed into associations about everyone's childhood feelings of restriction and freedom along with their fears. . . [Still,] everyone was highly involved in what [Mel] was saying and the *focus was strongly with her*.

[Mel's feelings had *resonance* to more than just her]

This then led on to them speaking about fathers. Sam [talked about] the death of her mother, the struggles with her stepmother and her subsequent recognition that father was to blame for this. This was linked to her stepmother, who treated her cruelly, and her father not protecting her. By this time she had moved completely away from needing to oscillate between the enacted clown imagery and was reflective and tearful. At one point *I suggested that she and others seemed to be having a lot of difficulties with mixed feelings* about either pertinent people in their lives or particular events in their childhood. Focusing on Sam, I suggested that she moved between putting her father on a pedestal and the difficulty in experiencing anger towards him, or even expressing it.'

'It was as if *people were working a lot out through her*.'

[*Interpretations* Parallels were drawn between the group members' real fathers and the two male therapists. The therapists were put on a pedestals in order to fulfil the dependency needs of the group but at the same time they were seen as bad for either oppressing or not protecting them. Placing the therapists/fathers on pedestals did not allow group members to express their anger towards them]

Authors' wording in [brackets]

3. Taking responsibility for one's actions.

4. Death is inevitable; but the nothingness of this can gives meaning to life.

5. We are each engaged in a creative search for individual patterns that will give meaning to our existence. (Aveline & Dryden 1988, p. 45)

Waller (1993) accepts these principles and describes relevant applications within AT group work, thereby moving from a group analytical to an interpersonal and existential rationale. Interpersonal and existential thinking, although not as extensively used as psychoanalytic/psychodynamic approaches to AT in the UK, are becoming increasingly relevant to American practice. Moon (1995) for example, an American art therapist, adopts a clear existential perspective for his work. Nevertheless, he regards existentialism as a philosophy that can guide the therapist's thinking rather than a specific model of practice with specific techniques. According to Malchiodi (2003, p. 61), within existential AT approaches:

Art-making serves as stage for therapist–client dialogue about existential issues of freedom to choose, will to meaning, and the search for purpose, values and goals.

Malchiodi (2003) refers to a number of additional AT approaches with a humanistic orientation that are present in the American context, such as Gestalt and transpersonal perspectives, alongside client-centred and existential frameworks. Within the British AT literature, Gestalt and transpersonal perspectives are hardly ever mentioned. One of the few exceptions comes from Mottram (2000, 2001). In her eclectic model of brief AT assessment and treatment, Mottram (2000, 2001) makes reference to Gestalt therapy (see earlier in the chapter for references to Mottram's work in relation to the artistic approaches to AT). She discusses the value of working in the here-and-now and understanding clients' needs in terms of figure and ground, i.e. needs that are satisfied recede into the ground and new needs emerge in the figure. Another British-based AT practitioner who utilises principles from Gestalt therapy is Ford (J Ford, unpublished interview, 2002). He believes that Gestalt/psychodrama can be used effectively in conjunction with AT as a means of giving voice to introjected feelings and regards vocalisation as being as important as image-making. Directive techniques that are individually tailored are used to find a voice for these feelings, e.g. through vocalising a part of an image made by the client.

Another important perspective of AT, with possibly a wider use within the British context than humanistic models, is the developmental perspective of AT. On the one hand, developmental models can refer to a psychoanalytic/psychodynamic understanding of development as discussed in previous sections (e.g. Klein, Winnicott). On the other hand, developmental thinking may derive from cognitive models and Piaget's understanding of cognitive development particularly (see the 'Developmental Trend in Arts Therapies' section in Ch. 4). However, a very important framework of development for AT practice, in particular, is related to models of artistic development as presented by Lowenfeld (1957), Kellogg (1969) and to a lesser extent Gardner (1973). Lowenfeld's developmental frame is frequently used amongst British practitioners and consists of six stages: scribbling (2–4 years of age), preschematic (4–7 years of age), schematic (7–9 years of age), dawning realism (9–11 years of age), pseudorealism (11–13 years of age), period of decision (adolescence). When working with children, developmental models of this kind can become particularly relevant. However, they can also be relevant to working with adults as a means of understanding the level of skill and cognitive development (e.g. with clients with disabilities) or as a means of actively setting goals to be achieved (Malchiodi 2003). An example of a British practitioner who has researched and used models of art development in his work can be found in Dubowski (1990).

AT is also influenced by postmodern thinking; the presence of different theoretical models within the field is increasingly acknowledged and valued. The resulting eclectic/integrative models are seen as more able to address clients from different cultural backgrounds and also enable art therapists to work in increasingly diverse areas of employment. Byrne (1995, 2001) provides a good example of a leading figure within the AT field with a wide postmodern rationale for his practice. He refers to Foucault (1967) as particularly relevant to his practice, as well as phenomenological concepts and humanistic thinking. Byrne (P Byrne, unpublished interview, 2002) also draws upon Winnicott (1971) for the central place of creativity within his theory and for his emphasis upon interaction between two people. He regards the Winnicottian concept of interaction as bearing links with Foucault's concept of discourse and therefore as having relevance to his own AT practice. However, at the same time he questions psychoanalytic thinking for the set view of the self and its claims of absolute truths. Some of the major aims of his work are to manage fragmentation and stay split in the face of the threat of fusion with the imaginary and/or the 'other', to facilitate client's wishes and desires, and to collaborate in a practice aimed at giving the client the opportunity to create improved self-descriptions. Art is central in this approach and is based on the belief of 'doing as being'.

Summary

This chapter traced the development of AT in the UK from its roots in art education, psychoanalysis and the interest of psychiatrists in the artwork of mentally ill patients, via the establishment of the BAAT (currently the largest arts therapies professional body), to its current status as a modern profession recognised by the Health Professions Council. With reference to research, it was shown that the main focus of AT practice appears to be on clients with mental health issues followed by learning difficulties, and the predominant working environments are the health services, voluntary/private organisations and social services, although there are indications of growing interest in education. Some of the main approaches to AT, i.e. psychoanalytic/psychodynamic approaches and to a lesser extent artistic/creative and humanistic practices, were described and illustrated with reference to the literature, major practitioners and case vignettes. Interactive/interpersonal and existential, Gestalt, developmental and postmodern perspectives are additional, influential approaches which were also briefly presented.

References

- Adamson E 1970 Art and mental health. In: Creedy J (ed) The social context of art. Tavistock, London
- Adamson E (in association with Timlin J) 1984 Art as healing. Coventure, London

- Alvin J 1978 Music therapy for the autistic child. Oxford University Press, London
- Arieti S 1976 Creativity and magic synthesis. Basic Books, London
- Aveline M, Dryden W 1988 Group therapy in Britain. Open University Press, Milton Keynes
- Bion W R 1961 Experiences in groups. Tavistock/Routledge, London
- Bion W R 1964 Elements of psychoanalysis. Heinemann, London
- British Association of Art Therapists (BAAT) 2004a About BAAT. Online. Available: http://www.baat.org/aboutbaat.html 11 Dec 2004
- British Association of Art Therapists (BAAT) 2004b What is art therapy? Online. Available: http://www.baat.org/art_therapy.html 11 Dec 2004
- Burleigh L R, Beutler L E 1997 A critical analysis of two creative arts therapies. The Arts of Psychotherapy 23(5): 375–381
- Byrne P 1995 From the depths to the surface: art therapy as a discursive practice in the post-modern era, The Arts in Psychotherapy 22(3):235–239
- Byrne P 1996 Obituaries: Edward Adamson and the experiment. Inscape 1(1):32–36
- Byrne P 2001 Proposed new identities. In: Kossolapow L, Scoble S, Waller D (eds) Arts – therapies – communication: on the way to a communicative European arts therapy, vol 1. Lit Verlag, Munster, p 251–265
- Campbell J 1993 Creative art in group work. Winslow, Oxon
- Case C 1990 Reflections and shadows: an exploration of the world of the rejected girl. In: Case C, Dalley T (eds) Working with children in art therapy. Tavistock/Routledge, London, p 131–160
- Case C 2000 'Our lady of the Queen', journeys around the maternal object. In: Gilroy A, McNeilly G (eds) The changing shape of art therapy: new developments in theory and practice. Jessica Kingsley, London, p 15–54
- Case C, Dalley T 1992 The handbook of art therapy. Routledge, London
- Chilvers I, Osborne H, Farr D 1988 The Oxford dictionary of art. Oxford University Press, Oxford
- Dalley T 2000 Back to the future: thinking about theoretical developments in art therapy. In: Gilroy A, McNeilly G (eds) The changing shape of art therapy: new developments in theory and practice. Jessica Kingsley, London, p 84–98
- Deco S 1998 Return to the open studio group: art therapy groups in acute psychiatry. In: Skaife S, Huet V (eds) Art psychotherapy groups: between pictures and words. Routledge, London, p 88–108
- Dubowski J 1990 Art versus language: separate development during childhood. In: Case C, Dalley T (eds) Working with children in art therapy. Tavistock/Routledge, London, p 7–22
- Edwards D 2004 Art therapy. Sage, London
- Foucault M 1967 Madness and civilisation: a history of insanity in the age of reason. Tavistock, London
- Foulkes S H 1964 Therapeutic group analysis. Allen and Unwin, London
- Gardner H 1973 The arts and human development. Wiley, New York
- Gilroy A, Lee C 1995 Art and music: therapy and research. Routledge, London
- Gilroy A, McNeily G 2000 The changing shape of art therapy. Jessica Kingsley, London
- Greenwood H, Layton G 1987 An out-patient Art Therapy Group. Inscape (summer) 12-19
- Hill A 1945 Art versus illness. George Allen and Unwin, London
- Hill A 1951 Painting out illness. Williams and Norgate, London
- Hogan S 2000 British art therapy pioneer Edward Adamson: a non-interventionist approach. History of Psychiatry xi:259–271
- Hogan S 2001 Healing arts: the history of art therapy. Jessica Kingsley, London
- Karkou V 1999 Art therapy in education: findings from a nation-wide survey in arts therapies. Inscape 4(2):62–70
- Karkou V 2002 Report: from theory to practice. Unpublished report submitted to the University of Hertfordshire
- Karkou V, Glasman J 2004 Arts, education and society: the role of the arts in promoting the emotional well-being and social inclusion of young people. Support for Learning 19(2):57–64
- Kellogg R 1969 Analysing children's art. Mayfield, Palo Alto, CA
- Killick K 2000 The analytical art psychotherapy setting as a containing object in psychotic states. In: Gilroy A, McNeilly G (eds) The changing shape of art therapy: new developments in theory and practice. Jessica Kingsley, London, p 99–127

- Klein M 1975 Collected works of Melanie Klein, vols I, II, III, IV. Hogarth Press and Institute of Psychoanalysis, London
- Kramer E 1971 Art therapy with children. Schocken Books, New York
- Laing R D 1959 The divided self. Penguin Books, London
- Liebmann M F 1979 A study of structured art therapy groups. Unpublished MA thesis. Birmingham Polytechnic
- Liebmann M 1986 Art therapy for groups: a handbook of themes, games and exercises. Routledge, London
- Lowenfeld V 1957 Creative and mental growth, 3rd edn. MacMillan, New York
- McNeilly G 1983 Directive and non-directive approaches in art therapy, The Arts in Psychotherapy 10(4):211–219
- McNeilly, G 1987 Further contributions to group analytic art therapy. Inscape (Summer):8-11
- McNeilly G 1989 Group analytic art groups. In: Gilroy A, Dalley T (eds) Pictures at an Exhibition. Routledge, London, p 156-166
- McNeilly G 2000 Failure in group analytic art therapy. In: Gilroy A, McNeilly G (eds) The changing shape of art therapy: new developments in theory and practice. Jessica Kingsley, London, p 143–171
- McNiff S 1992 Art as medicine. Shambhala, Boston
- Malchiodi C A 1998 The art therapy sourcebook. Lowell House, Los Angeles
- Malchiodi C A 2003 Humanistic approaches. In: Malchiodi C A (ed) A handbook of art therapy. The Guildford Press, New York, p 58–71
- Mann D 1989 The talisman or projective identification? A critique. Inscape (autumn):11–15
- Molloy T 1988 'Letter'. Inscape(Spring):27–28
- Moon B 1995 Existential art therapy. Charles C Thomas, Springfield, IL
- Mottram P 2000 Assessment and treatment in brief art therapy. In: Wigram T (ed) Assessment and evaluation in the arts therapies: art therapy, music therapy and dramatherapy. Harper House Publications, Radlet, p 9–19
- Mottram P 2001 1+1+1+. . . a model of art therapy for an assessment and treatment unit for adults with learning disability and mental health illness. In: Kossolapow L, Scoble S, Waller D (eds) Arts – therapies – communication: on the way to a communicative European arts therapy, vol 1. Lit Verlag, Munster, p 199–206
- Mottram P 2002 Research into the skills and interventions used by British art therapists in their work with clients' images. Virtual International Arts Therapies Journal 1(Dec). The Virtual Arts Therapies Network. Online. Available: http://www.derby.ac.uk/research/vart/journal/archives/2002/articles/pmottram.html 22 Jan 2002
- Naumburg M 1966 Dynamically oriented art therapy: its principles and practices. Grune and Stratton, New York
- Payne H (ed) Handbook of inquiry in the arts therapies: one river many currents. Jessica Kingsley, London
- Rees M 1998 Drawing on difference: art therapy with people who have learning difficulties. Routledge, London
- Rogers C 1951 Client-centered therapy: its current practise, implications and theory. Constable and Company, London
- Sanderson P, Karkou V 2000 Art therapy in mainstream education. A case study. Research report. The University of Manchester, School of Education
- Schaverien J 1987 The scapegoat and talisman: transference in art therapy. In: Dalley T, Case C, Schaverien J et al (eds) Images of art therapy. Tavistock, London
- Schaverien J 1991 The revealing image: analytical art psychotherapy in theory and practice. Jessica Kingsley, London
- Schaverien J 1994 Analytical art psychotherapy: further reflections on theory and practice. Inscape 2:41–49
- Schaverien J 1995 Desire and the female therapist: engendered gazes in psychotherapy and art therapy. Routledge, London
- Schaverien J 2000 The triangular relationship and the aesthetic countertransference in analytic art psychotherapy. In: Gilroy A, McNeilly G (eds) The changing shape of art therapy: new developments in theory and practice. Jessica Kingsley, London, p 55–83
- Silverstone L 1993 Art therapy: the person-centred way, art and the development of the person. Autonomy Books, London

- Skaife S, Huet V Art psychotherapy groups: between pictures and words. Routledge, London
- Thornton R 1985 Review of Gerry McNeilly's article: directive and non-directive approaches in art therapy. Inscape (summer):23–24
- Waller D 1991 Becoming a profession: the history of art therapy in Britain 1940–1982. Tavistock/Routledge, London
- Waller D 1992 Different things to different people: art therapy in Britain – a brief survey of its history and current development. The Arts in Psychotherapy 19:87–92
- Waller D 1993 Group interactive art therapy: its use in training and treatment. Tavistock/Routledge, London
- Waller D (ed) 2002 Arts therapies and progressive illness: nameless dread. Jessica Kingsley, London
- Waller D, Gilroy A (eds) 1992 Art therapy: a handbook. Open University Press, Buckingham
- Winnicott D W 1971 Playing and reality. London, Routledge
- Wood C 1997 The history of art therapy and psychosis 1938–1995. In: Killick K, Schaverien J (eds) Art, psychotherapy and psychosis. Routledge, London

Chapter 7

Dramatherapy (DT)

Key issues:

- During the beginning of the 20th century, movements in the theatre and psychotherapy developed practices that used drama/theatre for therapeutic purposes. In the UK, drama education was even more significant in the emergence of DT. DT was officially established in 1976. Since 1999, DT has been regulated by the Health Professions Council.

- Dramatherapists work with clients with a range of difficulties, but primarily with clients with mental health and learning difficulties. Many also work as consultants for organisations or run workshops for the general public.

- Dramatherapists work in a wide range of settings including health and social services, schools, voluntary or private organisations. A relatively large number of dramatherapists also work in private practice.

- A wide range of practices and techniques can be found within a DT sessions stemming from the theatre and drama.

- DT draws primarily upon the humanistic therapeutic trend, eclectic/integrative approaches and artistic/creative influences.

- Therapeutic models/approaches are booming within current DT practice. Some examples of practice we refer to are theatre-based approaches, humanistic approaches, input from Child Drama and Jungian thinking and the Sesame approach. Psychoanalytically/psychodynamically informed practices, the role theory model, and developmental approaches are also briefly mentioned.

Introduction

Dramatherapy (or drama therapy – two words – as it is known in the USA) uses drama and theatre as the main therapeutic agents. Similar to other arts therapies, current developments are closely linked with a number of movements in the arts, education and psychology. In this chapter we will see how the field developed over time and expanded its scope in terms of numbers of practitioners, training courses and client groups. We will also look at some examples of the wide-ranging approaches that can be found in the field, their main theoretical premises and how they can be expressed within daily practice.

Brief DT history

The most comprehensive history of DT as a modern profession can be found in Jones (1996). Jones (1996) claims that certain theatre traditions have been of particular value for reframing artistic work into a therapeutic practice. Amongst them, Stanislavski from the Moscow Art Theatre is the most important figure. Johnson (2000a) claims that the most relevant ideas of Stanislavski's work for DT were his emphasis upon the psychological qualities of acting, 'emotional memory' and subconscious material. These ideas have influenced a number of theatre practices since then. For example, during the first half of the 20th century, Evreinov, a student of Stanislavski, was arguing for the value of 'theatrotherapy'. During the same period, and again influenced by Stanislavski's techniques, the Russian psychiatrist Iljine developed his own way of working with his patients, students with emotional difficulties and others in a theatre context. His work is known as the 'therapeutic theatre' approach.

However, Jones (1996) claims that neither Evreinov nor Iljine became particularly known in the UK or the USA. In contrast, Moreno (1972), the founder of the humanistic movement and psychodrama, seems to have a much stronger impact upon English-speaking countries and the USA in particular. During the 1920s, Moreno began experimenting in Austria with what he called the 'theatre of spontaneity'. When he moved to the USA, one strand of his theatrical experimentations evolved into what is currently known as psychodrama. Psychodrama is now a form of group psychotherapy with a number of similarities with DT, but also clear differences (see the section on 'Humanistic Approaches to DT' in this chapter for further discussion about similarities and differences between the two modalities). Despite the separate developments and distinctive professional identities of the two fields, psychodrama can be seen as an early expression of theatrical structures used for therapeutic change and thus an area of work that has prepared the ground for the emergence of DT.

Other psychotherapeutic traditions also started acknowledging the value of drama and theatre for therapeutic work. Freud, himself, acquired inspiration for his theories from the theatre (e.g. the Oedipus complex is one such example) leading to interesting cross-fertilisations across fields. But, as Jones (1996) argues, unlike humanistic perspectives, the degree to which enactment has been 'allowed' within traditional psychoanalytic practice is questionable. Enactment has been seen as 'acting out'; the dramatic potential of 'as if' situations has not been sufficiently explored, and physicality and the presence of the body have been ignored; we explore this point further in the following chapter in relation to dance movement therapy (DMT). Jungian thinking, seems, once again, to be much more open towards the theatre and drama and, as with other arts therapies disciplines, has offered a protective space for emergence of some of the early DT work. For example, Lindkvist (Pearson 1996), one of the pioneers of DT and the founder of the Sesame approach, has had a Jungian orientation.

After the Second World War there was an increase in drama work from members of staff within hospital settings. Jones (1996) testifies that one strand of this work in hospitals was undertaken by psychiatrists/psychotherapists who, in the typical way of the period, used dramatic activities as adjunctive to the therapeutic work, or as an aid for psychotherapeutic assessment, diagnosis or rehabilitation. Alongside them, occupational therapists discovered the benefits of using dramatic enactments within their work. Therapeutic drama was intensified in the 1960s and 1970s with the boom of humanistic therapies. As we have already seen (see Ch. 4), Gestalt therapy and transactional analysis are two such examples, with Gestalt drama and transactional psychodrama using techniques that favour enactments (BADth 2004). During the same period, behavioural therapists began to employ role-play as a useful way of developing social skills, while a number of psychoanalytically informed drama practices emerged, particularly in France, e.g. the 'Expression Scenique', 'analytical drama therapy' and 'integrated drama therapy'. Parallel to these movements we can find an increasing experimentation within theatrical circles of work that borders on therapeutic work, such as Peter Brook's (1968), Jerzy Grotowski's (1968) and Augusto Boal's (1979) work, and the spreading of relevant sociological theories such as symbolic interactionism and dramaturgy (e.g. Goffman 1959, Mead 1934).

Within a British context, however, the emergence of DT seems to be substantially enabled by drama education. The most important contribution for the DT field comes from Peter Slade (Slade 1954). Although he is better known for his child drama work, Slade used the term 'dramatherapy' for the first time in the UK as early as 1939. His lectures and workshops and the refinement of his originally educational ideas into the therapeutic value of drama enabled the emergence of DT in the UK as an independent field.

During the 1960s and 1970s, practitioners who recognised the therapeutic value of drama and theatre started coming together, first under the Remedial Drama Group forum (early 1960s) and eventually (1976) as the British Association of Dramatherapists (BADth). Despite these groupings, however, the majority of practitioners continued working independently, often with the 'blessing' and encouragement of the groups and centres they were affiliated with. For example, the Dramatherapy Centre, the forerunner of BADth, had, amongst other functions, the role to promote private consultancy (BADth 2004). With subsequent professional developments, i.e. the establishment of training courses, the definition of career and salary grading within the NHS, and registration with the Health Professions Council (HPC) (see Box 7.1), professional identity became clearer and stronger.

Box 7.1: Significant dates in the development of DT in the UK (BADth 2004, Jennings 1987, 1998, Meldrum 1994a, Sesame 2003)

Year	Development
Early 1960s	Sue Jennings and Gordon Wiseman form the Remedial Drama Group, later (1970) renamed the Dramatherapy Centre, a forerunner of the British Association of Dramatherapists.
1964	Marian (Billy) Lindkvist founds the Sesame course, a short training course in drama and movement therapy at the York Clinic, Guy's Hospital, London.
1976	Establishment of the British Association of Dramatherapists (BADth).
1977	The first full DT training course is established at St Albans, alongside the existing art therapy training course.
1978	A research fellow post in DT is established at the College of Ripon and York St John and a course in DT begins there at the same time.
1980	A third diploma course is initiated in the South Devon Technical College.
1987	The Institute of Dramatherapy begins as an independent theatre-based training course; in 1994 it moves to the Roehampton Institute.
1989	Dramatherapists working for the NHS join art therapists and music therapists as professionals awarded career and grading structure recognised by the Department of Health and Social Security.
1999	Registration with the Health Professions Council, alongside art therapy and music therapy.

Current DT professional development

Since DT established a separate professional identity, there have been a number of substantial developments in the field. There are currently at least five training courses in the UK: two in London, one in Derby, one in Exeter and one in Huddersfield (see Appendix 2). Although the philosophy of each course varies, set standards have been established across these trainings (Joint Quality Assurance Committee 2002).

DT practitioners have substantially increased in numbers. For example, Meldrum (1994a) reports that in 1991, the British Association of Dramatherapists (BADth) had around 200–250 members. During the time of our study (1996) the number had increased to around 300 members. By 2004, the number of qualified dramatherapists in the UK is reported to be over 400 (BADth 2004).

DT is now used with a number of different client groups (see Table 7.1).

Table 7.1 shows that dramatherapists work primarily with clients with mental health problems (emotional/behavioural) and learning difficulties. Some of the client difficulties discussed in the DT literature include children with challenging behaviour and autism, children who have been physically or

Table 7.1: Main DT client groups and differences from other arts therapies

Type of difficulty	% for DT	% for other arts therapies	Chi-square (x^2) value	Degrees of freedom (df)	P-value (p)
Emotional/ behavioural	58.3	60.3	Not significant		
Learning	23.6	22.7	Not significant		
None apparent	13.6	2.8	22.64	1	0.000**
Other	2.7	6.4	Not significant		
Multiple	0.9	3.9	Not significant		
Physical/sensory/ medical	0.9	3.9	Not significant		
Total	100.0	100.0			

**Accepted at the 0.01 level of significance
The table shows that emotional/behavioural difficulties (mental health) and learning difficulties were the most frequent types of difficulties faced by the main client groups of dramatherapists. The third largest group was people with no apparent difficulties.
Chi-square tests performed for the different client groups revealed one statistically significant difference between DT and other arts therapies. Dramatherapists tended to work more often with clients with no apparent difficulties than other arts therapists (p = 0.000).

sexually abused, adults with depression, prolonged bereavement, thought disorders, eating disorders, children and adults with trauma, offenders, etc. In the research registers compiled by Payne (1993) and Dent-Brown (2004), there are a number of, primarily qualitative, research studies completed with these different client groups, some of which are on a PhD level. There are only a few studies that use quantitative research methods and only few studies have a randomised controlled trial (RCT) design (one with clients with severe mental health problems and one with children at risk). Burleigh & Beutler (1997), in their critical analysis of empirical research work in art therapy (AT) and DT, describe and discuss a similar type of research activity undertaken in the USA context and urge for further developments.

According to results from our study, a relatively large proportion of DT practitioners in the UK are also working with people who do not present an apparent difficulty (more than 10%). This type of work is undertaken by dramatherapists with much more frequency than any of the other arts therapies professionals. It is not clear why this is the case. One reason might be the nature of DT per se. With drama being potentially more verbal than any of the other art forms, DT might be better suited to clients with some degree of cognitive/physical/emotional skill; severe learning difficulties or serious mental health problems might be less relevant to 'mainstream' DT practices, although several adaptations have been made to suit such clients. Independent work reported earlier (see the brief history section earlier in this chapter) may be another reason. Unlike other arts therapists, DT practitioners embark on consultation work with both individuals and groups/organisations facing difficulties, alongside more traditional therapy work with more vulnerable clients. They also become involved in management training in terms of running support groups and training groups (Meldrum 1994a).

This last point seems to be well connected with the working environments in which dramatherapists are most frequently found. Social services/community work is a very important area of work, as Table 7.2 shows. Private practice is another area in which a relatively large percentage of dramatherapists are demonstrated as working. Both social services/community work and private practice are areas of work that attract more dramatherapists than any other arts therapists. It is interesting to note that BADth is the only arts therapies professional association that, for years, has not restricted its members from private practice, i.e. there have been no requirements for seniority or other evidence of sufficient experience before dramatherapists can take up private practice. This policy, or better, lack of policy regarding private practice seems to fit within the overall trend of dramatherapists undertaking independent work, as discussed before.

Another important difference between DT and other arts therapies is in relation to employment within health services. Although this area of work is the most important one for DT practitioners, the proportion of dramatherapists

Table 7.2: Main DT working environments and differences from other arts therapies

Working environment	% for DT	% for other arts therapies	Chi-square (x^2) value	Degrees of freedom (df)	P-value (p)
Health	29.4	53.0	19.79	1	0.000**
Social service	22.0	9.6	12.99	1	0.000**
Education	17.4	16.3	Not significant		
Voluntary/private agency	12.8	12.6	Not significant		
Private practice	14.7	5.9	9.79	1	0.002**
Other	3.7	2.6	Not significant		
Total	100.0	100.0			

**Accepted at the 0.01 level of significance
Health services were the most frequently reported areas of work, followed by social services, education and voluntary/private organisations.
When chi-square tests were performed for these different working environments, three statistically significant differences were found between dramatherapists and non-dramatherapists. In proportion, more dramatherapists were found to be working in social services and private practice compared with other arts therapists, while fewer dramatherapists were found in health services. These differences were accepted at the 0.01 level of significance.

who are employed in such settings is much smaller than for other arts therapists. Historical reasons may, once again, explain this finding. While AT and music therapy (MT) became recognised NHS professions in the early 1980s, it was not until 1989 that DT joined them. Ambiguity amongst dramatherapists in terms of their health profession identity and concerns about joining mainstream establishments was echoed within BADth circles at the time. A fear that governmental registration would limit freedom and creativity versus the need to assure professional survival has been at the heart of the debate and resembles similar debates in other arts therapies associations (Waller 2001). Given that BADth finally decided to follow the route opened up by AT and MT, it is expected that future representation of DT in the NHS will be increased.

DT defined

As we have already discussed in Chapter 2, there are two definitions of DT in current use in the UK. One refers to DT as having its emphasis upon:

> . . . the intentional use of healing aspects of drama and theatre as the therapeutic process. It is a method of working and playing that uses action methods to facilitate creativity, imagination, learning, insight and growth. (BADth 2004, p. 1)

In this definition, accepted by BADth as the official one, the language used echoes older perspectives of DT as a 'healing' medium (e.g. see Meldrum 1994a). As an improvement from older definitions, however, not only does it refer to an intentional, rather than a general, use of drama and theatre but it also clarifies this intention further, i.e. facilitating creativity, imagination, learning, insight or growth.

Another definition of the modality that is in frequent use in the UK refers to DT as a form of creative psychotherapy and is formulated by the American dramatherapist Johnson (1982, p. 83):

> Dramatherapy, like the other creative arts therapies (art, music and dance), is the application of a creative medium to psychotherapy. Specifically, dramatherapy refers to those activities in which there is an established therapeutic understanding between client and therapist and where the therapeutic goals are primary and not incidental to the ongoing activity.

As we have already stated, this definition has been used as part of the DT documentation for UK governmental registration (Jenkyns & Barham 1991 cited in Meldrum 1994a). Words such as 'healing' are dropped in favour of psychotherapeutic language. Affiliation with psychotherapy has probably been reinforced in an attempt to raise professional status.

The presence of different definitions reflects different opinions and practices held within the field. Both Meldrum (1994a) and Valente & Fontana (1993) testify to a wide diversity of practices as a characteristic of the field. Therapeutic techniques used within the DT field are similarly diverse. The nature of drama and theatre per se perpetuate such methodological diversity. For example, different art forms are used within a theatre performance. Theatre work assumes the existence of visual components (i.e. lighting and scenery) and music and dance alongside character formation and role enactments. An actor is expected to be able to sing and dance as well as act in front of an audience, while the director will guide the process until the final outcome. Similarly, within a DT context, the client may often assume an acting role, while the therapist assumes that of a facilitative director (Meldrum 1993, 1994a).

Therapeutic drama is another important source for DT methods. In contrast to work that is theatre-related, drama does not assume the production of a performance, but merely the presence of a pretended reality. DT methods that relate to drama can range from using scripts, stories and myths to using objects, toys, masks and puppets. Jones (1996) talks also about the body in a dramatic form (e.g. the body disguised), and role-play with created or scripted characters. Within what is known as the anthropological or shamanistic perspectives to DT, rituals are also valued as rites of passage that can be re-enacted within a DT session (Jennings 1995, Jones 1996, Meldrum 1994a).

There are a number of publications that refer to dramatic activities. Some such publications come from dramatherapists such as Jennings (1986) and Andersen-Warren & Grainger (2000). However, activities can be borrowed from a number of different sources such as drama education and community theatre. DT practitioners agree that the distinguishing factor between them being activities with an educational, social or other function, and being therapeutic methods, is the presence of a trained therapist and a therapeutic intention. Jennings (1998) claims that these activities need not be treated as mere tasks but as parts of a therapeutic process. Furthermore, she argues for the need to undertake extensive training and supervision in order to safeguard vulnerable clients from potential harmful results. Dramatherapists are clearly moving away from the notion that the use of dramatic activities per se has therapeutic benefit.

A session structure that is frequently referred to within the DT literature consists of: warm-up, focusing, main activity, closure and de-roling, completion (e.g. Jones 1996). However, although clear session structures are suggested, most dramatherapists follow such structures flexibly by adapting them to the needs of the clients. With a few exceptions (e.g. Mitchell 1994a, 1996) the work takes place primarily in a group context. Jennings (1998) claims that, although one-to-one DT is expanding, DT is of particular value in a group situation. This opinion seems to be holding firmly within the field until the present time.

Main therapeutic trends within DT

As Table 7.3 shows, the most relevant psychotherapeutic school of thought for this group of arts therapists is the humanistic school; and although principles from this tradition are also very important for other arts therapists, DT practitioners seem to place greater value on it than their other arts therapies colleagues. Humanistic thinking appears to offer either overall theoretical back-up or just relevant therapeutic principles and methodological ideas for DT practice.

Also apparent in the findings in Table 7.3 is the tendency of dramatherapists to affiliate their work with eclectic/integrative thinking. The wide diversity in the field, discussed before, seems to be relevant not only for the field as a whole but also for individual practices. Valente & Fontana (1993), in particular, caution for this tendency; they claim that it bears the danger of an amorphous practice without clear rationale. Discussing this point further, Jones

Table 7.3: Main DT therapeutic trends and differences from other arts therapies

Therapeutic trends	Mean for DT[1]	Mean for other arts therapies[1]	t-test value	Degrees of freedom (df)	P-value (p)
Humanistic	4.03	3.86	3.26	578	0.001**
Eclectic/ integrative	3.80	3.66	2.07	578	0.039*
Artistic/creative	3.27	3.10	2.54	146.31	0.012*
Psychoanalytic/ psychodynamic	3.27	3.36	−1.99	578	0.047*
Developmental	3.23	3.21	Not significant		
Active/directive	3.11	3.07	Not significant		

[1]The higher the score, the stronger the agreement with this group of statements (a five-point scale was used ranging from strongly agree = 5 to strongly disagree = 1)

**Accepted at the 0.01 level of significance

*Accepted at the 0.05 level of significance

As the table shows, dramatherapists demonstrated the strongest agreement with the humanistic group of statements and least agreement with the active/directive group. Statistically significant differences existed between DT and other arts therapies in relation to the humanistic, the eclectic/integrative, the artistic/creative and the psychoanalytic/psychodynamic group of statements. In the first three cases, dramatherapists showed stronger agreement with these groups of statements than their colleagues, while the opposite was true with the statements relating to psychoanalytic/psychodynamic thinking.

(1996) talks about a booming of therapeutic models to epidemic proportions that stem directly from attempts to define the field. There are references, for example, to the creative/expressive, learning and insight/psychotherapeutic models (Jennings 1983). Meldrum (1994a) talks about the theatrical, therapeutic drama, role theory and anthropological/shamanistic models. Under these broad categories, there are examples of a number of different approaches; one would claim as many as there are practitioners involved.

According to Jones (1996), most of the so-called 'models' do not constitute comprehensive theoretical frameworks. Instead, they stress a particular idea and area of work over another. Alternatively, he attempts to define what is common across different approaches using primarily the language of drama and theatre. He suggests nine core processes, otherwise known as 'therapeutic factors', that are relevant to all DT approaches: dramatic projection, therapeutic performance process, empathy and distancing, personification and impersonation, interactive audience and witnessing, embodiment, playing, life-drama connection and transformation.

Similar pre-occupation with defining the field through the language of the dramatic/theatrical form is also apparent in the official definition of the discipline and the writings of other leading figures in the field, such as Jennings (1998) and Mitchell (1990, 1994a,b, 1996). It is therefore not surprising that DT practitioners who participated in our study appeared to place strong value upon artistic/creative principles, much stronger than other arts therapists did (see Table 7.3). Equally unsurprising is our finding that dramatherapists seem to be in less agreement with psychoanalytic/psychodynamic thinking than other arts therapists. When other arts therapists turned to psychoanalytic/psychodynamic thinking in an attempt to acquire theoretical justification and professional status, the majority of dramatherapists turned to theories of theatre and drama, sociology and social anthropology.

This does not mean that psychoanalytic/psychodynamic thinking cannot also be found in the field. However, it does mean that DT is much more strongly rooted within the art form. Given the diversity and complexity of the art form itself, the DT field is similarly diverse.

Theatre approaches to DT: starting with Nikolai Evrenov and Vladimir Iljine

The DT literature makes a number of references to leading figures in the world of theatre as playing a significant role in the development of DT in the 20th century, such as Stanislavski, Artaud, Brecht, Ionesco, Beckett, Grotowski, Boal and Brook. Amongst them Stanislavski might be the most important figure because of the emphasis he placed upon studying the inner psychological ensembles of a character and developing improvisatory techniques that would enable the actor/actress to release the creative powers of his or her subconscious (Carlson 1993, Johnson 2000a). His work is also important because it gave rise to some early expressions of DT practice. Nikolai Evreinov and his 'theatreotherapy' is one such example. According to Carlson (1993), Evreinov defined theatre as a human instinct that is directly linked with life. As such, theatre is not just a pastime, but a human necessity. Linked with this is the idea that transformation is at the heart of theatre practice and its ultimate goal. Interestingly enough, Evreinov's emphasis was upon the theatrical process itself rather than the performance, a characteristic of most contemporary DT practices. Although he did not develop specific methodological suggestions, his ideas made clear links between theatre and personal change (Jones 1996).

Iljine and his 'therapeutic theatre' is another example of an early expression of DT that stems directly from the theatre. Jones (1996) offers a very good description of Iljine's approach, which started in pre-revolution Russia (1908–1917) and developed further during Iljine's travelling in Europe. During this travelling time, Jones (1996) claims that Iljine came across Ferenczi in Hungary and became familiar with 'active techniques' in psychoanalysis. Role-play was one of them. In Iljine's own work there were improvisatory training sessions and therapeutic theatre performance meetings. Improvisatory training involved drama games and exercises with the aim of encouraging spontaneity, flexibility, expression, communication and sensitivity. Iljine believed that these qualities could be lost with people who experience mental health problems. He would also emphasise the body and voice as an agent for emotional expression and exploration. By being able to use the body and voice, clients could become able to also express emotions in the therapeutic theatre performance sessions and eventually in life.

During the therapeutic theatre performance meetings, certain stages were followed as described in Table 7.4. The duration of these stages would vary considerably depending on the clients; each stage could take more than one

Table 7.4: Stages of therapeutic theatre – summary of Vladimir Iljine's work by Jones (1996, pp. 59-61)

Needs of clients
[Primarily people with mental health problems]

Aims
[To identify, work on and resolve emerging issues and memories through ongoing alteration of enactments and reflection]

Stages of therapeutic theatre

1. Theme identification
[At the beginning a theme would be identified which had to have the potential for improvisation. Some of the ways of identifying a themes were: looking at the client's case history, using diagnostic tests and/or encouraging group discussion (when groups were involved)]

[The] 'process of choosing themes was seen as giving diagnostic information to the therapist/s. This concerned the identification of issues, which troubled clients, but could also involve the interpersonal dynamics which emerged during negotiations. The therapist/s would give interpretations or make interventions which aimed to stimulate the selection process.'

2. Reflection on themes
[The therapist and the client or the group] 'discussed the choice of theme, its relevance, the key areas of conflict contained within it and the ways in which it might be expressed and explored through drama. . . . Other means of reflection could be used in addition to verbal discussion; for example, group members might paint or draw a picture in relation to the theme.'

3. Scenario design
[Based on the theme a scenario was designed which was a brief outline that could be used for enactment] 'A scenario design would include: the theme, key words, details about roles and the characteristic roles attached to the roles, a short series of basic situations or scenes to be focused upon, and the location or locations.'

4. Scenario realisation
'A stage and materials such as masks and costumes can be used, or the work can take place within a defined space in a room using only some chairs to sit in. . . . A series of improvisation training exercises could be used prior to enactment, aiming to warm up the participants to the situations and characters they were to portray. . . . The scenario [was] then enacted. . . . [Emphasis was placed] upon the importance of a high level of emotional and imaginative involvement for those taking part.'

5. Reflection/feedback
'Each person discussed how they felt whilst in role. . . . The belief was that issues from the life of the player could become connected to the enactment they were making.' [If there was more than one scene, then there would be reflection after each one of them. Reflection was regarded as essential in order to deepen the exploration in the following scene]

Authors' wording in [brackets]

session to complete. It was important to develop flexible scenes, which could be worked and re-worked until the underlying issue was finally resolved.

Despite the clarity of this approach and its use in DT training in Germany and the Netherlands, Jones (1996) claims that Iljine's work did not become known in the UK until recently. The main reason for this has been the lack of translations of this work into English. Despite its limited application to the British context, Iljine's approach remains a very good early example of theatre-based approaches to DT that needs to be acknowledged.

More contemporary influences upon DT practice that come directly from the theatre are: Grotowski's Laboratory Theatre (1968), Brook's 'Empty Space' (1968), Boal's 'Theatre of the Oppressed' or Forum Theatre (1979) and the more recent Playback Theatre (Fox 1994), amongst others. Although it is outside the scope of this book to cover this type of work, some common aspects of all of them involve the introduction of new ideas that highlight improvisatory techniques, question the supremacy and value of fixed scripts and make explicit links between the theatre and personal/social change. For example, Mitchell (1994a,b), a dramatherapist who acted for years as the director of the DT training course at the Roehampton Institute, makes explicit references to influences from Grotowski and Brook. His work is regarded as an important theatre approach to DT, and is known by different names, e.g. the 'therapeutic theatre' approach and the para-theatrical model to DT. However, the most prolific writer of the theatre model for DT and perhaps one of the most important pioneers of DT in the UK is Sue Jennings. An outline of her work follows.

A theatre approach to DT applied to a forensic setting

Sue Jennings' approach to DT is wide-ranging and particularly rich. As a pioneer of DT, she was the founder of the first DT professional group in the UK, established training courses in the UK and abroad, and has written extensively. Over the years, a number of names have been attached to her work: it is known as 'developmental', 'anthropological/shamanistic', 'ritual theatre of healing', 'theatre of health and healing'; the bottom line of all of these versions of her work is that it is a truly artistic practice.

Primarily a dancer and an actress, Jennings began working with movement and drama in psychiatric hospitals and special schools as early as the 1960s. With the Remedial Drama Group she co-founded with Gordon Wiseman, she toured extensively in the UK and Europe, working directly with patients and offering workshops to members of staff. In the 1970s she studied social anthropology in an attempt to create a frame for her work. As part of her doctoral studies she stayed with the Temiar people in Malaysia, studying their children's rearing and rituals (Jennings 1994a). Her social anthropology studies have had a significant impact upon subsequent work; for example, there is a wide understanding of drama practices across different cultures and an emphasis upon ritual as a useful dramatherapeutic concept. According to Jennings (1994b, p. 95):

Dramatic ritual is a set of performed actions involving metaphor and symbol which not only communicates to us about change, status and values but also affects us.

Rituals have an impact upon participants at a number of different levels: physical, emotional, cognitive, imaginative and metaphysical. Within DT they often take the form of a dramatic reality as opposed to everyday reality. Moving to a dramatic reality somehow involves an altered state of mind. In Jennings' (1994b) terms this is a type of 'trance' and the dramatherapist can be seen as a type of modern shaman. Within primarily American writings the shamanistic approach assumes that the dramatherapist takes the role of the actor/shaman and the client that of the spectator (Johnson 1992). Jennings' view of these roles is different, reflecting uneasiness amongst British dramatherapists with practices in which the client is not in charge of the drama-making process. According to Jennings (1994b), the dramatherapist, as a modern shaman, is seen solely as having an assisting role that can enable clients' 'transit' from the everyday reality to the dramatic reality and back, rather than one where the therapist is the main actor of a dramatic enactment.

Despite influences from social anthropology, however, theatre art remains the main source of structures, techniques and themes for Jennings' practice. For example, Jennings (1987) makes direct references to the Greek theatre and the Dionysian versus Apollonian theatre, and acknowledges the contribution of Grotowski and Brook to DT. She refers to the 'as if' principle discussed by Stanislavski as a key concept for creating dramatic reality and consequently enabling therapeutic change within DT. She also discusses extensively the idea of the dramatic or aesthetic distance within DT, a concept also borrowed from the theatre and Brecht in particular. Jennings explains that, paradoxically, the fact that drama provides such distance, i.e. the clients in DT do not have to work on their own issues directly, means that new perspectives are offered into their own life issues. Other relevant principles to Jennings' practice of DT come from Artaud himself. According to Jennings (1994b), Artaud's ideas that have relevance to DT are:

- *The search for new language through sound and movement.* Jennings argues that new languages of voice and movement may enable the expression of difficult things. Searching for these new languages should not be restricted to one system of movement, e.g. Laban-based or Yoga or Alexander or Balinese theatre (notice how Lindkvist, another pioneer of DT in the UK [discussed later in association with the Sesame approach], draws upon Laban's theory of movement in particular).
- *The use of 'larger than life' images and effigies.* Artaud referred to 'cruelty', i.e. harsh gestures and movement that can give a sense of danger. Jennings talks about being involved in artistic expressions that exaggerate the 'life-size' or daily experience. Such practices can take people beyond their ordinary limits in a way that new ways of communication are created. It is important that people are challenged with the new without putting their defences in danger.
- *The dialogue of opposites and reconciliation.* Through 'larger than life' practices polar opposites can be explored and particular stereotypes can be clarified before transformation can take place. Given the 'larger than life' context, it is possible to make new connections away from the stereotypical and the banal and thus reach 'artistic authenticity' that enables movement and change.

Thematically, Jennings (Jennings 1992, Jennings et al 1997) will often utilise Shakespearian stories, e.g. *A Midsummer Night's Dream* or *King Lear*. She finds Shakespearian complexity of character formation as offering a unique insight into human psyche and, as such, of particular value for DT practice. Within this primarily theatrical model, Jennings incorporates a developmental methodology that is seen as offering a useful and safe structure for people to engage in drama work. This is known as the EPR developmental paradigm, which consists of the three stages of embodiment, projection and role enactment:

- *Embodiment* involves gestures, exploration of body parts and whole body movement, and is equivalent to children's sensory play (first year of life).
- *Projection* is about images being projected onto drawing, painting, sculpting, masks and any other objects outside the self. This stage is equivalent to projected play and can also incorporate sensory components (14 months to 2/3 years of age).
- *Role enactment* consists of drama games, role-play, rituals and masked dramas. This is similar to children's dramatic play (2–3 to 5 years of age). It incorporates opposites such as good/bad and light/dark.

According to Jennings (1996, p. 206), these stages:

. . . should not be seen in a linear way, but as life stages that will continue to be re-visited throughout life. Increasingly the individual is able both to play a variety of roles as well as being able to socialise with a variety of roles.

The final outcome of the developmental process is therefore an ability to acquire and interact with a variety of roles. Similarities with Landy's (1986, 1993) role theory model are apparent on this point. Jennings (S Jennings, unpublished interview, 2002) explains that 'artistic construction', which is fundamental in the EPR model and Jennings' work in general, is a process that resembles 'social construction'.

Table 7.5 illustrates briefly some of the main components of Jennings' approach (for a fuller account of this work and research undertaken in this setting, see Jennings et al 1997). Relevance of the humanistic school of thought is apparent in a number of points made in the above case; for example her emphasis upon working with the healthy parts of clients and in the here-and-now. Further discussion of this affiliation can be found in Jennings (1992, 1996). In contrast, Jennings (1987, 1996) seems to be opposing psychoanalytic/psychodynamic thinking as raising issues of questionable power dynamics and blurred distinctions between the dramatic and the everyday reality. As a result of this 'anti-psychoanalytic/psychodynamic' position, in her own work, she avoids interpretations, believing that the drama speaks for itself directly to the clients. Her approach can therefore easily be regarded as an 'oblique' approach, i.e. an approach where meaning is created within the artistic form without seeing a necessity for verbalisation. This belief is common in other DT approaches (e.g. the Sesame approach) as well as other arts therapies approaches (e.g. see 'The Creative MT Approach' in Ch. 5).

Table 7.5: The theatre of healing approach with clients in a forensic setting – Sue Jennings (adapted from example provided to V Karkou for 'Arts Therapies: from Theory to Practice' study [Karkou 2002; reproduced with permission])

Description of process	Comments from the authors
Needs of clients within specific setting	
'Closed institution, forensic setting.' [The clients have *limited choices and social skills*]	[*Initial assessment* involves an interview and an open workshop. Assessment tools used are: EPR for developmental assessment. BasicPh (Lahad 1992): using a six-piece story that assesses a person's strengths]
Main aims/main assumptions [The clients] 'need to "engage"; explore "*fixed roles*" through characters.'	[Influences from the *role model* in DT (Landy 1986)]
Beginning of DT process 'Discussion, establishing contract, demonstration, open sessions – commitment to time frame.	
Habituation to *methods*: movement, drawing/painting, games, improvisation, stories, text work, masks.	[Methods follow the *EPR paradigm*, i.e. embodiment, projection and role enactment]
[There is an emphasis upon the] "*dramatic reality/everyday reality*".'	[Clients are encouraged to shift from the everyday reality to the dramatic reality and vice versa]
Development of DT work 'Choosing main *text/story* – negotiation where possible, structuring exploration of themes and characters through EPR. [The client becomes a] performer, designer and director.	[Text/story can be taken from *Shakespearian plays* such as *King Lear* or *A Midsummer Night Dream*] [Masks can be used as *larger than life effigies* that can enable moving away from the stereotypical and integrate opposites. Over-identification with the masks should be avoided]
Integration through *masks*.	
Staying with the metaphor rather than interpretation.	[*Interpretation* is seen as questioning dramatic distance]
Initial *choice of character* were characters who had been violent to women. Their second choice after 6 months work showed a variety of choice and a greater flexibility and less violent "inevitability".'	[Landy's (1993) *role taxonomy* is used as evidence of progress]

Continued

Table 7.5: The theatre of healing approach with clients in a forensic setting – Sue Jennings (adapted from example provided to V Karkou for 'Arts Therapies: from Theory to Practice' study [Karkou 2002; reproduced with permission])—cont'd

Description of process	Comments from the authors
Completion of DT work 'Closure of themes and stories, creation of a closure mask, *reflection of journey* through the sessions.'	[*Final evaluation* of the work involves feedback and self-evaluation; EPR final assessment of developmental progress is used and any other observed changes in dramatic work and choices]

Authors' wording in [brackets]

Jennings' teaching and writing has been particularly influential amongst British dramatherapists. An example of a theatre approach to DT with a similar conceptualisation can be seen in the following section.

A theatre approach to DT with an adult in prolonged bereavement

Madeline Andersen-Warren is another dramatherapist with a clear theatre/drama bias. Having practised for over 15 years in the NHS and currently acting as a co-convenor of the Northern Trust for DT, one of the DT training courses based in the north-west of England, her work involves a range of client groups (e.g. adult survivors of sexual abuse, people with psychotic disorders, the elderly) and DT perspectives. She argues for the need for DT to be flexible and adjustable to the needs of the client rather than to expect the client to fit into a rigid therapy framework. As part of exploring flexible therapy practices, alongside her more conventional DT work, she has explored the overlap between theatre and therapy in performance productions with her NHS clients (Andersen-Warren 1996).

The influence of Jennings' work upon Andersen-Warren's practice is apparent. Similarly to Jennings, Andersen-Warren: talks about dramatic/aesthetic distance and utilises Jennings' EPR methodological structure; finds inspiration for her DT work from historical drama (e.g. Elizabethan/Jacobean theatre, melodrama); addresses spiritual elements, as is apparent in the clinical example in Table 7.6.

In addition to influences from Jennings, however, Andersen-Warren (M. Andersen-Warren, unpublished interview, 2002) also makes references to existential psychotherapy as particularly relevant to working with people with bereavement, and values political theatre as relevant to offering ways of addressing social and political oppression. There are therefore explicit links with humanistic perspectives. DT approaches with predominantly humanistic rationales are further discussed in the following section.

Table 7.6: A theatre approach of DT with an adult in prolonged bereavement – Madeline Andersen-Warren [adapted from example provided to V Karkou for 'Arts Therapies: from Theory to Practice' study [Karkou 2002; reproduced with permission]]

Description of process	Comments from the authors
Needs of clients within specific setting	[*Initial assessment* can last for four to five 1-hour sessions and is about:
'Client stuck in *prolonged grief reaction*. Multiple bereavements. Trying to move away from a stern Catholic upbringing and find a merciful God to give her comfort. Viewed God as punishing and lacking in compassion and humour. Client ashamed of bodily functions. No affect, feelings of hopelessness and numbness.'	• finding out whether the two can work together, and whether a long-term or brief intervention group or individual work, DT or another form of therapy, is relevant
	• setting goals, establishing metaphors and symbols that are most potent for client, identifying images they use to describe feelings and finding genre of story or text that has resonance for them.
	• Jennings' (1996) EPR developmental assessment is also used]
Main aims/main assumptions	[The client's *spiritual viewpoint* is respected and taken on board alongside the therapist's assessment of needs
'To assist to *create a compassionate God*. She wanted to believe in the God she had heard about – a loving God;	
To readjust her view of the body;	
To assist her to express her feelings.	
She was so divorced from her feelings that direct intervention could be overwhelming. Therefore to work with *text as a container* for her expression and to work with the body.'	Dramatic reality creates *dramatic distance* that is useful for containing overwhelming feelings and offers a starting point for body work]

Continued

Table 7.6: A theatre approach of DT with an adult in prolonged bereavement – Madeline Andersen-Warren (adapted from example provided to V Karkou for 'Arts Therapies: from Theory to Practice' study [Karkou 2002; reproduced with permission]]—cont'd

Description of process	Comments from the authors
Beginning of DT process 'In this case we looked for images of God that had resonance for the client. [We chose to work with] some *medieval paintings* as she had mentioned these [before]. These contained images of Hell and were bleak and frightening. I talked about the *Mystery Plays* and she was quite interested. We worked dramatically with the role of The Virgin Mary as she was portrayed as gentle and loving. This started to help the client to embody in a slow and tender manner. Mary was also viewed as a messenger to God.'	*[Projection]* *[Mystery Plays are a form of early medieval drama* that grew under the sponsorship of the church. Initially they were significant sections of the mass, which were elaborated until they became short *liturgical dramas.* The selection of Mystery Plays is based on the client's initial images]
Development of DT work 'The work developed through the texts of the Mystery Plays (Mary, Jesus). She viewed it as safe to play these characters through a play text but would have seen it as blasphemous to have improvised these roles. The work developed through one of the plays performed by itinerant players, *Mankind.* She played Mercy and the characters who mock God and Mercy. *Playing the roles allowed her to experiment with gross body movement, humour and anger.* Playing Mercy allowed her to find mercy and love for herself. She saw the character of Mankind as herself and was able to improvise 'his' responses to Mercy and the other characters. Mary from the Mystery Play was always our 'safety net' and 'she' would often comment on the action.	'*Mankind* is a morality play that contains frequent references to excretion and is often irreverent, although the character of Mankind does find the true way of God by the end of the play.' *[Embodiment and Role enactments]*

I only played roles she had created and would copy her movement so they were not my creations.'	[The therapist's main interventions are those of the director. In one-to-one work, sometimes the therapist can also 'hold' roles so that the client can have a co-actor]
Completion of DT work 'She had acknowledged the God she had created through the character of Mankind and found compassion for herself. *She had reinvested in life* and could accept her body and right to express a range of emotions.'	[The client will *monitor progress* and changes and both client and therapist will examine helpful and unhelpful interventions, and monitor the effectiveness of DT. Relevant information is often passed on to managers and other interested parties]
Authors' wording in [brackets]	

Humanistic approaches to DT: starting with Jacob Moreno

The founder of humanistic thinking and, some would argue, one of the 'grandfathers' of DT, is Jacob Moreno. During the turn of the 20th century and as a reaction to the flourishing movement of psychoanalysis, Moreno, a qualified psychiatrist, started experimenting in Vienna with what he called the 'theatre of spontaneity'. After moving to the USA in 1925, Moreno developed these ideas further (Moreno 1972). One strand of his work developed into what is now known as psychodrama, a structured form of group therapy with a defined theoretical frame. Another strand involved sociodrama, a theatre practice with a similar rationale to psychodrama but with a slightly different emphasis (i.e. in sociodrama the emphasis is upon the group as a whole; it is often used with large groups, organisations or businesses and according to Moreno, aims to 'heal all of mankind' [Sternberg & Garcia 2000, p. 198]).

According to Garcia & Buchanan (2000), the main theoretical concepts that underlie psychodrama are:

- *Role theory*: each person is the construct of the roles he or she plays. These roles can be psychosomatic (roles manifested physically due to physical or psychological reasons), social (those enacted in relation to other people) or psychodramatic (roles that are enacted within people's heads). Dysfunction is seen as a lack of social or psychodramatic roles and function as a balance of both. When a new role is learnt, there is a specific development that people follow: to start with they take roles, then they learn to play roles and eventually they can create roles.
- *Sociometry*: the assessment of social choices people make in relation to at least one defined criterion. Connected with sociometry are also sets of tools developed by Moreno to facilitate social change such as the sociogram, the social atom, the role diagram, etc.
- *Spontaneity/creativity theory*: the two concepts are seen as linked with spirituality and interlinked with each other. The former is about readiness for action, while the latter is about the idea to act. Functionality is related to a sufficient amount of both of these. Dysfunction in the realms of spontaneity can be caused by paralysis, impulsivity or reactivity, while in creativity it can be related to pathological creativity (i.e. a compulsive drive for the new), inability to create new roles, or becoming overwhelmed by the number and complexities of social choices.

The above ideas have strong relevance to contemporary DT. Role theory and spontaneity/creativity are important concepts within many different approaches to DT, while sociometry has offered useful tools extensively used within DT practice as a means for assessment/evaluation (see Jones 1996 in relation to the use of the social atom within DT). Chesner (1994) adds to the above: the central role of drama in both approaches, the value placed upon the body and movement, a similar use of the space that is at the same time therapeutic as well as theatrical, and a similar emphasis upon externalising the 'drama of the inner world' (p. 116).

Methodologically, psychodrama assigns certain roles to the participants: the director (psychodramatist), the protagonist (one of the group members is selected each time), the auxiliary egos (group members playing certain roles assigned to them by the protagonist that have to do with either the protagonist's different parts of him or herself or with significant others), the audience and the stage. The common structure for a psychodrama session is the warm-up, action, and sharing as Table 7.7 shows.

Although some of the techniques described in Table 7.7, such as role-reversals and doubling, are also extensively used within DT, the methodology and structure of psychodrama is very specific. This constitutes a major difference between psychodrama and DT. Psychodrama has specificity in its techniques, while DT relies on a much wider methodology (Chesner 1994, Jones 1996). Another major difference between the two fields is, of course, the fact that psychodrama comes directly from the work of Moreno (1972), while DT owes its existence to more than just him and a lot to the theatre as we have seen in the previous section. It is interesting that in Lewis & Johnson's (2000) American publication, both psychodrama and sociodrama are presented as two of the current approaches to DT. The profound impact of Moreno's work upon American DT practice is apparent. Although such classification is not common within the UK context, the discussion between the two fields regarding areas of overlap and distinctive practices continues (e.g. Bannister 1995, Chesner 1994, Davies 1987, Jones 1996).

At the same time, the influence of humanistic schools of thought such as the Rogerian person-centred therapy, Gestalt and transactional analysis remain strong upon British DT practices (Valente & Fontana 1993). Existential thinking, another perspective that is often seen as associated with the humanistic tradition, can also be found within current British DT practices as the following example demonstrates.

A strategic, existential approach to DT; working with bereavement

Alida Gersie is well known in association with the therapeutic use of storymaking within DT (Gersie 1991, 1993/1994, Gersie & King 1990). Through her writings, workshops and her role as the Director of Studies on the Hertfordshire course, she has trained many dramatherapists in her storymaking approach. Over the years, she has selected numerous myths and traditional stories that come from a number of different cultures. Her belief is that myths and stories that survive from one generation to another bear universality of human existence and reveal themes that can have resonance with personal experiences. Gersie suggests a number of different structures that make the basic elements of a myth/story relevant for use within a DT context. Myths and/or stories are used as starting points for clients to create their own stories, their personal narratives. A basic structure of Gersie's storymaking approach to DT consists of: a landscape, the main character, a dwelling place, an obstacle, the helpmate and the resolution. This structure has been used as both a storymaking device for therapeutic use as well as an assessment tool (Meldrum 1994a,b).

However, another important strand of her work is related to brief DT and the conceptual links of her work with existential philosophical thinking. Gersie (1996) identifies three stages that are embedded within what she

Table 7.7: Session structure of 'classical' psychodrama – adapted from summary of Jacob Moreno's work by Garcia and Buchanan (2000, pp. 181–190)

Needs of clients

[Emotional growth, stress or phobias, mental health problems, children and adolescents with emotional difficulties, addictions, eating disorders, offenders]

Aims

[To achieve catharsis, i.e. deep emotional expression; to practise new ways of handling situations; to achieve insight and reorganise perceptual patterns in an 'action-based way' to achieve spiritual connections]

Session structure

1. Warm-up

[It can be structured or unstructured aiming to assist the emergence of a theme. A protagonist is then selected through: (a) the system, i.e. the setting/institution may determine that certain individuals may have to become protagonists, e.g. in order to assess the strengths and weakness of this individual, whether to discharge him/her, etc; (b) the director makes the selection; (c) a group member volunteers for this role; (d) the group chooses the protagonist]

2. Action

'After the protagonist is selected, the director and protagonist walk side by side in a circle and discuss the contract of the drama. [This] serves to deepen empathy between the director and the protagonist, to clear up any distorted expectations, to warm up the protagonist and group to the drama, and to establish a contract for the drama.'

[The contract is clearly restated in front of the group and usually the protagonist with the help of the director assigns roles to group members ('auxiliary egos'). Training for these roles and scene setting begins. Group members selected receive verbal descriptions of physical and psychological characteristics of the character and a role demonstration from the protagonist. The location, age of the protagonist, time and duration of the scene is clarified. The protagonist arranges objects in the room in a way that represent the scene as they want it to be and explain what they stand for in the imaginary scene.]

[The scene is enacted]

Some techniques used are:

(a) soliloquy: 'the protagonist is asked to . . . [walk] in a circle and [speak] aloud the thoughts and feelings in his head'. [This process is equivalent to free association but with movement]

(b) aside: 'the protagonist is instructed to turn his head to the side (an aside) [while action continues] and speak his thoughts he is thinking but not saying'. [The aside technique is used when the protagonist's body language and words do not match]

(c) double: 'an individual chosen by the protagonist literally reflects the protagonist's physical posture and brings a voice to underdeveloped domains. There are many kinds of doubles: affective, cognitive, somatic and amplifying and containing doubles . . .'

(d) role reversal: '. . . the protagonist reverses with another and becomes the other'.

(e) mirror: 'the protagonist is asked to step out of the scene and choose someone to take his role. The protagonist then observes his 'mirror' enact the scene'. [The protagonist can then see himself as others see him]

[Other techniques used are: the empty chair (later popularised by Perls within Gestalt therapy, future projection, 'psychodrama a deux' (i.e. psychodrama for two))]

3. Sharing

[After action, the protagonist deconstructed the scene and both him/her and the group members were asked to de-role. Thoughts and feelings about issues and concerns explored in the drama were shared. Identification with the protagonist was encouraged over criticism, judgement or advice]

Authors' wording in [brackets]

calls, 'long dramatisations' (that is dramatisations that are connected with clients' life experiences and that are not mere warm-up exercises): (1) a dilemma, possibility or problem that give rise to action, (2) the action itself that may involve a crisis or a turning point of some kind, (3) the solution or release that brings integration. Within the context of brief DT, there is a 'trouble' focus and group membership is arranged with common 'troubles' in mind. For example, prolonged bereavement is the common issue shared by the members of the group described in Table 7.8. Gersie calls this type of brief work 'strategic' and refers to 'problematisation', i.e. the process during which complex experiences that the client previously regarded as having no solutions are revisited and treated as difficulties with possible solution. It is interesting that although within a humanistic perspective that advocates working with clients' strengths, Gersie refers directly to problems the client faces through the 'emancipatory and conscientising aspects of DT' (A Gersie, unpublished interview, 2002, p. 1). Goals are agreed collaboratively with the clients in such a way that therapy is guided and motivated and clear criteria for the evaluation of outcomes are identified. According to her:

> The approach also focuses on unhelpful aspects of a client's accommodation to dysfunctional communication. Unhelpful aspects of such accommodation are reworked through strengthening the client's narrative, creative-expressive and performative capacity and by re-awakening his/her 'will to curiosity' and 'courage to encounter'. (A Gersie, unpublished interview, 2002, p.1)

The link between strengthening clients' narratives and Gersie's earlier writings on story-making is apparent and clearly framed within an existential philosophical position. Gersie (1996; A Gersie, unpublished interview, 2002) refers to her work as an existential DT approach and draws, amongst others, upon May (1961) and Yalom (1970). In *Dramatic Approaches to Brief Therapy*, Gersie (1996) also discusses the relevance of Marcel (1949) and Frankl (1963) to her work (i.e. existential theorists, who highlighted the value of articulating the nature of being and identifying the meaning of suffering).

The relevance of this orientation for clients facing complex bereavement can be further traced in Table 7.8.

Although existential thinking adapted for brief therapy is the strongest theoretical perspective for the above work, in the characteristic tendency of the field, Gersie draws upon more than one theoretical frameworks. For example, Bowlby's (1969) attachment theory is also seen as relevant to her work. She talks about the need for a holding environment and a strong therapeutic relationship, principles of work that are particularly important in psychodynamically-informed practices. Finally, she argues that her understanding of the 'self' incorporates both 'psycho-dynamic' and 'socio-dynamic' perspectives of human development and interaction.

Child drama and Jung in DT: starting with Peter Slade

The influence of the American educator Dewey upon the educational philosophy of English-speaking countries is already acknowledged in relation to

Table 7.8: Strategic, existential DT with a group of adults with complex bereavements – Alida Gersie [Adapted from example provided to V. Karkou for 'Arts Therapies: from Theory to Practice' study [© A. Gersie 2002, reproduced with permission]

Description of process	Comments from therapist and authors
Needs of clients [Brief DT group (12 sessions) consisting of 8 members who experienced *bereavements*. Amongst the members of the group there were:] '*Myra*, a childless woman in her mid-forties, who had experienced her husband's slow death from cancer about 12 months previously. *Joe* who was a burly man in his late thirties. He lived alone. His marriage had recently broken down after the death, a year earlier, of his 8-year-old daughter Laura who had died beneath the reversing wheels of Joe's own truck. His two surviving teenage children lived with their mother. When Joe joined the group his knowledge of life was based on a desperate, angry assessment that its burden was greater than he was able and willing to bear. . . . He had thought about various ways to *violently end his life* in excruciating detail and had committed himself in the silence of his heart to a steady, purposeful self-destruction.'	'During complex bereavements clients encounter *multiple concrete complex changes* in their lives. They often experience lack of understanding by important others, great pain and loss and disorientation.' [These] 'two clients represented the group's dominant *modes of dealing with grief:* (a) [Myra's] primary way of surviving her pain was through withdrawal, silence and isolation. (b) Joe rushed from one pub to another, trying not to think, not to remember that fatal moment.' 'He echoed *Camus*' words that there is but one truly serious philosophical problem and that is suicide.'
Main aims 'Restoration of function, education regarding symptoms, symptom relief, support, catharsis, socialisation, life-goal and life-philosophy clarification.'	
Beginning of DT process [The beginning of the work involved establishing] 'a clear contract and identifiable goals that can be evaluated (process- and final-evaluation).	

Continued

Table 7.8: Strategic, existential DT with a group of adults with complex bereavements – Alida Gersie ([Adapted from example provided to V. Karkou for 'Arts Therapies: from Theory to Practice' study [© A. Gersie 2002, reproduced with permission]—cont'd

Description of process	Comments from therapist and authors
[Also, building] a group that can work together and with the dramatherapist.	
At this stage all *exercises* [were] relatively short and purposefully sequential. They [invited] cooperation and [matched] the clients' needs and concentration-span.	*Each exercise is very carefully chosen as it must achieve multiple aims.*
When Joe and Myra first met in the group, they appeared to have *little in common*. Her mouse-like quality and his ferocious verbal style alienated them from each other. The witnessing of her husband's agonisingly gradual death at age 50 seemed so very different from the violent shock of his child's fatal accident at age 8. Though Myra struggled with her beliefs, she was at her core a devout Christian who believed that her husband, Martin, awaited her in after-life. Joe was convinced religion was mere illusion.'	'It is . . . vital to welcome and validate the *uniqueness of each person's history* and experiences, to model active respect for difference and the ability to tolerance intense emotions, contradictions, ambiguities and uncertainty. . . . I ensure that each client in the group receives the same amount of "timed" attention, no more but also no less.'
Development of DT work 'During the fifth session Joe and Myra both spoke with strong feelings about God's and Life's uselessness. The group responded to their despair by sheltering in tough silence. After some talk and reflective interpretations, I suggested that we might do a role-play provisionally called: "*The trial of life*". In this role-play "Life" would be on trial for its supposedly unfair cruelty. Intrigued, the group noted that this required the roles of a prosecutor, a judge, and various witnesses. I suggested that we also needed roles called "Life" and "its advocate". I placed two chairs in the enactment area to represent their "presences".	[In this case the starting point is not a pre-existing myth or story. The idea for *dramatisation* comes from a group theme and roles are identified primarily by the group-members]

Continued

Once the enactment area was set up each group member wrote a *witness statement or testimony* that outlined his/her case against "Life".
Their writing addressed:
The losses they had experienced.
Why these were unjust.
I suggested that their statement could refer to actual people and events, and be no longer than two sides of an A4 sheet of paper.

[*Personal narratives are re-constructed and shared*]

For the enactment of the "testimonies" I designed a *rotation-role-play*. Here each client plays each role in a predetermined, sequential pattern. In this case: the role of Witness for the prosecution, the role of Judge and finally the role of the Prosecutor. When the Prosecutor leaves the enactment area, the others change role. A new person then enters in the role of Witness and the same sequence begins. In each role I invited the clients to use a distinct performative move, such as the beating of a gong and some text-echoing. Additionally the Prosecutor was asked to use the closing statement: "Your honour I rest my case." These moves provided further containment.

[The role sequence was the result of] 'a very carefully considered therapeutic, *strategic decision*.'

I carefully *discussed this rotation-role-play and the performative moves with the group-members.*
A moving sequence of mini-scenes was soon established. The returning sentence: "Your honour, I rest my case" was spoken with increasing dignity and outrage. During the final scene Myra was in the role of judge. Joe went to the witness place. A client named Peter, was the Prosecutor. Joe crumbled the piece of paper with his written statement in his hand. With a surprisingly strong and kindly voice Myra said: "Joe, the court wants to hear you speak. Please tell us your story." Joe

[*Role of drama*]
'Drama serves not only as pleasure, but also as protection to bring a certain part of a chaotic world under control. I aimed to construct such a protective order through the conscious use of stage setting, rhythmicity and predictable punctuation. Thereby to safeguard and to enhance individual's involvement. The establishment of shared understanding of the "dramatic how" of intense work substantially increases clients' authority over involvement in the enactment. The "imaginative rehearsal" also establishes mutually understood boundaries and clarifies expectations regarding the dramatherapist's whereabouts and function during the enactment.'

Table 7.8: Strategic, existential DT with a group of adults with complex bereavements – Alida Gersie (Adapted from example provided to V. Karkou for 'Arts Therapies: from Theory to Practice' study [© A. Gersie 2002, reproduced with permission])—cont'd

Description of process	Comments from therapist and authors
groaned: "I can't. I can't." With my encouragement Myra held steady in her role. The other group-members watched quietly. I now asked Joe if Peter, in the role of Prosecutor might read the statement for him. With tears trickling down his face Joe nodded his sad consent. The final words were: "That moment . . . that moment my daughter died." Looking at Myra, the Judge, Peter repeated: "His daughter died. Your honour . . . I rest my case." Then he burst into tears. On hearing Peter sob, Joe shouted: "It's no bloody use." He made ready to leave the enactment space, ready too to embrace the feeling that there was no way out. I asked Joe to wait a little and to ponder whether leaving the enactment space, and therefore not hearing himself speak the words he had written, was really what he needed and wanted to do. He sat a while, shaking his head. Then he said: "I don't know how I can." Peter offered to stand next to him. With Peter at his side Joe then read his own words, softly and quite steadily. At the end of the statement he added these crucial words: "I killed my daughter. I murdered her." There was a long, long silence. Into that silence Myra's voice emerged. *She spoke as if to an unknown presence: "There is no easy answer . . ." Then, she continued: "He is not guilty of murder." And turning to Joe: "You are not guilty."* I cannot find the words adequately to describe the change that came over Joe's face when he heard her words. He repeated with a voice trembling with hesitant wonder: "Not guilty . . .?"	'The accumulative effect of the previous mini-scenes and her own recent playing of the role of witness contribute somewhat to Myra's action in her *role as Judge.*'

I asked Myra and Joe to freeze in role for a brief moment. To hold the same posture for a little while. Then I requested that Peter beat the gong three times. As agreed this would signal the play's overall ending. The gong sounded. *Then the three players fell in each other's arms and wept.* After a while they thoughtfully crossed the boundary from enactment to group space. The enactment space with its five chairs and one gong faced the group in all its post-performance emptiness. Words came slowly. The group took its time to de-role and de-brief the enactment space. Finally I invited each client to touch the chairs that represented "Life" and its "Advocate", and to make one closing statement. Everyone participated in this exercise. Addressing "Life" Myra said: "You didn't give me what I wanted". Joe tasted the words: "Not guilty?" A calmer and paradoxically somewhat happier group of people left the session that day. . . . *A new strength and intimacy had been established.'*

[Dramatisation had a strong cathartic outcome]

'The group had dared to become publicly unreconciled and thereby infinitely stronger in their awareness of grief.'

Completion of DT work

'During this session the group grew beyond the paralysis of stuck mourning, where each person's sorrow is isolated and kept apart from life even though it is enacted in life. Grief's dark, vibrant centre could now be shared. The group's . . . solution to felt pain had been [to maintain] silence about that which mattered most. The *dramatic structure of the rotation-role-play and its theme had contributed to its successful reworking.'*

[Endings]
'In bereavement groups the ending of the group is present from the beginning. Group-members learn constructive ways of dealing with themes of beginning, being together, ending and letting go in each session and each activity. The actual ending phase of such dramatherapy groups takes about a third to a quarter of its overall time. During this phase it is acknowledged that an important bond exists and that the ending of the group will unavoidably alter this bond. This allows group-members to re-work the done and to work through what must still be done. Clients are further encouraged to share their fears, delights and plans for anticipated and the hoped for future events as well as the preparation for likely difficulties.'

Authors' wording in [brackets]

the other arts therapies. Also acknowledged is the shift of education, and arts education in particular, towards a child-centred practice. Within a drama education context, names such as Heathcote (1991), Courtney (1980) and others are firmly linked with the emerging child-centred drama education (Meldrum 1994a). These people have acknowledged the value of dramatic play, especially in relation to work with children, have outlined developmental processes, and have given rise to therapeutic approaches to drama, either within the remits of DT or play therapy. Ann Cattanach is one example of a dramatherapist/play therapist who has been extensively influenced by theoreticians in education drama of the 1960s and 1970s (Cattanach 1993, 1994a,b, 2003). However, amongst the drama educators, the person who deserves most attention is Peter Slade, as he was the first to coin the term 'Dramatherapy' (in 1939) and to make a direct contribution to the emergence of DT in the UK.

Slade's starting point was an approach to educational drama with a strong client-centred character. Children's creativity and engagement to drama was seen as often disturbed and controlled by adults. His message was that we – adults – had to listen to our children (Meldrum 1994a). His work very often fell between what is currently considered an overlap of education and therapy. For example, he claimed that his role was about facilitating children's 'free-play' and regarded his child drama approach as offering children the benefits of emotional and physical control, confidence, ability to observe, and toleration and consideration of others (Slade 1954). Thirty years later he described DT as 'therapy for educational purposes' (Schattner & Courtney 1981, p. 78).

However, even before his book on child drama was published (1954) and before the Second World War, Slade was experimenting with bringing his drama approach to adults within a much clearer therapeutic context (Jones 1996). During 1937–1939, he worked in a collaborative manner with a Jungian analyst called Kraemer. Kraemer would work with clients on dreams in a Jungian way, while Slade would play through these dreams with them or engage them in improvisatory enactment of situations. Both Kraemer and Slade were working on a one-to-one basis with clients. Although Slade (in an interview with Jones 1996) acknowledged that he did not have enough psychotherapeutic knowledge and experience and it was important to work alongside a qualified doctor, he also witnessed a number of breakthroughs that clients had with him in drama enactments in a way that verbal analysis was not achieving. Slade's explanation for this was that verbal analysis was working with 'projective play', while his drama enactments were to do with 'personal play'. He regarded a combination of both as important. Slade reports on one of these 'breakthroughs' for a client he was seeing with Kraemer as follows:

> I remember a man who had some difficulty over getting into trains and he didn't quite know why it was and in his work with Kraemer this kept coming up, this business of the train. He came to me and we were doing trains together. We would be sitting here and 'You're in a train and I'm in a train and perhaps we're having breakfast together'. I would say, 'Have you seen the paper today?' or something like that, and that would start him off. Then I would choose something that was in my pretend paper, probably trying to get closer to his mind, and so on and then something would come out of that. This man suddenly said, 'My God! The crash!' I said, 'no, I don't think we are in a crash. That's something that

happened somewhere else'. 'My God, you're bloody right! Yes!' And he remembered the crash and that was why he was afraid to get into trains. It was somebody he had loved very much, they had died in a crash.' (Interview with Jones 1996, p. 85)

As a result of Slade's collaborative work with Kraemer, a number of Jungian concepts became increasingly relevant to child drama and the application of this work to children and adults. Active imagination was one such idea (Jones 1996). Identifying characteristics of children's play that were innate rather than socially imposed was another; his observations regarding children's play often resembled Jung's ideas of the existence of a collective unconscious and the presence of archetypes (Pearson 1996).

Although Slade's work is not that popular anymore, his emphasis upon play and child development, and his suggestion that Jungian thinking offers a relevant theoretical framework for drama/theatre work, has been taken on board by a number of contemporary DT practitioners (Valente & Fontana 1993). Furthermore, his ideas have influenced a number of the pioneers of DT in the UK, including Jennings, and even more profoundly, Lindkvist, the founder of the Sesame approach, as we will see in the following section.

The Sesame approach to DT with abused children

Marian (Billy) Lindkvist's initial work involved offering workshops to occupational therapists in the use of movement and drama. As early as 1964, she met Slade who recognised the links of this early work with child drama and the psychological implications of her approach. He encouraged her to develop further the psychological side of her work. Although initially this suggestion was met with despondence (Lindkvist regarded herself primarily as an artist), she became increasingly informed by Slade's child drama ideas. She also pursued psychotherapeutic justifications of her practice through Jungian analytical psychology, an area of work Slade himself was familiar with. In order to acquire a language and a theoretical frame for using movement and dance, Lindkvist also drew upon Laban's movement theory as the third main influence upon her practice.

By 1975, the initial workshop-based training became a full-time advanced level course established at the Kingsway Princeton College before it moved to its current location at the Central School of Speech and Drama. The strong experiential and movement/dance aspects of Lindkvist's approach have been retained up to the present day and are particular to the Sesame approach to DT. Another important characteristic of Sesame work is its oblique approach to therapy. This means that its practitioners see difficulties as expressed through metaphor and symbol without the need for verbal confrontation and exposure (see similar positions discussed in Jennings's theatre model, and in 'The Creative MT Approach' in Ch. 5). In summary, some of the main assumptions of the Sesame approach are:

- Drama and movement in a safe environment enable people suffering in mind, spirit or body to find ways of expressing difficulties spontaneously and naturally.
- The emphasis is upon the creative and expressive use of the imagination.

- Symbolic material offered by the client in drama and movement can act as a bridge between the conscious and the unconscious.
- The dramatic or movement context and the session structure can act as containment that channels and holds the release of inner/unconscious needs.
- Coming to terms with aspects of the unconscious, developing personal strengths and working with the person as a whole through the creative expression is likely to have real and lasting effect on a person. (Sesame 2003)

The influence of Jungian analytical theory (Jung 1990) is apparent in the above principles and reflected in the Sesame course curriculum (Sesame 2003) and recent publications (e.g. Pearson 1996). Similarly to other Jungian-informed practices in arts therapies (e.g. Champernowne in AT and Whitehouse in DMT) the client is encouraged to engage in the art-making process in a 'natural' way, i.e. without interference from the therapist, while the therapist's role is to act as a 'midwife'; someone who assists the birth and rebirth of the art and/or the client. Laban-based movement work (Laban 1975) and Lindkvist's work on 'movement with touch' (a set of exercises that resemble Sherborne's [1990] work on developmental movement) are encouraged, alongside voice work, story telling/making (traditional stories are frequently used), mime that relies on gesture, Slade-informed dramatic play and straightforward dramatic enactments. Sesame practitioners work with a wide range of clients including the elderly, people with disabilities, psychiatry and forensic psychiatry, and children facing all sorts of difficulties including autism and challenging behaviour. Some of this work has been researched by Lindkvist herself, especially regarding people with schizophrenia, autism and adults with learning disabilities (Sesame 2003).

Current Sesame practice places an emphasis upon creating a safe environment in order to open up the possibility for play. According to Pearson (1996, p.12):

> The space is held by the session leader who is responsible for bringing people into the inner space by way of some kind of warm-up and bridging activity, being firmly present and in charge while the group experiences the symbolic reality of the shared inner space, and then bringing them back to a sense of the here and now at the end of sessions.

Despite the emphasis of the above extract upon the role of the leader, a lot of the work undertaken by Sesame workers (often referred to as drama and movement practitioners) involves more than one facilitator, as the example in Table 7.9. One of the Sesame workers involved in this example is Marian Lindkvist herself, referred to and known amongst her colleagues as 'Billy'.

The movement components of the approach are not described in the example in Table 7.9. Nevertheless, Pearson (1996) describes movement exercises as integral to the session, often in terms of bridging between children's initial unfocused energy and the need for focused attention during story telling/making. In other cases, movement might be the main focus for a number of sessions and the work might resemble DMT practices more closely (e.g. Smail 1996). Consequently, at times, Sesame work can be seen as a

Table 7.9: An example of Sesame work with 'disturbed' children – Jenny Pearson (1996, pp. 184–189) [Adapted]

Description of process	Comments from therapist and authors
Needs of clients within specific setting [*Children* who were physically or sexually abused. The setting was a small therapeutic community] 'Jason was an 8-year-old boy who was very absent-minded, – could neither read nor write and didn't seem to be able to learn. [He] was described as "borderline", though it was also felt that his symptoms could be the result of severe trauma.'	[Work with adults may also take place. One-to-one work is also a possibility]
Main assumptions '. . . *story* is giving [children] an entry to places within themselves that they didn't know were there, so that they begin to surprise themselves and us with powers of imagination and communication.' [*Movement*] 'serves as a "bridge" leading from the wild, unfocused movement of children on arrival into a quieter, more focused place where there it becomes possible to tell and enact a story.'	[*Traditional fairy tales and myths* from different cultures are primarily used in order to call up personal feelings and energies with a universal quality] [*Movement with touch* exercises are often used when working with children as an introduction/physical warm-up. Special attention is placed upon the use of touch with this client group]
Beginning of process [Jason joined an existing DT group soon after he arrived in the centre in which there was more than one Sesame practitioner and a number of other children]	

Continued

Table 7.9: An example of Sesame work with 'disturbed' children – Jenny Pearson (1996, pp. 184–189) [Adapted]—cont'd

Description of process	Comments from therapist and authors
'One day, when the small group in his drama session was embarked on a ship, Jason suddenly came out of his trance and took command. He continued to engage in the drama sessions that followed, usually contriving to seize a part in which he could exercise *control*.	[This behaviour is seen as] *'a sensible precaution for someone needing to protect himself and his feelings.'*
When he required someone to carry out his orders, one of us would quickly get into that role and be *exaggeratedly subservient.* Then he began to suggest *original twists to some of the [group] stories. . .'*	[It is important that the child can *see and enjoy* the humorous side of what is going on] [Original contributions are seen as showing *active imagination at work*]
Development of work 'One day came when he announced that *he had a story that he wanted to enact . . .* We encouraged him to tell his story. . . Jason asked us to sit around him and told the following story:	[*Suggestions from the group members are taken on board. Story is heard without promises that it will be enacted as they are not always 'actable']*
There was a boy called Jack who found a stone with a dark hole in it. He looked inside and found two snakes, a Mummy snake and a Daddy snake, who began to chase Jack. They moved quickly, but he managed to get away because he could move at the speed of light. After he got away he came to the woods and a Woodcutter looked after him. One day the Woodcutter and Jack were in the woods and they saw a brown thing and a spotted thing in the shape of trees. The Woodcutter saw eyes in the trees looking down at them and he realised that they were	

the snakes. He grabbed a very sharp axe and cut the snakes in half. After that Jack was safe and went home to his parents.

We were all amazed at the story.

As we prepared to enact it . . . [Jason] spoke firmly to Billy [i.e. Marian Lindkvist] telling her "You be Jack!" Billy said "I can't run fast enough. I'm too old." "You don't have to", said Jason. "You can pretend like this!" And he showed her.

In fact, [another member of the Sesame team] took the part of Jack and Billy chose to be the Woodcutter.

We enacted the story for Jason while he sat on a table and watched. As the Woodcutter, Billy contributed an *important detail*: after cutting the snakes in half, the Woodcutter skinned them and asked Jack to help her make something from their beautiful skins."

Completion of work

'Jason went on constructing stories with shapely plots and traditional imagery for the rest of his time at the [Centre], not every week, but frequently. Coinciding with this development, we were informed he had *begun to make progress* with his reading and writing.'

Authors' wording in [brackets]

[*Facilitators' response* Stories created by children can be appreciated for their structure and content, as well as the degree to which they show original imagination and personal material. In this case, the fact that Jason had problems with his learning made his story even more impressive, as it suggested very clear thinking and learning potential.]

'*It is a basic rule that people choose what parts they play.*'

[In most cases, *both children and Sesame facilitators are involved in the enactments*]

'This kind of *resolution through making or growing* at the end of a story that has expressed angry, even murderous feelings, is a form of containment frequently used in Sesame.'

[*Therapeutic benefit*]

'It has been noticeable that . . . children who have found a unique, creative voice in drama and movement sessions have simultaneously begun to change and blossom in their lives outside.'

hybrid practice between DT and DMT. And although this 'hybrid' nature created ambiguity in the past regarding professional affiliations and course accreditation, the Sesame approach is now a clearly-established approach to DT with a specific ethos and practice.

Other approaches to DT

There are a number of other approaches to DT that have not been covered so far. One important contribution comes from Ditty Dokter, a dramatherapist and dance movement therapist with lengthy involvement in DT and DMT training for several years. Dokter (D Dokter, unpublished interview, 2002) regards her work as a developmental approach based on psychodynamic principles. She uses Jennings' EPR developmental model for her clinical practice, i.e. she places an emphasis upon projective and movement work as ways of accessing drama and role. She also values dramatic play and the concept of appropriate emotional distance for achieving therapeutic outcomes. However, unlike Jennings, the wider resonance of her work comes from psychodynamic frameworks (object relations and group analytic schools of thought) in which the main agent of therapeutic change is attributed to the relationship between the client and the therapist or between the client and the group. Dokter (D Dokter, unpublished interview, 2002) will acknowledge and work with transference and countertransference issues, she will make psychodynamic interpretations and, if appropriate, she will feed back these interpretations to the clients. She also encourages links between feelings evoked during dramatic enactments and both past experiences as well as current life situations. Thus, dramatic work is seen primarily as a reflective tool rather than as sufficient in itself to generate therapeutic change. Dokter has written about her clinical work with a range of client groups including those with eating disorders (Dokter 1994, 1996), immigrants and refugees (Dokter 1998, 2000), and about research studies in related topics (e.g. Dokter 1993, Dokter et al 2002). With her current role as a course convenor of the Roehampton course, her perspective is expected to be particularly influential in the future development of DT in the UK.

Other important approaches to DT come from an American context and are becoming increasingly influential upon British DT practice. For example, Johnson's (2000b) approach to DT is highly regarded amongst his British colleagues. Johnson (2000b) advocates a developmental perspective, what he calls a 'developmental transformations' approach, that has as its essence 'an embodied encounter in the playspace' (p. 87). Johnson (2000b) argues for the relevance of the following sources in the conceptualisation of this approach: theatre (particularly Grotowski and Spolin), cognitive development, psychoanalytic thinking (particularly free association), object relations, client-centred therapy, DMT, existentialism and deconstruction next to the spiritual perspective of Buddhism. However, at the same time he encourages the therapist to act in the session in an a-theoretical way in order to become able to really experience what takes place with the client.

Another influential approach to DT, again originating in the USA, is Landy's role theory model (1986, 1993, 2000). According to Meldrum

(1994a), role and role-play is also extensively discussed within British practice. However, it is primarily American DT (and Landy in particular) that has articulated role theory in the most eloquent and comprehensive manner. Landy's (2000) theory is rooted in the theatre (e.g. Brook, alongside Stanislavski and Brecht) as well as in social psychology, symbolic interactionism and dramaturgy in particular (e.g. Mead 1934 and Goffman 1959). Links with Jung (1990) are also made. In Landy's (1986) role model, the aim of the therapy is to help clients increase the number of roles they have and to make flexible transitions from one role to another. The therapeutic outcome involves clients becoming skilled performers in their everyday life. The process of achieving this aim, involves working with an identified 'role', a 'counter role' and a 'guide'. It also involves the application of Landy's (1993) taxonomy of roles for assessment and evaluation.

Lewis & Johnson (2000) mention a number of other approaches to DT within the American context. Amongst them, the following might be of greater relevance to British practice: the psychoanalytic approach (Irwin 2000), the integrative five-phase model (Emunah 2000), narrative approaches (Dunne 2000), developmental themes approach (Lewis 2000a) transpersonal DT (Lewis 2000b) and family dynamic play approach (Harvey 2000).

Summary

DT was the third arts therapies discipline to form an association and achieve professional status following the example of MT and AT. However, the roots of the profession can be traced back to the turn of the 20th century in the work inspired by leading figures in the theatre such as Stanislavski, Artaud and Brecht. Before and after the Second World War, the interest expressed by health professionals in the use of active techniques in therapy and work carried out in child drama, were additional contributors to the emergence of DT as a modern profession. Current professional development is evident in the establishment of several training courses; as well as a wide expansion in areas of employment and client groups, which includes consultancy work for organisations and workshops for the general public. Dramatherapists use a wide range of techniques stemming from the theatre and drama and show preferences for humanistic, eclectic/integrative and artistic/creative therapeutic trends. Some of the examples of current practice that were presented in this chapter include: the theatre model, a strategic existential approach and the Sesame approach. Parallels between these models and important pioneers in the field were drawn. For example, we found conceptual links between the work of Evrenov and Iljine and the theatre model, the work of Moreno and DT practices with a humanistic orientation, and the contributions of Slade and Jung with the Sesame approach. Other practices were also briefly described such as psychoanalytically/psychodynamically-informed DT, the developmental transformation approach and the role theory model. The first is a growing type of practice within the British context; the other two originate in the USA, but are becoming increasingly influential upon British DT through good-quality publications and workshops.

References

- Andersen-Warren M 1996 Therapeutic theatre. In: Mitchell S (ed) DT: clinical studies. Jessica Kingsley, London, p 108–135
- Andersen-Warren M, Grainger R 2000 Practical approaches to DT: the shield of Perseus. Jessica Kingsley, London
- Bannister A 1995 Images and action: dramatherapy and psychodrama with sexually abused adolescents. In: Jennings S (ed) Dramatherapy with children and adolescents. Routledge, London, p 169–186
- Boal A (McBride M L, trans.) 1979 Theatre of the oppressed. Urizen Books, New York
- Bowlby J 1969 Attachment and loss, vol I. Hogarth Press, London
- British Association of Dramatherapists (BADth) 2004 About dramatherapy. Online. Available: http://www.badth.org.uk/therapy.html 11 December 2004
- Brook P 1968 The empty space. Penguin Books, London
- Burleigh L R, Beutler L E 1997 A critical analysis of two creative arts therapies. The Arts of Psychotherapy 23(5):375–381
- Carlson M 1993 Theories of the theatre: a historical and critical survey, from the Greeks to the present day. Cornell University Press, Ithaca
- Cattanach A 1993 Play therapy with abused children. Jessica Kingsley, London
- Cattanach A 1994a The developmental model of dramatherapy. In: Jennings S, Cattanach A, Mitchell S et al (eds) The handbook of dramatherapy. Routledge, London, p 28–40
- Cattanach A 1994b Dramatic play with children: the interface of DT and play therapy. In: Jennings S, Cattanach A, Mitchell S et al (eds) The handbook of dramatherapy. Routledge, London, p 133–144
- Cattanach A 2003 Introduction to play therapy. Brunner-Routledge, London
- Chesner A 1994 DT and psychodrama: similarities and differences. In: Jennings S, Cattanach A, Mitchell S, et al (eds) The handbook of dramatherapy. Routledge, London, p 114–132
- Courtney R 1980 The dramatic curriculum. Drama Book Specialists, New York
- Davies M H 1987 DT and psychodrama. In: Jennings S (ed) Dramatherapy: theory and practice 1. Routledge, London, p 104–123
- Dent-Brown K 2004 UK research register for DT. Online. Available: http://www.badth.org.uk/register.html 8 October 2004
- Dokter D 1993 Dramatherapy across Europe: cultural contradictions. In: Payne H (ed) Handbook of inquiry in the arts therapies: one river many currents. Jessica Kingsley, London and Philadelphia, p 79–90
- Dokter D 1994 Fragile board – arts therapies and clients with eating disorders. In: Dokter D (ed) Arts therapies and clients with eating disorders: fragile board. Jessica Kingsley, London, p 7–22
- Dokter D 1996 DT with clients with eating disorders: fragile board. In: Mitchell S (ed) DT: clinical studies. Jessica Kingsley, London, p 179–193
- Dokter D (ed) 1998 Arts therapies, refugees and migrants: reaching across borders. Jessica Kingsley, London
- Dokter D (ed) 2000 Exile: refugees and the arts therapies. University of Hertfordshire, Hertfordshire
- Dokter D, Karkou V, Burchell et al 2002 Supporting student placement learning: the tutor's role. Presented at the Hertfordshire Integrated Learning Project (HILP) Annual Conference, July 2002
- Dunne P 2000 Narradrama: narrative approach in DT. In: Lewis P, Johnson D R (eds) Current approaches in drama therapy. Charles C Thomas, Springfield IL, p 111–128
- Emunah R 2000 The integrative five-phase model of drama therapy. In: Lewis P, Johnson D R (eds) Current approaches in drama therapy. Charles C Thomas, Springfield, IL, p 70–86
- Fox J 1994 Acts of service: spontaneity, commitment, tradition in the non-scripted theatre. Tusitala Publishing, New Paltz
- Frankl V 1963 Man's search for meaning. Beacon Press, Boston
- Garcia A, Buchanan D R 2000 Psychodrama. In: Lewis P, Johnson D R (eds) Current approaches in drama therapy. Charles C Thomas, Springfield, p 162–195
- Gersie A 1991 Storymaking in bereavement: dragons fight in the meadow. Jessica Kingsley, London

- Gersie A 1993/1994 On being both author and actor: reflections on therapeutic storymaking, Dramatherapy 15(3):2–11
- Gersie A (ed) 1996 Dramatic approaches to brief therapy. Jessica Kingsley, London
- Gersie A, King N 1990 Storymaking in education and therapy. Jessica Kingsley & Stockholm Institute of Education Press, London
- Goffman E 1959 The presentation of self in everyday life. Doubleday, New York
- Grotowski J 1968 Towards a poor theatre. Simon and Schuster, New York
- Harvey S 2000 Family dynamic play. In: Lewis P, Johnson D R (eds) Current approaches in drama therapy. Charles C Thomas, Springfield IL, p 379–411
- Heathcote D 1991 Collected writings on education and drama. Northwestern University, Evanston, IL
- Irwin E 2000 Psychoanalytic approach to drama therapy. In: Lewis P, Johnson D R (eds) Current approaches in drama therapy. Charles C Thomas, Springfield IL, p 27–49
- Jennings S 1983 Models of practice in DT. Dramatherapy 7(1):3–6
- Jennings S 1986 Creative drama in groupwork Winslow Press, Oxon
- Jennings S (ed) 1987 Dramatherapy: theory and practice 1. Routledge, London
- Jennings S 1992 Reason in madness; therapeutic journeys through King Lear. In: Jennings S (ed) Dramatherapy: theory and practice 2. Routledge, London, p 5–18
- Jennings S 1994a Theatre, ritual and transformation: semoi temiar. Routledge, London
- Jennings S 1994b The theatre of healing: metaphor and metaphysics in the healing process. In: Jennings S, Cattanach A, Mitchell S et al (eds) The handbook of dramatherapy. Routledge, London, p 93–113
- Jennings S 1995 Dramatherapy for survival: some thoughts on transitions and choices for children and adolescents. In: Jennings S (ed) Dramatherapy with children and adolescents. Routledge, London, p 90–104
- Jennings S 1996 Brief DT: the healing power of the dramatised here and now. In: Gersie A (ed) Dramatic approaches to brief therapy. Jessica Kingsley, London, p 201–215
- Jennings S 1998 Introduction to dramatherapy: theatre and healing, Ariadne's Ball of Thread. Jessica Kingsley, London
- Jennings S, McGinley J D, Orr M 1997 Masking and unmasking: DT with offender patients. In: Jennings S (ed) Dramatherapy: theory and practice 3. Routledge, London, p 83–112
- Johnson D R 1982 Principles and techniques of drama therapy. The Arts in Psychotherapy 9:83–90
- Johnson. D R 1992 The dramatherapist in role. In: Jennings S (ed) Dramatherapy: theory and practice 2. Routledge, London, p 112–136
- Johnson D R 2000a History of drama therapy. In: Lewis P, Johnson D R (eds) Current approaches in drama therapy. Charles C Thomas, Springfield, p 5–15
- Johnson D R 2000b Developmental transformations: towards the body as presence. In: Lewis P, Johnson D R (eds) Current approaches in drama therapy. Charles C Thomas, Springfield IL, p 87–110
- Joint Quality Assurance Committee (JQAC) 2002 Handbook. Unpublished document produced by the Arts Therapies Board, APMT, BAAT and BADth
- Jones P 1996 Drama as therapy: theatre as living. Routledge, London
- Jung C G (ed) 1990 Man and his symbols. Arkana, Penguin Group, London (first published by Aldus Books 1964)
- Karkou V 2002 Report: from theory to practice. Unpublished report submitted to the University of Hertfordshire
- Laban R 1975 Modern educational dance. MacDonald and Evans, London
- Lahad M 1992 Storymaking: an assessment method for coping with stress. Six-piece Storymaking and the BASIC Ph. In: Jennings S (ed) Dramatherapy: theory and practice 2. Routledge, London, p 150–163
- Landy R 1986 Drama therapy: concepts and practices. Charles C. Thomas, Springfield, IL
- Landy R 1993 Persona and performance: the meaning of role in drama, therapy and everyday life. Jessica Kingsley, London
- Landy R 2000 Role theory and the role method of drama therapy. In: Lewis P, Johnson D R (eds) Current approaches in drama therapy. Charles C Thomas, Springfield IL, p 50–69
- Lewis R 2000a The developmental themes approach in drama therapy. In: Lewis P, Johnson D R (eds) Current approaches in drama therapy. Charles C Thomas, Springfield IL, p 129-161
- Lewis R 2000b Recovery and individuation: two stage model in transpersonal drama therapy. In: Lewis P, Johnson D R (eds) Current approaches in drama therapy. Charles C Thomas, Springfield IL, p 260–287

- Lewis P, Johnson D R (eds) 2000 Current approaches in drama therapy. Charles C Thomas, Springfield, p 50–69
- Marcel G (Harari M, trans.) 1949 The philosophy of existence. Collins Harvill, London
- May R 1961 Existential psychology. Basic Books, New York:
- Mead G H 1934 Mind, self and society. University of Chicago Press, Chicago
- Meldrum B A 1993 Theatrical model of DT. Dramatherapy 14(2):10–13
- Meldrum B 1994a Historical background and overview of dramatherapy. In: Jennings S, Cattanach A, Mitchell S et al (eds) The handbook of dramatherapy. Routledge, London, p 12–27
- Meldrum B 1994b Evaluation and assessment in dramatherapy. In: Jennings S, Cattanach A, Mitchell S et al (eds) The handbook of dramatherapy. Routledge, London, p 187–208
- Mitchell S 1990 The theatre of Peter Brook as a model for dramatherapy. Dramatherapy 13:1
- Mitchell S 1994a The theatre of self-expression; a 'therapeutic theatre' model of dramatherapy. In: Jennings S, Cattanach A, Mitchell S et al (eds) The handbook of dramatherapy. Routledge, London, p 41–57
- Mitchell S 1994b The dramatherapy venture project. In: Jennings S, Cattanach A, Mitchell S et al (eds) The handbook of dramatherapy. Routledge, London, p 145–165
- Mitchell S 1996 The ritual of individual DT. In: Mitchell S (ed) DT: clinical studies. Jessica Kingsley, London, p 71–90
- Moreno J L 1972 Psychodrama. Boston House, New York
- Payne H (ed) 1993 Handbook of inquiry in the arts therapies: one river many currents. Jessica Kingsley, London
- Pearson J (ed) 1996 Discovering the self through drama and movement: the Sesame approach. Jessica Kingsley, London
- Schattner G, Courtney G 1981 Drama in therapy, vols 1, 2. Drama Book Specialists, New York
- Sesame 2003 Leaflet. Sesame Institute, London
- Sherborne V 1990 Developmental movement for children. Cambridge University Press, Cambridge
- Slade P 1954 Child drama. University Press, London
- Smail M 1996 Moving through a block in psychotherapy. In: Pearson J (ed) Discovering the self through drama and movement: the Sesame approach. Jessica Kingsley, London, p 175–180
- Sternberg P, Garcia A 2000 Sociodrama. In: Lewis P, Johnson D R (eds) Current approaches in drama therapy. Charles C Thomas, Springfield, p 196–217
- Valente L, Fontana D 1993 Research into dramatherapy theory and practice: some implications for training. In: Payne H (ed) Handbook of inquiry in the arts therapies: one river, many currents. Jessica Kingsley, London and Philadelphia, p 56–67
- Waller D 2001 Come back Professor Higgins – arts therapists need you! The importance of clear communication for arts therapists. In: Kossolapow L, Scoble S, Waller D (eds) Arts – therapies – communication: on the way to a communicative European arts therapy, vol 1. Lit Verlag, Munster, p 244–256
- Yalom I D 1970 The theory and practice of group psychotherapy. Basic Books, New York

Chapter 8

Dance Movement Therapy (DMT)

Key issues:

- Although dance movement therapy (DMT) is the most recently established of the arts therapies in the UK, progress has been rapid. For example, in 2004 DMT was accepted as a profession to be regulated by the Health Professions Council.

- Research indicates that mental health difficulties are the major focus of DMT practice, followed by learning difficulties. The main working environments for dance movement therapists are education, health services and work in the community.

- Improvisational movement and dance is central to DMT practice and is encouraged in a number of different ways in order to promote emotional, cognitive and social integration in the person.

- Research evidence shows that DMT is based on the same principles as for other arts therapies, e.g. humanistic; eclectic/integrative; psychoanalytic/psychodynamic. However, compared with the other arts therapies, a higher value seems to be placed upon humanistic principles.

- Stemming from pioneering work in the UK and USA, current DMT practice in the UK includes movement-based, interactive or psychoanalytically/psychodynamically-informed approaches. Case examples illustrate some theoretical and methodological principles inherent in these approaches.

Introduction

Dance movement therapy (DMT) (or dance/movement therapy as it is known in the USA) is the youngest of the arts therapies disciplines to be established as a distinctive modality. Despite its newness, the field has its own history, ways of working and certain tendencies for practitioners to engage with certain client groups in specific environments. In this chapter, we will provide an historical overview, describe current practice within the DMT field in the UK, and identify prevalent areas of work. Wherever relevant we will also highlight differences from other arts therapies.

Brief DMT history

Although evidence for the therapeutic application of movement and dance can be found in the early part of the 20th century, it was not until 1982 that DMT became a professional grouping (see Box 8.1). The relative delay in the establishment of DMT in the UK mirrors the delayed emergence of dance as an established art form and academic discipline (Sanderson 2001, 2002). For instance, the recognition of dance as a major art form has occurred, for the most part, only within the past 30 years, and the opportunity to undertake dance studies within a university as recently as the 1980s. Both Sanderson (1996, 2001) and Meekums (2000) suggest that such phenomena may be connected with the prevailing view in the UK that dance activity is a pursuit suited mainly to women. It is also suggested that the focus on the body, more so than in any of the other three arts therapies, has been an additional limiting factor in the growth of DMT. The Descartesian dualism, whereby the body is seen as inferior to the mind, has only recently been seriously challenged.

Box 8.1: Significant dates in the development of DMT in the UK (Meekums 2000, 2002, Payne 1992a, 1994a)	
Year	**Development**
1976	Laban Certificates in special education and community led by North and Meier.
1982	Association of Dance Movement Therapists (ADMT) is formed as the first DMT association by Payne, Krane and Garvie; currently renamed ADMT UK
1985	First DMT training at the Laban Centre 'imported' from Hahnemann University in the USA.
1987	Second American-led training course at Roehampton Institute directed and taught by Marcia Leventhal.
1988	First UK-validated DMT training at Hertfordshire College of Art and Design.
1996	Registration of qualified dance movement therapists with ADMT UK; ADMT UK officially becomes a professional body rather than a group of practitioners.
2004	Application of ADMT UK for professional registration is accepted by the Health Professions Council

The growth of feminist studies, input from social psychology and postmodern theory are currently at the frontline of challenging dualism and re-instating a value for the body alongside the mind (Finfgeld 2001, Gergen 1991, Grentz 1996, Lyotard 1984).

Despite the difficulties encountered in establishing DMT in the UK, pioneers such as Payne (1994a), and Meekums (2000, 2002) suggest two periods of significant development: the first starting in the 1940s, paralleling that in the USA, and the second during the 1970s which continues.

The first period refers mainly to work in psychotherapy and education, with few documented accounts of the work of actual DMT practice. Within this period an early example of the use of the body as a means of therapeutic change can be found in body psychotherapy introduced by Reich (1960). Reichian therapy is based on the argument that the body reflects psychological processes and, furthermore, uses 'character armouring' as a means of 'freezing' emotions. The aim of the therapeutic process is to liberate these emotions. Reichian therapy gave rise to a number of body-orientated therapies such as bioenergetics (Lowen 1975), the Feldenkrais technique (Feldenkrais 1972, 1985) and structural integration (Rolf 1975).

Although Reichian therapy's emphasis on the body has a close resonance with some aspects of current DMT practice and overlaps are frequently acknowledged (Levy 1988, Payne 1992a), DMT has not derived from it directly. The pioneering work of Rudolf Laban who came to England in the 1930s as a refugee from Nazi Germany presents a closer link with the development of DMT in the UK (Karkou & Sanderson 2001, Sanderson 1984, 1996). Laban's major contribution rests with his comprehensive theory of human movement that offers methods of movement observation and analysis, as well as a precise system of movement notation. His work, which was developed further by his pupils, notably Lamb (1965), Preston-Dunlop (1963) and Sherborne (1990), had a major impact on physical and dance education programmes between 1945 and 1980 in the UK, especially those for female teachers and pupils (Sanderson 1986, 1996, 2001, Sanderson & Meakin 1983). Sherborne's (1990) application of Laban theory (1975) in her work with special needs children provides an early link between the child-centred creative dance education of the Laban approach and the early development of DMT.

Those prominent in the second wave of DMT development continued to refine Laban's theory and make relevant applications to the emerging DMT field. North (1972), for example, one of Laban's 'disciples', was among the first to study links between movement preferences and personality traits. According to Meekums (2000), the 'New Dance' movement of the 1970s also had a significant effect upon the development of DMT, as it questioned the idealised versions of the body presented in some forms of dance, and the exploitation of the body in others. 'New Dance' paralleled the growth in humanistic psychotherapies and the review of preconceived ideas about the body and the self. Within this context, practitioners working with movement in a therapeutic way began to use the term 'therapy' as a means of describing their practice. American dance movement therapists visiting the UK supported these tentative steps of British practitioners, enabling them to define their DMT practice as a distinctive discipline and to start moving towards professionalism (Payne 1992a). In 1985 the first DMT training course began as an imported scheme from the USA that was based at the Laban Centre in London, followed by two more training courses, one of which was also American-led initially (see Box 8.1).

Since the 1990s, DMT has entered a new phase of development, in that all recognised training courses became validated by UK higher education institutions. Similarly, the Association of Dance Movement Therapists (ADMT) has grown from a small group of professionals that met in order to offer training and mutual support, to an organised professional body with registered members, disciplinary procedures and training accreditation rights in place. The association (now known as ADMT UK) is currently represented in arts therapies groups and committees and, following the example of other arts therapies disciplines, it applied and was accepted for professional registration with the Health Professions Council (HPC) (See Box 8.1). Full registration is expected to take place in 2008.

Despite the progress of the profession in the UK towards maturity, the American DMT influences remain strong. These influences include DMT pioneers such as Chace and Whitehouse. They also include Laban's ideas which, having been developed independently in the USA, have been re-introduced into the UK context by means of visiting American dance movement therapists and imported training courses. At present there is an harmonious development of Laban's theories in both countries (e.g. Bartenieff & Lewis 1980, North 1972). The co-existence of American and UK influences upon current practice will be apparent in the following sections.

Table 8.1: Main DMT client groups and differences from other arts therapies

Type of difficulty	% for DMT	% for other arts therapies	Chi-square (x^2) value	Degrees of freedom (df)	P-value (p)
Emotional/ behavioural	48.8	60.7	not significant		
Learning	26.8	22.6	not significant		
No apparent	9.7	4.5	not significant		
Physical/sensory/ medical	4.9	3.2	not significant		
Multiple	4.9	3.2	not significant		
Other	4.9	5.8	not significant		
Total	100.0	100.0			

The table shows that emotional/behavioural (otherwise known as mental health) was the most frequent type of difficulty faced by DMT clients, followed by learning difficulties and 'no apparent' difficulties (i.e. clients otherwise labelled as 'normal neurotic'). Although Table 8.1 shows differences in the percentages presented for DMT and the other arts therapies, these differences are not statistically significant.

Current DMT professional development

Compared with the other arts therapies, ADMT UK remains a fairly small group of around 200 registered practitioners. In 2004, two training courses were available at the University of Surrey-Roehampton and at Goldsmiths College, London; a further two courses gained accreditation from ADMT UK in Derby and Bristol (see Appendix 2), and there is currently the prospect of others being developed in Yorkshire and Scotland.

Dance movement therapists are involved with different client groups and in different settings. Both Table 8.1 and Table 8.2 present these areas of work and compare them with those of other arts therapies.

Although work with learning difficulties continues, mental health remains the major focus of current practice (Table 8.1). This could be a consequence of the emphasis placed on this area in DMT training courses, in placements for instance, as well as the continuing influence of USA pioneers such as Chace, who developed her DMT approach while working with people with chronic mental health problems (e.g. schizophrenia).

However, meta-analysis conducted in the USA on randomised controlled trials (RCTs) by Ritter & Low (1996, 1998) and recalculated by Cruz & Sabers (1998) provides evidence for the effectiveness of DMT with clients with a wide array of symptoms. The studies that have been included refer to DMT work with clients with chronic and severe disabilities and mental health

Table 8.2: Main DMT working environments and differences from other arts therapies working environments

Working environment	% for DMT	% for other arts therapies	Chi-square (x^2) value	Degrees of freedom (df)	P-value (p)
Education	40.0	14.7	17.20	1	0.000**
Health	27.5	50.1	7.60	1	0.006**
Voluntary/private organisations	12.5	12.7	Not significant		
Social service	10.0	12.1	Not significant		
Other	7.5	2.5	Not significant		
Private practice	2.5	7.9	Not significant		
Total	100.0	100.0			

**Accepted at the 0.001 level of significance

Dance movement therapists participating in this study reported education and health work in the community (either voluntary/private organisations or social services) as the most important main working environments. Interesting statistical differences were found between DMT and the other arts therapies regarding the two first settings: dance movement therapists were, in comparison, more frequently located in education and less often in health services.

issues, people with alcoholism, breast cancer and a number of clients with no apparent difficulties such as students in DMT training and psychiatric nursing students. A particular effect upon reducing anxiety has been reported. In the UK, small-scale qualitative research studies have been completed with a number of client groups (e.g. mothers and toddlers, adolescents with challenging behaviour, survivors of sexual abuse, people with dementia and Parkinson's disease, chronic pain, brain injury and eating disorders) and referred to by Payne (1993). Abstracts of the most recent of these studies are available in the research register compiled by Karkou (2003). In this research register, two RCTs are included that have been completed by large research teams with clients with schizophrenia and/or enduring mental health problems, both of which provide evidence of positive effects of DMT interventions with this client group. Further research activity has been reported on a European level, e.g. Germany, Sweden, Spain and Portugal, with varying client needs.

We have already discussed the considerable influence of Laban-based educational work on the development of DMT. It is evident that this link continues since many DMT practitioners are working in an educational environment, more so than their other arts therapies colleagues (Table 8.2). The NHS remains an area where few DMT practitioners are employed, a situation which needs to be addressed by the ADMT UK, especially as pioneering work began in this sector at least 30 years ago (Holden 1990, MacDonald 1992). Meanwhile, a major reason for the poor representation to date in the NHS is that DMT is the last of the arts therapies to gain registration with HPC. Now that the application for accepted HPC registration has been it is expected that more posts in the NHS will become increasingly available for DMT practitioners.

In the remaining areas of social services and voluntary or private organisations, there are similar patterns of employment with other arts therapies. In the case of DMT, however, higher education institutions such as the Laban Centre in London may have stimulated further interest in community work through their 'dance and community' courses. DMT in the community is currently expanding as indicated and further discussed in Karkou (in press).

DMT defined

According to ADMT UK (2004), DMT is defined as:

> . . . the psychotherapeutic use of movement and dance through which a person can engage creatively in a process to further their emotional, cognitive, physical and social integration. (p. 1)

This definition, which was presented and discussed in Chapter 2, reflects the continued American influence and presents DMT as a form of psychotherapy. This signifies an important departure from the previous, movement-based definition of DMT that was used during the early days of the profession. The affiliation of DMT with psychotherapy suggests that the field is distinct from dance as an art form, therapeutic dance or dance education. It also gives DMT a strong theoretical base, supporting its pursuit of general recognition as a form of therapy. Furthermore, this definition has resulted in the adoption of the term 'movement psychotherapy' by a number of DMT practitioners as an appropriate description of their work.

As the definition above suggests, an overarching aim for all dance movement therapists is to bring together the emotional, cognitive and the social through physical engagement. In order to achieve this, DMT practitioners use a number of body/movement/dance techniques that are adapted to individual needs. Improvisational movement and dance – often based upon Laban's (1949, 1975) principles – with or without music, are central to most DMT approaches. The most common starting point for these improvisations is spontaneous movement, although subsequent development varies considerably. Penfield (1992), for example, outlines a number of developmental techniques for individual work, such as touch, mirroring, exaggeration and organised movement sequences. Similarly, Payne (1990) outlines a developmental sequence when she refers to the use of simple movement, symbolic movement and communicative dance as areas of work within DMT sessions. She also suggests several creative movement and dance ideas relevant to DMT group work with special needs populations and children. Other movement ideas can be found within resource books such as Bloom & Shreeves (1998) and within publications describing specific DMT approaches such as MacDonald (1992) and Meekums (2000, 2002).

It appears however, that although these movement ideas can be utilised in varying degrees within DMT sessions, the majority of British dance movement therapists draw upon techniques developed by Marion Chace (Chaiklin & Schmais 1986) when working with groups. Chace's work values the circle as an optimal form of group communication through movement. Within the circle, movements initiated by an individual are supported by the therapist and followed by both therapist and members of the group, with leadership changing periodically, thereby promoting autonomy, self-esteem, communication and group cohesion. There are currently many variations on Chace's circle, but the fundamental ideas are still in wide use due to the belief that it is a simple but robust structure. Chace's work is examined more closely in a later section.

When working one-to-one, and with highly functioning individuals in particular, the theoretical and technical approach developed by Whitehouse (Pallaro 1999) often becomes a more relevant model for DMT practitioners. Those influenced by Whitehouse encourage a somatic awareness of polarities (physical, emotional and psychological), and work extensively with images, symbols and metaphor. A practitioner with such an approach encourages the client to improvise personal material, while the therapist acts as a witness of the clients' movement exploration.

Techniques within DMT can therefore be summarised as: those that highlight the movement/dance (based mainly on Laban's work); relational aspects (as a result of 'Chacian' influences); or personal (as in the 'authentic movement' approach of Whitehouse). Further discussion of these techniques and their respective therapeutic models will be included in later relevant sections in this chapter.

Main therapeutic trends within DMT

The research evidence presented in Table 8.3 suggests that DMT practice draws upon the same therapeutic trends as other arts therapies, i.e. humanistic, eclectic/integrative, psychoanalytic/psychodynamic, developmental, artis-

Table 8.3: Main DMT therapeutic trends and differences from other arts therapies

Therapeutic approaches	Mean for DMT[1]	Mean for other arts therapies[1]	t-test value	Degrees of freedom (df)	P-value (p)
Humanistic	4.08	3.88	2.47	578	0.014*
Eclectic/integrative	3.83	3.68	Not significant		
Psychoanalytic/ psychodynamic	3.33	3.35	Not significant		
Developmental	3.32	3.21	Not significant		
Artistic/creative	3.23	3.12	Not significant		
Active/directive	3.12	3.07	Not significant		

[1]The higher the score, the stronger the agreement with this group of statements (a five-point scale was used ranging from strongly agree = 5 to strongly disagree = 1).
*Accepted at the 0.05 level of significance
Dance movement therapists valued mainly humanistic, eclectic/integrative and psychoanalytic/psychodynamic approaches. The first group of statements received statistically stronger agreement from dance movement therapists than from other arts therapists (p = 0.014). Although differences between the two groups (DMT and non-DMT participants) were also present in the mean score of other therapeutic approaches, these differences were not statistically significant.

tic/creative and active/directive. The order with which these trends appear within DMT is also similar to other arts therapies. However, it seems that dance movement therapists place a higher value upon humanistic principles than other arts therapists. This is a characteristic of the field as a whole, and is matched only by dramatherapy (DT) (see Chs 7 and 9). Reasons for this humanistic preference may lie in historical associations with humanistic therapies (e.g. Reichian therapy) and also the child-centred focus of the Laban approach to dance education referred to earlier. DMT continues to value the humanistic principle of addressing the 'whole person' as fundamental to practice and an ultimate therapeutic aim.

However, since the emergence of DMT as a profession, there has been an increased influence upon DMT practice from psychoanalytic/psychodynamic thinking. It can be argued that in many cases psychoanalytic theory helps explain what is happening in a session, while humanistic principles guide the actual practice, particularly in terms of the presentation of the therapist's self and his or her relationship with the client. At the same time, pioneers of DMT in the UK and USA such as Laban, Chace and Whitehouse, often adopted and significantly adapted psychotherapeutic principles to movement and dance, and created a distinctive body of knowledge. Along with other arts therapies, overlaps amongst DMT approaches are the rule rather than the exception, and eclectic/integrative approaches are commonplace. Eclectic/integrative approaches enable DMT practice to adapt to the client, the stage of therapy, overall culture of the setting, and are congruent with current postmodern thinking. Flexible practices are also essential strategies for professional survival.

Movement-based DMT approaches: starting with Rudolf Laban

Rudolf Laban was an architect and a painter who became interested in dance during the early years of the 20th century (Levy 1988). Laban's major contributions include the development of a detailed movement notation system (Labanotation) and a comprehensive movement theory that consists of 'choreutics' or 'space harmony', as well as his concept of 'effort'. 'Effort' was subsequently developed into 'effort-shape' by Lamb (1965) and has been widely applied in areas such as industry, business, recreation, physical education and dance. Laban's movement theory was developed separately in the USA and the UK, e.g. by Bartenieff (Bartenieff & Lewis 1980) and North (1972), respectively. However, when the Hahnemann training was introduced to the UK at the Laban Centre in London, the work of Bartenieff and that of North was integrated, resulting in the current generic term of 'Laban movement analysis' (LMA).

Important movement categories within LMA are: body, space, shape and effort. The last of these, the 'effort' category, is probably most widely used amongst dance movement therapists in the UK. According to Stanton-Jones (1992), the effort category refers to the qualitative nuances of movement and is something fairly internal. Figure 8.1 shows that the effort category consists of four 'factors': weight, space, time and flow. The theory associates each one of these factors with certain psychological traits, and has affinities with the broad movement categories of body, space, shape and effort (Kaylo 2003). Each factor consists of two elements.

Variations in the words and terms used in Figure 8.1 occur to some extent, according to the tradition employed, i.e. that of the British or American tradition. Although the meaning of each one of these concepts remains essentially the same, the Bartenieff DMT protégées, for example, see effort elements as being presented in a dynamic continuum, rather than as a static

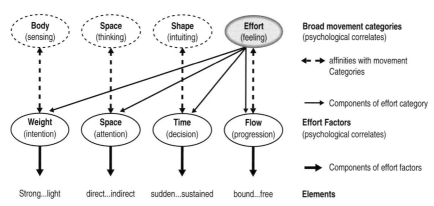

Figure. 8.1: *LMA concepts frequently used within UK DMT practice. (Sources: Bartenieff & Lewis 1980, Kaylo 2003, North 1972, Stanton-Jones 1992)*

manifestation of inner attitude: increasing/decreasing pressure (weight), direct/indirect (space), accelerating/decelerating (time) and binding/freeing (flow). In addition they make more extensive use of all four movement categories within their DMT practice. They may also utilise the 'Bartenieff fundamentals', i.e. specific body exercises, which aim to integrate body feelings with emotional feelings (Kaylo 2003).

LMA offers an essential tool to dance movement therapists to understand the client's movement and the corresponding psychological issues. LMA becomes increasingly complex when the dance movement therapist incorporates more aspects of the system into his or her practice, such as the components of the effort category (i.e. factors and elements) with the components of the body, space and shape categories. Detailed movement profiles of clients can be drawn, often with the aid of video recordings. Therapeutic changes are then monitored through changes in the client's movement profile. More often, however, LMA is used informally as a guide for planning interventions before the session, as a means of informing interactions with the client during the session and as a tool for reflection afterwards. When LMA is used in a more formal way, it often provides an important conceptual base for DMT and a theoretical framework for the work. When it is used more informally, LMA is perceived as an additional tool for practice; in these cases, the overall conceptual framework is primarily borrowed from psychotherapeutic thinking.

A movement-based DMT approach with an adult with phobias

The fundamental principle of LMA within DMT is the belief that there is body–mind connection and that changes in the client's movement 'vocabulary' may facilitate changes in the psychological state. An early expression of this principle within a British DMT context is the work of North (1972). The relationship between movement, feelings and attitudes is characteristic of North's early contribution to DMT. North supports her views by reference to her empirical research work with children, which involved movement observations, teachers' reports and tests of IQ, apperception and maladjustment. Although this work has been heavily criticised on issues of validity, reliability and other methodological flaws (e.g. by Whiting 1973), it provides a useful theoretical model that is firmly rooted in clinical observation.

A summary of a case example of North's essentially movement-based approach to DMT is presented in Table 8.4.

As Table 8.4 shows, North (1972) draws heavily upon her initial observations in order to develop movement-based therapeutic guidelines. She believes that with appropriate guidance from the therapist, the unique movement repertoire of the client can provide 'building blocks' for further positive growth. In the example provided, her work has strong directive elements. The therapist suggests movements and sequences that the client 'practises' until she learns them. The aim is to change the client's existing habitual movement patterns. Although attempts are also made to 'interest the patient to create her own sequences of movements', the movement content on the whole is primarily therapist-led. Links between these ideas and behavioural thinking are apparent, albeit not explicitly referred to. Nevertheless, North (1972) herself agrees that so much structure and direction from the part of the therapist is

Table 8.4: A movement-based DMT approach with an adult with phobias – Marion North (1972, pp. 104–114) [Adapted]

Description of process	Comments by the authors
Needs of client *Psychological issues* [A 34-year-old female patient, referred to as J, was suffering from intense feelings of deadness, negativity, remoteness, and unreality, compounded by intense fears to the point of phobias. She felt stuck inside herself and wanted desperately to get out]	[LMA is a comprehensive system to describe movement behaviour and a way of correlating various *movement preferences* with *personality characteristics*. LMA is therefore used for personality assessment and for establishing body movement treatment goals]
Movement presentation 'J looked fairly healthy with no restrictions or physical deformities. There was mobility in the centre of her *body* but lack of integration or connection between the movements of the upper and lower body parts.	[*Body category*]
The use of *weight* and *flow*, which [were] basic in her make-up, had come to be used in its negative aspects, strong tension and bound flow, inwardly oriented . . .'	[*Effort category*: factors of 'weight' and 'flow' are associated with intention' and 'progression', see Fig. 8.1]
Aims [DMT's *aim* for this patient was to break] into the habitual response pattern revealed in her movement, and helping to release the tensions.'	[*Movement-based goals* deriving from the use of LMA to act as guidelines (however, not necessarily to be followed rigidly)]
Beginning of work 'The first concern over the initial sessions was to give the patient *confidence in the person with whom she was working*. . .	[Establishing the client's *trust* in the therapist]

Continued

Table 8.4: A movement-based DMT approach with an adult with phobias – Marion North (1972, pp. 104–114) [Adapted]—cont'd

Description of process	Comments by the authors
A strict pattern was chosen, one which gave room both for some immediate achievement and some obvious failure . . .: gathering in – a grasping, losing movement, contrasted with a scattering opening movement. [This aimed at confronting and/or engaging the conflict J experienced over the tendency to go 'inside herself' rather than 'getting out'] The *initial session* produced mainly a feeling of frustration and inability, but also a challenge to master the movement.'	[Interventions ranging from very *directive movement suggestions* to less directive interventions. In this case it appears that the therapist made specific movement suggestions] [*Confrontation and engagements with conflicts via movement tasks*] [Usually it is necessary to provide '*entertainment*' and a sense of achievement as a starting point. This is not the case with the case example provided]
Development of work [As the therapeutic work developed, client and therapist engaged in *different aspects of movement* including:] ' . . . the achievement of expressive positions, to be held securely in space and in sequence . . . The sequence included: • A rising, lifting movement to high; • An advancing, extending movement forward; a closing, covering movement backward and down; and • An opening, spreading sideways.' [Each of these movements *was worked through over a period of time* and had certain significance for the client, presenting higher or low difficulty.]	[*Acute observation is necessary* in order to detect a changing situation and to respond, as appropriate. The therapist offers encouragement, guidance, comment, or suggests a new task, while concurrently cooperating with the patient in the therapeutic process] [*Mastering movement sequences*]

'There was *an attempt to interest the patient in creating her own sequences of movement*, but apart from the contribution of a hesitant phrase, there was obviously no confidence or desire for this at this stage . . .

[Encouraging *client to initiate his/her own movements*]

After a considerable build up of security of movement in space, the patient was ready to *tackle more precisely the rhythmical and accent aspects of her movement*. Again this was introduced through a simple spatial pattern of movement . . .'

[Tackling *precise aspects of movement*]

Completion of work

[Eventually isolated *achievements in movement* became integrated into J's movement repertoire, e.g. the 'inward-flowing mood of release' became 'efficient choice of action']

[Movement is seen as a help to understand issues and to act upon them through release of tension, re-formation and regaining of natural responses]

'Gradually, she could only manage to come [to the sessions] every other week, and the telephone calls between sessions became fewer and fewer. Both she and I are sure that she received great help from the movement, both in understanding and in direct action on helping her to release tensions and reform and regain her natural responses.

not required with all clients and in all cases. The particular needs of the client (e.g. someone faced with phobias) can partly explain the type of approach adopted. Another explanation for the choice of such an approach can be the fact that North (1972) was an early pioneer of DMT in the UK when psychological reasoning stemming from psychoanalytic/psychodynamic thinking and/or humanistic psychology was not as yet fully integrated within DMT practice.

A number of dance movement therapists have used a similar starting point to North, i.e. LMA, but developed their practice slightly differently. For example, we have seen how Lindqvist (Pearson 1996) incorporated Laban's movement principles within a dramatic and Jungian perspective (this work eventually developed into the Sesame approach to DT; see Ch. 7). Sherborne (1990) has been particularly influential upon the practice of dance teachers and DMT pioneers with her developmental movement approach to teaching mainstream and special needs children, while Meier (1997) for many years applied Laban principles within a dance education and DMT training context at the Laban Centre. Finally, Marie Ware, who still works at the 'Bristol DMT school', utilises Laban principles with a humanistic orientation and works predominantly with children with learning difficulties.

The interactive DMT approach: starting with Marian Chace

Marian Chace is regarded as both the founder of DMT in the USA and as making a significant impact upon group DMT practice in the UK. Starting as a dancer and choreographer, she studied at the Denishawn School, which favoured connections between dance and folk traditions as well as valuing the role of music and drama. Chace's approach evolved from dance teaching, through dance as communication, to a form of dance therapy, when she started working with clients with schizophrenia at the St Elisabeth's Hospital. It is reported that her DMT approach developed a strong relational and social character as a result of influences from Sullivan (1955), an American psychiatrist who founded the interpersonal school of psychotherapy, and was working at the same time in the same hospital. According to Levy (1988), however, Chace's DMT work has also obvious roots in her original dance training: for instance, there are structures and principles utilised in folk dancing, especially the circle, and incorporation of dramatic and musical forms.

Chaiklin & Schmais (1986), Chace's protégées, have classified her work into four major areas: body action, symbolism, therapeutic movement relationship, and rhythmic activity.

- *Body action*. Dance is seen as a means of structuring and organising muscular activity that expresses emotion. Change comes not by merely practising a movement within a dance, but by allowing oneself to experience this action in the body.
- *Symbolism*. Problems can be worked through via pure symbolic action without requiring interpretation or analysis. Once symbolic release of conflicts is accepted and established through empathetic support, issues behind symbolic work can emerge into consciousness. Symbolic work

involves mobilising imagery, fantasy, recollection and enactment, and can be facilitated through the use of visualisation, verbalisation and dance activity.

▪ *Therapeutic movement relationship.* The basis for establishing a client–therapist relationship is empathy expressed within a DMT situation in the form of 'mirroring'. The therapist, taking the non-verbal language of the client seriously, embodies this language and reflects it back to the client, enabling him or her to expand and/or clarify issues. The aim is to acknowledge, understand and affirm the client.

▪ *Rhythmic activity* (according to Levy 1988: Group Rhythmic Movement Relationship). This is valued by Chace in that it enables her clients to express themselves in an organised way. Those who are withdrawn are drawn into action through the contagious quality of rhythmical activity and those with extreme or bizarre behaviour are enabled to modify their movement through the organised dance. Symbolism is often elicited during this time and verbalisations may take place.

Chace's methodological input is summarised by Levy (1988) and present- ed in Table 8.5. References to unconscious material and inner conflicts included in the description of Chace's work suggest an acknowledgement of psychoanalytic/psychodymanic concepts in her work. However, her approach is more closely placed within humanistic thinking and the interpersonal school of psychotherapy in particular, following influences from Sullivan in the early development of her work. Furthermore, she places an overall emphasis upon the healthy aspects of the clients (e.g. their ability to use dance as communication), the empathetic response of the therapist and his or her active involvement within the therapeutic process reflecting strong humanistic underpinnings. Finally, Schmais (1985), one of Chace's followers, draws parallels between the Chacian model and Yalom (1970), an interper- sonal/existential group psychotherapist. Yalom (1970) has articulated a num- ber of therapeutic factors of working with groups in verbal psychotherapy, e.g. the development of socialising techniques, learning through imitation, a corrective recapitulation of a family group, group cohesiveness, catharsis and the recognition of the universal nature of emotional experiences. Schmais (1985) regards these factors as relevant to group DMT approach- es with a Chacian orientation and adds some DMT-specific therapeutic fac- tors such as synchrony, expression, rhythm, vitalisation, integration, cohesion and symbolism. Although these factors are insufficiently researched within DMT, they are concepts that are relevant to a Chacian approach to DMT with a possible applicability and value for other DMT approaches as well.

An interactive DMT approach with mental health clients living in the community

Chace's work is perceived as a robust approach to working in groups with a number of different clients and has a wide applicability to the work under- taken by British-based dance movement therapists. Karkou illustrates the use of fundamental principles of Chace's work in the case example presented in Table 8.6. In this example, the clients present problems similar to many of

Table 8.5: The structure of interactive DMT sessions – summary of Marian Chace's approach by Levy (1988, pp. 26–31) (Adapted)

Needs of clients
[Mainly adults with schizophrenia, but currently applicable to group DMT with a wide range of client needs]

Aims of session
  [I. To mobilise and connect with clients, to build trust and openness in the group, to develop a full body movement and arouse a sense of pleasure and enjoyment of body action.
  II. To focus and clarify emotive themes and conflicts in the group and enable patients to enter into a deep exploration of these themes and conflicts.
  III. To offer a supportive closure that gives a sense of satisfaction and resolution]

Structure of session
  I. 'Warm up
    A. Initial contacts
      1. Mirroring [or empathetic reflection]
      2. Clarifying and expanding the movement repertoire
      3. Movement elicitation/movement dialogue.'
[These were overlapping interventions with Chace moving back and forth between them in a similar way to conducting a verbal dialogue. The therapist was interacting with one client at a time but kept attuned into the whole group atmosphere]

    B. 'Group development – gradual formation of circle'
[The therapist would move from interacting with individual clients into encouraging the formation of a circle; she would position and lead the group from the circle itself]
    C. 'Group rhythmic expression/physical warm up'
[The therapist would initiate simple rhythmical movement taking into account certain physical tensions in the group and enable the group to develop expressive movements that involved the whole body. Preliminary themes would emerge but have not as yet been dealt with in depth.]

  II. 'Theme development
    A. Picking up on non-verbal clues [e.g. a simple movement that may appear to have an unconscious intention]
    B. Broadening, extending and clarifying actions
    C. Use of verbalisation and imagery
    D. Various other theme oriented possibilities (e.g. role playing, symbolic action, group themes).'
[There would be a continuation from the previous section but the therapist would encourage further clarity and focus through picking up a simple movement with a potential unconscious intention, intensifying it in her own body and reflecting it back to the group. In order to encourage the group to relate to this emergent theme, while still engaged in rhythmical activity, she could also say a word and make a sound that seemed to be reflecting this movement. Questions to the group would shed light on underlying issues and evoke material for further movement work, role playing and/or symbolic action.]

Chace's clients (i.e. clients with schizophrenia with issues relating to lengthy institutionalisation). However, Karkou's clients are outpatients, i.e. people who live in the community, following changes of mental health policies away from hospital-based care provision.

Like Chace, Karkou's initial training has been in folk dance. Influences from this training are apparent in the example presented in Table 8.6 (although not necessarily as apparent in Karkou's work with other client groups). For example, folk formations and concepts underpin the use of the circle and rhythm and the encouragement of group cohesion. In line with Chace, Karkou also draws heavily upon interpersonal psychotherapeutic frameworks (Yalom in particular) and regards empathetic responses, active presence, and at times personal disclosures on the part of the therapist, as contributing factors for therapeutic change. In the case of the group described in Table 8.6, she acknowledges psychoanalytic concepts (e.g. transference/countertransference), but similarly to Chace, she also avoids making verbal interpretations within the session.

This approach also presents a number of differences from Chace's work. Karkou works with another therapist in the session; they both share therapeutic responsibility as co-therapists. The interpersonal emphasis of this approach as a whole starts from the presence of these two therapists. The clients live in the community in supported accommodation rather than in an institution and attend the DMT group at a day centre run by a voluntary organisation. Given the recent transition of most of these clients to the community and the sense of anxiety and chaos experienced as a consequence, the beginning of the sessions is much more structured than Chace's approach advocates. The therapists introduce movement ideas that can offer some kind of structure, offer a safe physical warm-up, encourage movement qualities that are not readily forthcoming and stimulate 'vitalisation', i.e. one of the therapeutic factors described by Schmais (1985) as relevant to group DMT.

However, as the therapeutic process unfolds, the session becomes much more client-led. For example, movements are entirely initiated by the clients, while therapists' interventions are limited to encouraging the clients to (1) make concrete connections between these movements and words and (2) develop relationships amongst members of the group. Given the forthcoming ending of the group, the clients initiate themes of intimacy and loss. These themes are expressed through symbolic movement and verbalisations. Certain clients initiate rhythm through clapping and the whole group

Table 8.6: Interactive DMT with clients with continuing mental health problems who live in the community – Vassiliki Karkou and K Hyvonen, unpublished clinical notes, 2001)

Description of session	Comments by the authors
Needs of members of the group [This DMT group took place within a day centre based at a voluntary organisation. There were five members in the group with a wide age range (34–75 years); all had a diagnosis of *psychosis and/or schizophrenia*. Verbal capacity: Two of these clients had limited ability to communicate verbally. The other three, although highly articulate, were often talking in a very incoherent way. Movement preferences: Most group members shared a preference for moving body parts rather than engaging in whole body actions. Their movement seemed disconnected from the rest of the body and from what was taking place before and after in the session. They often engaged in the same repetitive movements that lacked clarity of 'inner attitude'. It appeared easier for them to follow than initiate movement]	[People who move from lengthy institutionalisation to the community require *ongoing support at personal and relational level*. The move to the community is a major disruption in the lives of these clients. Given that they are faced with severe mental health issues they are often regarded as inappropriate for counselling or other talking therapies. They therefore often lack an opportunity to express loss of the familiar environment, fear, anger or find opportunities for intimate interactions. Furthermore, life in the community requires a much wider range of social skills than hospital-based environments; people often find themselves insufficiently equipped to deal with this change]
Aim [It was the 10th session in a block of 12 sessions. At that point it was uncertain whether DMT provision would continue in that centre. The *specific aim* was therefore to prepare the group for the forthcoming ending]	[The *overall aim* of DMT was to enable clients to deal with the transition from the hospital to the community and offer integrative physical, personal and relational experiences]

Beginning of session

'The therapists [there was a co-therapy arrangement] *acknowledged the length of time the group had been together and the time left*, and explained that it was not certain whether the group would continue.

[*Verbal introduction*: Practicalities are often discussed (e.g. ground rules, time frame, transport) and initial checking takes place (e.g. how has their week been, how are they right now emotionally and/or physically)]

All clients were sitting down and with encouragement by the therapists, *leg and arm movements were initiated by group members*. Torso *movements were initiated in a playful manner by one of the therapists*. Participants tried the therapist's movement and started laughing (response to the playfulness of the therapist? Weird sensation of using their torso given their preference for peripheral movements?).

[*Physical warm-up*: The therapists would draw upon *minimal movement clues* and would try to expand or minimise these movements; at this stage therapists also *initiate movements* that are useful for a physical warm-up and different from what the clients would bring in (e.g. torso movements suggested by one of the therapists in this example)]

One of the members of the group initiated a movement with his hands *tapping on his knees* (people were still sitting down). This lasted for some time with all joining in.'

[*Rhythmical activity* is useful for creating a sense of togetherness.]

[Further *verbal themes* were generated during the physical warm up:]

[Movement and verbal themes are raised at this stage but *not necessarily dealt with in depth*]

Participants showed an interest about the therapists' origins (both were non-UK nationals) and their families. The therapists responded with a *brief personal disclosure*.

[*Disclosure* of personal information by the therapists may take place if it seems appropriate (e.g. in this case the fact that the therapists' families were far away was meeting the group feelings around the forthcoming loss of the group and other losses experienced throughout their lives)]

One client claimed that one of the therapists *looked like his sister* (*a very supportive twin sister*) and that he would be supporting the therapist's national team in the football match shown on TV that night.

[*Transferences* are noted but verbal interpretations are avoided with this client group]

Continued

Table 8.6: Interactive DMT with clients with continuing mental health problems who live in the community – Vassiliki Karkou [Example from V Karkou and K Hyvonen, unpublished clinical notes, 2001]—cont'd

Description of session	Comments by the authors
Development of session	
[The therapists encouraged the group to *create the 'dance for the day'*. One of the quietest members of the group, a frail old woman in her 70s,] *'initiated a movement* with her hands starting from her chest and moving out in a light and sustained quality. [With the therapists' intervention] this movement was *enlarged and repeated a number of times*. She was *encouraged to add words* that may describe it. She uttered the words "heart" and "group". [In general she avoided talking in the group; at times when the therapists or other members of the group addressed her verbally, she used to show surprise or confusion]	[A *'dance'* is created which consists of clients', often very, simple movements]
	[Picking up on *non-verbal clues*]
	[*Broadening, extending and clarifying actions*]
[The therapists encouraged other members of the group to also attach words to the movement. It was eventually renamed as the 'broken heart' movement, understood by the therapists to stand for the sadness of the group coming to an end. This was followed by member discussion about families, funerals, dead and alive relatives. The therapists felt deep sadness but at the same time a strong sense of intimacy and cohesiveness that was not experienced in this group before.]	[*Using verbalisation and imagery* while moving. When client's ability to verbalise is minimal, other members of the group or the therapists may add 'voice' to these movements]
'Other group members initiated their own movements for the dance. Two members stood up and *a circle was formed*. The movements initiated by different clients were: moving in and out the group with different body parts (e.g. legs and arms). The "broken heart" movement initiated by the old woman earlier was repeated a number of times in a number of variations becoming eventually an "offering" for the group. As arms moved towards the centre of the circle one member noticed differences in the hands and pointed out the presence of rings. The group became more	[*Chacian circle/shared leadership*]

cheerful with free movement explorations under the *rhythm* of the clapping of one member.

The dance finished with a *circle dance*, in which all held hands and moved around in the circle. The group members stayed close together while performing this circle dance. [The therapists] encouraged them to find a name for the dance. The word "ring" came up again and all members agreed that this was an appropriate name for the dance (it appeared as an appropriate reference to the close circular formation of the group and the corresponding bonding between the members).'

[*Integration* within each of the group members and *cohesiveness* between different members of the group can be created within DMT sessions. Rhythmical activity and circular formations are often linked with individual integration and group cohesiveness]

Completion of session
'Despite encouragement [from the therapists], the members did *not seem willing to let go from moving together in the circle.*
[The therapists] suggested that clients chose the most important parts of the dance and repeated them. On completion of the prearranged number of repetitions of the dance all group members cheered and laughed congratulating each other and shaking hands.'

[*Closure*
Clients often sit back in their chairs and either say or draw something about their 'dance'. A communal movement or gesture is also encouraged as the final closure for the session]

[There seemed to be no further need to reflect on this session verbally. Clients had managed to share their feelings of loss (see also loss associated with transition from the hospital to the community) and got close to each other before the group ended. Two more sessions followed that did not have the intimacy of this session. On the final review of the group, the 'ring' dance was remembered and raised by a number of clients. Strong relationships developed between some of the clients of the group and continued long after the group ended]

Authors' wording in [brackets]

engages in synchronised movement that suggests group cohesiveness. The therapeutic factors outlined by Schmais (1985) as relevant to DMT with a Chacian orientation are apparent in this example (e.g. self-expression, integration, symbolic work, rhythm, synchronicity, cohesiveness). Vitality that is initially encouraged by the therapists is demonstrated by clients towards the end of the session through their lack of desire to stop moving and the celebratory manner with which they finally finish their dance. Ultimately, the intervention is seen as useful for these clients because it addresses their tendency for fragmentation, strengthens their interpersonal skills and offers support for their adjustment to community life. For further description/discussion of this work, see Karkou (in press).

Psychoanalytically/psychodynamically-informed DMT approaches: starting with Mary Whitehouse

A very different approach to the interactive emphasis of the previous approach is apparent in what is known as 'movement-in-depth'. This approach was developed originally by Mary Whitehouse (Pallaro 1999), another American pioneer practising during the early days of the DMT profession. Whitehouse was, like Chace, initially a professional dancer and a dance teacher. She trained with Wigman, the German dance expressionist, and later engaged in her own Jungian psychoanalysis. These two areas have played an important role in the development of her DMT approach. According to Levy (1988), Whitehouse's (1979) theoretical contribution evolves around issues of kinaesthetic awareness, polarities, active imagination, authentic movement (a term that nowadays also stands for the approach itself), and therapeutic relationship/intuition.

Kinaesthetic awareness

'Kinaesthetic awareness' is the internal sense of the individual's physical self. This concept highlights the difference between the mechanical use of the body as an object and the subjective understanding of how it feels to move in a certain way. For some people kinaesthetic awareness is refined and attuned, while others need to awaken, develop and encourage it. Kinaesthetic awareness is fundamental for the type of movement improvisation that takes place within this approach.

Polarity

'Polarity' is a concept closely linked with the Jungian perception that opposite drives (i.e. polarities) are often manifested in many different aspects of life and emotions. Conflict between the chosen and the rejected polarity may create conflict and exert pressure. Polarities can be worked through since for every movement there is often an opposite one (e.g. up and down, forward and backward). Ultimately, the aim is the integration of these polar opposites.

Active imagination

'Active imagination' is another Jungian concept adapted to DMT practice, which is linked with freeing conscious and unconscious associations.

Chodorow (1991), one of Whitehouse's students, claims that 'active imagination' is different from 'creative imagination', in that the former has an inward aim towards the development of the personality, while the latter has an outward direction towards the environment and the surrounding culture. With active imagination the therapist attempts to relax ego defences against spontaneous expressions by offering a supportive environment, movement vocabulary and facilitation. Active imagination enables the unification of the personal unconscious with the universal or 'collective unconscious' and places the ego in the role of the observer who allows physical expression of such unconscious processes without censoring or controlling them.

Authentic movement

'Authentic movement' takes place when consciousness withdraws from a controlling and directive role and is often defined as opposite to the 'invisible' movement. The latter fails to convey underlying emotions and thoughts, is often stylised and can be repeated and performed, while the former involves surrendering into a movement that 'cannot be explained, repeated exactly, sought for or tried out' (Whitehouse 1979, p. 57). The latter involves the phrase 'I move', while the former refers to 'I am moved'. According to Levy (1988), the two can be seen as the polarities of the conscious and the unconscious self and both have a place within an approach that values the integration of different aspects of the self as a final aim of therapy (see the definition of DMT presented earlier in the chapter).

Therapeutic relationship/intuition

'Therapeutic relationship/intuition' is the last concept outlined by Levy (1988). Whitehouse favoured a client-centred approach to this relationship by suggesting that therapists need to: meet clients where they are, feel comfortable with 'not knowing' and trust that client will evolve and find their own solutions. On the other hand, she suggested that therapists will have to make interventions based on their intuition, which may or may not be accepted by clients. The therapeutic relationship is, therefore, formed by knowing when to intervene and when to wait patiently for clients to find their own way.

Table 8.7 outlines Whitehouse's methodology as summarised by Levy (1988). Whitehouse (1979) herself claimed that she developed a *style of intervention*, rather than a method or a practical guide to conducting therapy and, congruent with other arts therapies approaches, she fluctuated from being directive and externally prompted, to being less directive and internally prompted.

The contribution of Whitehouse to British DMT practice is considerable, especially when highly functioning clients are involved and one-to-one work takes place. Dance movement therapists who work with this approach such as Lavendel, Payne, and Stromsted, tend to draw either directly upon Whitehouse and/or upon her followers (e.g. Adler 1999, Chodorow 1991). For example, the therapist may guide clients through warm-up exercises that enable them to gradually pay attention to their inner self. Clients often keep their eyes closed and wait for an image to move them. The therapist becomes

Table 8.7: The movement-in-depth DMT approach – summary of Whitehouse's (1979) approach by Levy (1988, pp. 69–74)

Needs of clients

[Mainly highly functioning adults (e.g. dance students) on a one-to-one DMT, but also applicable to groups]

Overall aim of therapy

[To integrate the polar opposites within the individual]

A. Beginning of work

[1. Offering a choice of starting position]

'Whitehouse often started a session by offering a quick choice to the client, for example "What would be most comfortable, easiest – lying, sitting, standing?"'

[2. Giving a client a feeling of self-confidence and greater kinaesthetic awareness]

'Another way Whitehouse began sessions was by teaching dance technique and/or simple movement tasks or ideas . . . For example, she might suggest that the client work first only with specific body parts (arms, legs, face) or she might encourage using only the right side or left side of the body for a certain movement theme.'

B. Development of work

[1. *Assessing the client's ability to allow movement ideas to flow freely*]

'. . . Intuition [guided] the therapist in deciding whether or not intervention is needed and if so, what kind of intervention would be most helpful.'

[2. *Providing unstructured or structured environment*]

'If she saw that the client was capable of allowing a free flow of thoughts and feelings in movement, she then provided an unstructured environment within which the client could make all of his/her own movement decisions. When this was not possible she would provide movement themes or broad creative structures within which the client could project thoughts and feelings through movement.' [She used music, metaphors and projective techniques (e.g. 'If you were in a cocoon, would it be large or small, stiff or soft, unyielding or flexible?')]

[3. *Adding more personal levels of content to initial use of imagery*]

[She would suggest certain concepts and add possible personal symbolism or meaning to certain movements]

[4. *Observing (witnessing) and talking*]

'Whitehouse rarely (if ever) spoke while the client was involved in a movement improvisation. . . . During . . . pauses in the movement improvisation, Whitehouse stressed the importance of talking in order to understand and integrate verbally the psychomotor events. . . . Although Whitehouse did not actually dance with her clients, she did move towards them at moments when support was needed. Aside from these moments she basically stayed on the periphery . . .

When she stood observing and experiencing with her client, she acted as the mediator between the individual's opposing drives, e.g. the drive to express versus the drive to repress thoughts and feeling . . . Whitehouse [was] a patient, empathetic observer. . . . Her role was one of being "with" the client as he/she encountered his/her personal experience in both thought (imagery) and muscular (movement) themes.'

C. Completion

[1. Utilising material surfacing to structure a new or continuing theme] an observer, otherwise referred to as the 'witness' to the client's 'authentic movement' journey; i.e. the therapist becomes a non-intrusive and empathetic companion who will often receive projections and/or transferences. Countertransference reactions are therefore monitored and form a basis for establishing trust between the client and the therapist. Eventually the client's unconscious material, which is projected into the movement and the therapist, is re-introjected within the individual and polar opposites are brought together in an integrated manner.

Other psychoanalytically/psychodynamically-informed DMT approaches

Jungian thinking and the developments made by Whitehouse are not the only psychoanalytic/psychodymanic inputs to DMT. Kestenberg (1975) and Siegel (1984) provide further examples of DMT approaches that draw upon psychoanalytic/psychodynamic thinking, including Freudian psychosexual development and object relations theory. Both of these examples can be seen as developmental approaches to DMT with a psychoanalytic/psychodynamic orientation.

Kestenberg (1975) and her followers (e.g. Kestenberg-Amighi et al 1999, Loman 1998, Loman & Foley 1996, Loman & Merman 1996) have expanded the effort-shape theory of Laban, and have provided an influential movement profile applicable to children and adults. According to Loman (1998), this model serves not only as a useful diagnostic tool, but also as a way of thinking while involved in therapy. 'Attunement in tension-flow' (matching changes of muscles tensions that parallel Freudian stages of development) and 'adjustment in shape flow' (matching body shape) are important concepts within this DMT approach (Loman & Foley 1996). Levy (1988) considers that these two concepts address a fundamental principle of the therapeutic process beginning with an 'empathetic' response to the client's movement ('attunement') and developing into Winnicott's concept of 'holding' ('adjustment').

Siegel (1984) also makes clear references to Freudian thinking and draws on object relations theoreticians (e.g. Mahler et al 1975, Spitz 1965). Siegel (1984) argues that movement ('motility') is one of the human drives that is situated within the 'id'. Viewing movement as an expression of both conscious and unconscious material, rather than an expression of either sexuality or aggression, offers strong support for the use of movement within therapy. Furthermore, Siegel (1984) argues that constricted motility is an indication of repression that is influenced by a specific period in the client's early development; motility develops through the Freudian psychosexual stages and also relates to Mahler's (Mahler et al 1975) normal autistic, normal symbiosis and the separation–individuation phases.

Additional publications that utilise psychoanalytic/psychodynamic thinking include Sandel & Johnson (1983). Although they advocate an 'interactive' approach to DMT similar to that of Chace, they discuss concepts often found within the psychoanalytic/psychodynamic literature of groups, particularly that of Bion (1961) (e.g. basic assumptions of dependency, fight/flight responses and pairing). When working with clients with schizophrenia, they talk about the 'nascent' group, which consists of three phases:

1. High hopes, in which there is a social façade and a tendency to please the new therapist (Bion's basic assumption of dependency)
2. Struggling for relatedness, in which there is a collapse of the previous social structure and gestation begins, which may develop into sharing a degree of intimacy (Bion's fight/flight responses may take place in order to protect the group from the fear of merging)
3. Termination, which is often association with a sense of dissolution in which there is a rapid return to the previous fragmented stage.

Sandel & Johnson's (1983) 'nascent' group theory presents DMT as an approach that may offer support, prevent atrophy and maintain functioning, rather than a therapeutic intervention that aims to eliminate problems and achieve deep personality changes. Their ideas are particularly relevant to working with clients with schizophrenia in a group situation.

These DMT approaches, originating in the USA, are frequently referred to by British practitioners as a source of direct and, more often, indirect influence upon their work. Most British dance movement therapists who draw heavily upon psychoanalytic/psychodynamic thinking do not necessarily prescribe to any one of them. One such example is found in Penfield's contribution to British DMT practice.

Kedzie Penfield trained originally in the USA, but has practised in the UK for a number of years and is regarded as one of the British pioneers. Although Penfield (1992) acknowledges that Reichian and Gestalt Therapy have lent techniques and concepts to DMT (e.g. she refers to the 'cathartic' potential of movement), her work is increasingly informed by psychoanalytic/psychodynamic thinking. This is particularly evident in Penfield's more recent publications (e.g. Penfield 2001). Conscious and unconscious processes are acknowledged as parallel to verbal and non-verbal communication. Transferences and countertransferences are considered, looked at and actively worked through via movement improvisations. Direct affiliation with a single psychoanalytic/psychodynamic theorist or a specific American-based DMT practice is not apparent. Within Penfield's approach (termed 'movement psychotherapy'), the meaning of movement is seen as multifaceted. For example, Penfield (1992) talks about the concepts of 'simultaneity' and 'transmutation', whereby the same movement is seen as encapsulating more than one meaning and/or holding different meanings. The potential of movement to carry multiple and different meanings depending on the context is a characteristic of many psychoanalytically/psychodynamically-informed DMT practices in the UK. Although Penfield's approach is rooted in LMA, it signifies a departure from Laban-based approaches where there is much stronger reliance upon specific movement-personality associations (e.g. see North's approach presented earlier in the chapter).

A similar use of Laban's movement theory is apparent in the examples in Tables 8.8 and 8.9. In both cases, Laban's work is perceived as a baseline that is placed within a wider psychoanalytic/psychodynamic framework. The first example, addresses children and incorporates developmental aspects of psychoanalytic/psychodynamic thinking. The second describes an approach with adults with mental health problems and has a broad psychoanalytic/psychodynamic conceptualisation (e.g. object-relations theory and Jungian principles).

Group movement psychotherapy with children in a mainstream school

In Table 8.8 Sue Curtis (Karkou 2002) provides an example of a psychoanalytically-informed DMT approach (called 'dance movement psychotherapy') with children within a mainstream school context. Her approach is influenced by Freud, the British object relations theory (e.g. Klein and Winnicott), as well as attachment theory (Bowlby) and developmental psychology (Stern). She also considers developmental movement (Sherborne), play therapy (Axline) and Laban movement analysis to be important aspects of her work.

As the example in Table 8.8 shows, there is minimal structure within the session: an initial warm-up and a final movement closure, both of which are designed specifically for, and with, each group and that are based on group themes. Sessions can therefore be seen as guided thematically rather than structurally (see Bruscia's [1988] distinction between different types of improvisational MT sessions). The overall aim is to enable children to transform uncontainable feelings into manageable, organised and acceptable expressions that eventually allow them to also progress with their learning. Some of the therapeutic tools are:

- organising children's body and movement preferences into sequences, games, symbolic and role-playing
- trusting and relating with an adult within the therapy context which becomes a cornerstone for also developing better relationships with the teachers
- interpreting transferential material in an age-appropriate way.

A short-term DMT approach with a group of people with mental health problems

Another example of the use of psychoanalytic/psychodynamic thinking within DMT is the case (Table 8.9) provided by Nina Papadopoulos. The example refers to a short-term group with adults with varied mental health problems. The clients are seen as sharing an overall need for stability and facing underlying conflicts. According to Papadopoulos (N. Papadopoulos, unpublished interview, 2002), one of the fundamental principles in her work is the belief that: 'the unconscious plays an important role in the psychological dynamics within intrapsychic and interpersonal contexts' (p. 3). Although this therapist also makes references to systemic theory, her overall understanding and guidance arise from a broad psychoanalytic/psychodynamic thinking that includes the Jungian concepts of symbolic work and polarities, issues of transference and countertransference and assumptions from group analytical work (e.g. the belief that that healing factors will be activated within the group). It is interesting that despite the bias of this approach towards psychodynamic thinking, the intervention is short-term (only 16 weeks), a practical decision informed by lengthy waiting lists and limited funding.

The case example in Table 8.9 presents DMT sessions as having a five-fold, flexible structure that consists of an initial check in, a physical warm-up, a

Table 8.8: Group movement psychotherapy with children in a mainstream school – Sue Curtis [Example provided to V Karkou for 'Arts Therapies: from Theory to Practice' study [Karkou 2002, reproduced with permission]]

Summary of session	Comments by the therapist and the authors
Description of needs	
'Small group of four boys (aged 6–7 years) all of whom have *difficulty containing their temper and aggression.*	'Children with *emotional/behavioural difficulties* or learning difficulties within mainstream and/or special schools.'
Tend to get into fights – cannot sit in a chair in class and run in and out of class.'	
Aims/expectations/assumptions	'To help children *find manageable form of expressing feelings* and to make links with their ability to learn in classroom, e.g. develop self-esteem, confidence, assertion and attention, help them initiate ideas, build social skills and develop meaningful relationships.
'To help them *develop their own boundaries.*	
To *contain aggression* by giving them other forms to express it (i.e. through movement and imaginative play – role play, characterisation).	
I assume that the group will start chaotically; I believe that *we find ideas to build upon.*'	Initial *aims are clarified* as the work progresses. Teachers' expectations are taken on board.'
Beginning of session	'There is a minimal *structure at the beginning and the end of the session* . . . [which involves] developing their own rituals within the group setting . . . [and] negotiating how to use the time and movement activities.'
'All four boys *came into the room,* raced around, went under tables/on tables, argued over the music, etc.	
I got the sense of them being like lottery balls bouncing around, hitting against each other, being unable to listen to each other. They had full energy but no boundaries or sense	*[Countertransference]*

of safety. They wanted to do everything (e.g. use all the props), go wild bodily, all at the same time.

We started by finding *large movements (energetic) and ways of moving all our body (i.e. jumps), but on the spot*. Then I suggested we *see how strong we are* and do four of everything (they did push ups, etc.). After a few minutes they started rolling around, so I gave them a focus of rolling across the room, then challenged them to roll fast – then slow – then in a line. They lined trying to roll in a line together. We developed small movement sequences with explosive (but safe) endings, i.e. rolling, jumping, then running into a huge jump at the end.'

'I am *structuring* what is already there . . . I use developmental milestones, gross motor and existing movement qualities as themes for structure.'

'I will introduce *challenges* (especially for boys).'

Development of session

'We used stretch cloths to find other ways of testing strength, i.e. pulling each other in twos. This developed into a *fisherman's game* where they caught each other (i.e. each other) in cloth to give to me to eat. I would then *put the fish in a big pot and pretend to eat them*. This in turn introduced symbolic play ideas and the opportunity for *simple interpretations*.'

[I will name] 'activities with them – building on movement and imaginative play repertoire.'

[*symbolic play*]

[*Interpretations of symbolic play are often made*]

The "pulling each other" developed into other games, i.e. horses, aeroplanes, etc. I would help them make scene/setting focusing on who we were, how we felt, helping them to think of and name details, i.e. 'flight no 426 going to Jamaica, stopping in Portugal (to pick up another boy) and going on holiday. We all *swapped roles and tried out* how it was like to be captain, passengers, stewardess, etc., and what you had to do bodily to be good at it, what you had to do verbally to be good at it, etc.

[I am] trying to *bring the body into learning* (creativity).

Continued

Table 8.8: Group movement psychotherapy with children in a mainstream school – Sue Curtis [Example provided to V Karkou for 'Arts Therapies: from Theory to Practice' study [Karkou 2002, reproduced with permission]]—cont'd

Summary of session	Comments by the therapist and the authors
As the theme developed and different relationships emerged both in the group and in the play, I asked them to *find a way to show when we were ready to start the play*, after the warm-up. One boy shouted: "we are amigos!" and raced and put his hand in the centre. We all joined hands (like musketeers) and shouted it too. The same boy continued explaining that "amigos" was Portuguese for "friends" and I reflected that that's what we had become . . .	Some of the *ritual* developed within one session might be repeated.
Completion of session 'At the end of every session we remind ourselves before we leave that we are "amigos" and do our ritual movement.'	'The work comes to an end . . . (usually about one and a half years, once a week) when group members can experience, know and contain their feelings sufficiently and they 'act out' less in class. By experiencing being held emotionally and physically in the therapy, building trusting relationships and developing friendships, they can have more support in themselves and with each other to manage better in the classroom situation. In turn their academic work progresses as they take in more and learn to organise their thoughts and ideas.'

Authors' wording in [brackets]

Table 8.9: A short-term DMT approach with a group of people with mental health problems – Nina Papadopoulos [Adapted from example provided to V karkou for 'Art Therapies: from Theory to Practice' study [© N. Papadopoulos 2002, reproduced with permission]

Description of process	Comments by the therapist and the authors
Description of needs '[This is] a Short Term closed DMT Group (ST-DMT-G) with Adult Mental Health patients within an NHS Trust Psychological Therapy Service (PTS). These *patients suffer from a variety of mental health/psychiatric problems* and they do not represent one coherent diagnostic category; these problems include panic attacks, depression, ME, and anxiety as well as trauma from abuse. Therefore, although their specific needs are varied, all are in need of psychological assistance, which would enable them to lead a functional life . . .'	*'Referrals* are made via the PTS service and potential patients are interviewed by me. In this *intake interview*, potential group members have the opportunity to identify their particular problems and specific therapeutic goals as well as their concerns about entering therapy in the form of a ST-DMT-G.'
Aims/expectations/assumptions 'The initial aim of the group is to offer a space for change within a tangible context of safety. . . . Within each patient there are dynamic conflicts, tensions and motivations, some conscious and others unconscious. The therapeutic process enables the patients to connect with and *address these inner conflicts* within the containing frame of the group; in turn, these *conflicts need to be related to the demands of the patients' external realities*. Moreover, it helps patients perceive the actual creative potential of these conflicts over and above their destructive and crippling impact.'	'Through movement and verbal interactions, patients are encouraged to explore their psychological world (both *intra-psychically* and *interpersonally*).'

Continued

Table 8.9: A short-term DMT approach with a group of people with mental health problems – Nina Papadopoulos [Adopted from example provided to V Karkou for 'Art Therapies: from Theory to Practice study [© N Papadopoulos 2002, reproduced with permission]—cont'd

Description of process	Comments by the therapist and the authors
Beginning of group	[Each session consists of a flexible structure that has five parts:]
'The first sessions usually *start off with extreme tension and anxiety* as patients meet each other for the first time. Consequently, I interpret the complex range of their contradictory feelings and expectations; also, I explain that each session will have a clear structure and that they will always have the opportunity to make choices within each session and decide whether to go along with the suggested structure or not.	[(i) *General check-in*]
Patients are encouraged to *focus as much as possible on their bodies*, with special emphasis on their anatomical structure, their breathing and the movement potential in each of the major joints. This generally helps the patients to feel grounded and more in control of themselves.	[(ii) *Physical warm up*]
In the second phase of the session, *I suggest that patients create movements that other group members may mirror, or make sculpted shapes.* These movements or shapes reflect themes or feelings that patients have experienced during or before the session. At all times during this phase, *I am as reassuring as possible to the patients,* confirming that there is not a "right" or "wrong" response to these creative opportunities, but rather that these activities offer a *possibility of experiencing or trying out something new about themselves or embodying something they may feel.*	[(iii) *Movement tasks/creative movement*] 'Often, at this early stage the *group does not feel solid and bonded together* – in fact quite the contrary – it often feels fragmented and this can contribute to a sense of insecurity. However, as the work progresses more realistic hope emerges which is often interspersed by negative feelings, such as despondence, despair and depression.' 'Throughout, I am trying to assist the patients to *differentiate their feelings, develop a reflective position on themselves* and thus diminish their fear of being overwhelmed by their difficulties.'
Following this experience, patients are invited to reflect verbally about their perceptions and responses. Then, a closure . . . may take the form of a *relaxation, grounding or breathing exercise.*	[(iv) *Reflections*] [(v) *Movement or verbal closure*]
Development of group	'As the work develops and the patients become more familiar with each other as well as with the group structure itself, they begin to feel much safer; yet, at the same time, as the therapeutic process deepens, within the
[Gradually patients enter] 'into a world of *symbolic and imaginative play* in which they may work through their inner unconscious conflicts and tensions at a deeper level. This is done through increasingly	

sophisticated forms of sharing movement, rhythm and dance together with other group members. Consequently, in order to assist in this process, I begin to employ additional props including balls, music, percussion instruments, balloons, etc.

After the warm-up the group may decide to use a prop to facilitate creative movement work. A multi-coloured parachute is often chosen and the group engages with it in a variety of ways. They may for example shake it, clothe themselves in it and become imaginary characters, float it in the air, bounce balloons or balls on top of it, create a tug of war with it, dance with it. The parachute becomes a vehicle for their imaginary symbolic play. Powerful *emotional responses* to this creative work are activated ranging from gentle, calming meditative feelings to violent and angry reactions both internally in themselves and in relation to each other. After the movement experience patients will reflect on their responses and not unusually they will connect the experience with their own personal difficulties and gain new insights about these.'

Completion of group

'At this stage, I encourage *verbal reflections* on the whole therapeutic process including assessment of any changes that patients have experienced either in relation to their bodies, their emotional expression, their relationships, their symptoms or their overall psychological state.

Finally, I *encourage the group to find a way to create an appropriate ending.* Often, the group develops such an ending by means of a shared ritual.

context of increased safety, they also access increasingly painful material. This contributes to the *further differentiation of their feelings and, in addition (paradoxically), they are likely to feel in a more tangible way the emergence of their creativity* and the healthy aspects of themselves.'

'Issues of *psychological change* are discussed and "moved" during this phase, highlighting both the excitement at the prospect and longing for change, as well as the fear and apprehension of change.'

'The final phase of the ST-DMT-G addresses *significant thematic material related to endings* and issues of loss, separation, abandonment, and/or relief and celebration. As always, these are explored through the media of both movement and verbal interactions.'

'A month or six weeks after the end of the ST-DMT-G each patient attends another *individual interview* with me in order to review the treatment process, to re-consider their therapeutic goals and to generally assess the effectiveness of the treatment. Follow up interviews continue on a three-monthly and then six-monthly basis.'

Authors' wording in [brackets]

middle section with creative movement/movement tasks, reflections and a movement or verbal closure. This structure is fairly common among British DMT practitioners (e.g. see example presented in Table 8.6). The example in Table 8.9, however, also presents DMT work progressing over the period of the 16 group sessions and outlines important themes that are pertinent at each stage of the therapy. Some of these themes are: concerns about entering therapy before the process starts, the initial sense of fragmentation and insecurity, the longing and fear of change in the middle stage, and issues of loss or celebration at the end of the group. Given the short-term emphasis of this example, the varied needs of the clients involved, and the overall psychoanalytic/psychodynamic orientation, these themes can be useful for a number of different therapeutic interventions (DMT or not). However, Papadopoulos (N Papadopoulos, unpublished interview, 2002) does not address these themes merely through making verbal interpretations (as a verbal psychoanalytic/psychodynamic therapist might have done), but through an extensive use of movement theory, the introduction of props and the provision of support to clients for creative explorations. The DMT specific outcomes of this process are summarised as, achieving a body–mind connection that gives clients a sense of being in control, and 'offers opportunities for change, mood elevation, anxiety reduction and increased creativity' (N Papadopoulos, unpublished interview, 2002, p. 6).

Another example of work by this therapist involves working with clients with schizophrenia within a directive body-oriented context. This work is part of a series of randomised controlled trials (RCTs) run by Priebe & Röhricht (2001) that compare movement interventions with verbal therapeutic treatments. Findings from this study will clarify further the role of movement in addressing the negative effects of schizophrenia.

Other DMT approaches

In contrast to psychoanalytically/psychodynamically-informed DMT practices described earlier, Bonnie Meekums, one of the pioneers of DMT in the UK, has long argued that DMT does not need justification through the use of neighbouring fields such as psychotherapy. The support for her work comes mainly from sustained research into her own practice, e.g. working with children and their mothers (Meekums 1990, 1992) and with adult survivors of sexual abuse (Meekums 1998, 2000). Although Laban's movement theory, developmental psychology (e.g. Stern), object relations theory (e.g. Winnicott and Mahler), humanistic psychotherapy (e.g. Rogers), and creativity theories (Hadamard, Poincaré), have informed her practice, she highlights the distinctive nature of DMT and regards her own work as a form of creative psychotherapy. This model was described in Chapter 4, as consisting of four stages that are developing in a spiral way: preparation, incubation, illumination and evaluation. When this model is specifically applied to DMT practice, Meekums (2002) stresses: the creative process as a 'workable model' and the 'metaphoric body' as an essential DMT tool.

Another important theoretician, researcher and practitioner in the field is Helen Payne. Payne (1994b) refers to her work as an 'integrative' practice and argues for the relevance of different schools of thought to her practice depending on the client, e.g. psychoanalytic/psychodynamic, humanistic, behavioural and transpersonal psychology. The needs of the clients determine the choice of one model over another, the clinical methodology and the level of direction, structure and active involvement of the therapist in the process.

Payne's selection of the model and methodology appropriate to categories of specific needs, is supported with reference to relevant research literature including Sandel & Johnson (1983) and Payne's research work with adolescents (1987, 1992b), eating disorders (1994b) and students in training (1995). Although originally trained in the Laban approach, Payne does not use movement analysis in her practice other than as an aid to observation. Influenced by her later training in Whitehouse's Jungian approach to DMT, her work with arts therapies students and with high functioning clients, Payne (2001) is currently emphasising 'authentic movement' as an intervention appropriate for many of her clients and as an important strand of her work.

Social construction theory appears as an additional therapeutic influence upon current arts therapies practice. As we have seen in Chapter 4, this perspective has close links with eclectic/integrative therapeutic trends in arts therapies. In both cases, the choice of the therapeutic framework is primarily determined by the clients' needs. However, unlike psychotherapeutic and other traditions in arts therapies, the social-constructionist viewpoint looks at identity, gender, and power relationships as its primary concerns. Allegranti (1997), Best (2000), and Best & Parker (2001) have discussed the impact of social construction theory on DMT. Allegranti (B Allegranti, unpublished interview, 2002), for example, insists that the therapeutic process involves addressing power issues, verbal/non-verbal interplay and integration, and connecting the internal world of the client with the external, social world. Although Allegranti (B Allegranti, unpublished interview, 2002) also mentions humanistic and psychodynamic approaches as potentially relevant to her practice when appropriate to clients' needs, she incorporates Chaplin's (1988) 'rhythm' model for feminist psychotherapy as an overall theoretical basis for her work. This model is perceived as permitting 'an ever changing space both between and inclusive of opposites' (B Allegranti, unpublished interview, 2002, p. 2).

Summary

Despite the newness of this arts therapies discipline, and the struggle faced by pioneers in the field to receive acknowledgement of their body-based practice as something of equal value to verbal/talking therapies, DMT is currently recognised as a health profession alongside the other arts therapies modalities. In the USA, the field emerged from the work of dancers and dance teachers, while in the UK there is a strong influence from American pioneers and Laban-trained practitioners. In its current form, the discipline has grown in terms of training courses, areas of work and client groups. Most dance movement therapists can be found working in education and to a lesser extent in hospitals and the community, while mental health and learning disabilities are the two clients groups that are currently receiving most frequent attention. Body/movement/dance techniques are used extensively, often within a strong humanistic frame. However, following the example of other arts therapies, eclectic/integrative, psychoanalytic/psychodynamic, and at times developmental principles, are particularly relevant. Some of the most important practices found within the field are: movement-based approaches connected with Laban, interactive approaches linked with Chace and psychoanalytic/psychodynamic practices initiated by Whitehouse and authentic movement. Other approaches to DMT briefly described in this chapter were the creative psychotherapy model, the integrative model and the social construction approach.

References

* Adler J 1999 Who is the witness? A description of authentic movement. In: Pallaro P (ed) Authentic movement: essay by Mary Starks Whitehouse, Janet Adler and Joan Chodorow. Jessica Kingsley, London, p 141–159
* Allegranti B 1997 Exploring the social construction of gender through movement improvisation. Unpublished Masters dissertation, University of Surrey-Roehampton
* Association for Dance Movement Therapy (ADMT UK) 2004 What is DMT? Online. Available: http://www.admt.org.uk/whatis.html 11 December 2004
* Bartenieff I, Lewis D 1980 Body movement: coping with the environment. Gordon and Breach Science Publishers, New York
* Best P 2000 Theoretical diversity and clinical collaboration: reflections by a dance/movement therapist. The Arts in Psychotherapy 27(3):197–211
* Best P, Parker G 2001 Moving reflections: the social creation of identities in communication. In: Kossolapow L, Scoble S, Waller D (eds) Arts – therapies – communication: on the way to a communicative European arts therapy, vol 1. Lit Verlag, Munster, p 142–148
* Bloom K, Shreeves R 1998 Moves: a sourcebook of ideas for body awareness and creative movement. Harwood Academic Publishers, Amsterdam
* Bruscia K E 1988 A survey of treatment procedures in improvisational music therapy. Psychology of Music 16:10–24
* Chaiklin S, Schmais D 1986 The Chace approach to dance therapy. In: Lewis P (ed) Theoretical approaches in dance/movement therapy, vol 1. Kendall/Hunt, Iowa, p 17–36
* Chaplin J 1988 Feminist counselling in action. Sage, London
* Chodorow J 1991 Dance therapy and depth psychology: the moving imagination. Routledge, London
* Cruz R F, Sabers D L 1998 Dance/movement therapy is more effective than previously reported. The Arts in Psychotherapy 25(2):101–104
* Feldenkrais M 1972 Awareness through movement. Harper and Row, New York
* Feldenkrais M 1985 The potent self. Harper and Row, San Francisco
* Finfgeld D L 2001 New directions for feminist therapy based on social constructionism. Archives of Psychiatric Nursing XV(3):148–154
* Gergen K J 1991 The saturated self. Basic Books, New York
* Grentz S 1996 A primer on postmodernism. William B Eermans, Grand Rapids, MI
* Holden S 1990 Moving together: the groups find a dance. Group Analysis 23:265–276
* Karkou V 2002 Report: from theory to practice. Unpublished report submitted to the University of Hertfordshire
* Karkou V 2003 UK research register for DMT. Online. Available: http://www.admt.org.uk/res_research.html 11 Dec 2004
* Karkou V in press. Dance movement therapy in the community: group work with people with enduring mental health difficulties. In: Payne H (ed) Dance movement therapy: theory, practice and research. Routledge, London
* Karkou V, Sanderson P 2001 Report: theories and assessment procedures used by dance/movement therapists in the UK. The Arts in Psychotherapy 28:13–20
* Kaylo J 2003 Unpublished workshop notes, ADMT UK workshop on Bartenieff's movement analysis
* Kestenberg J 1975 Children and parents: psychoanalytic studies in development. Jason Aronson, New York

- Kestenberg-Amighi J, Loman S, Lewis P et al 1999 The meaning of movement: developmental and clinical perspectives of the Kestenberg Movement Profile. Brunner-Routledge, New York
- Laban L 1949 Some notes on movement therapy, revised version: movement and dance
- Laban R 1975 Modern educational dance. MacDonald and Evans, London
- Lamb W 1965 Posture and gesture: an introduction to the study of physical behaviour. Gerald Duckworth, London
- Levy F 1988 Dance movement therapy: a healing art. American Alliance for Health, Physical Education, Recreation and Dance, Reston
- Loman S 1998 Employing a developmental model of movement patterns in dance/movement therapy with young children and their families. American Journal of Dance Therapy 20(2):101–115
- Loman S, Foley L 1996 Models for understanding the nonverbal process in relationships. The Arts in Psychotherapy 23(4):341–350
- Loman S, Merman H 1996 The KMP: a tool for dance/movement therapy. American Journal of Dance Therapy 18(1):29–52
- Low K G, Ritter M 1998 Response to Cruz & Sabers. The Arts in Psychotherapy 25(2):105–107
- Lowen A 1975 Bioenergetics. Coward, McCann and Geoghegan, New York
- Lyotard J F 1984 The postmodern condition. Manchester University Press, Manchester
- MacDonald J 1992 Dance? Of course I can't? Dance movement therapy for people with learning difficulties. In: Payne H (ed) Dance movement therapy: theory and practice. Tavistock/Routledge, London, p 202–217
- Mahler M, Pine F, Bergman A 1975 The psychological birth of the human infant. Basic Books, New York
- Meekums B 1990 Dance movement therapy and the development of mother-child interaction. Unpublished MPhil thesis. Faculty of Education, University of Manchester
- Meekums B 1992 The love bugs: dance music therapy in a family service unit. In: Payne H (ed) Handbook of inquiry in the arts therapies: one river, many currents. Jessica Kingsley, London and Philadelphia, p 18–38
- Meekums B V F 1998 Recovery from child sexual abuse trauma within an arts therapies programme for women. Unpublished PhD thesis. Faculty of Education, University of Manchester
- Meekums B 2000 Creative group therapy for women survivors of child sexual abuse. Jessica Kingsley Publishers, London
- Meekums B 2002 Dance movement therapy. Sage, London
- Meier W 1997 The teacher and the therapist. E-motion ADMT UK Quarterly IX(1):7–9
- North M 1972 Personality assessment through movement. Northcote House, Plymouth
- Pallaro P 1999 Authentic movement: essay by Mary Starks Whitehouse, Janet Adler and Joan Chodorow. Jessica Kingsley, London
- Payne H 1987 The perceptions of male adolescents, labelled delinquent towards dance movement therapy. Unpublished MPhil thesis. Faculty of Education, University of Manchester
- Payne H 1990 Creative movement and dance in groupwork. Winslow, Oxon
- Payne H 1992a Introduction. In: Payne H (ed) Dance movement therapy: theory and practice. Tavistock/Routledge, London, p 1–17
- Payne H 1992b Shut in, shut out: dance movement therapy with children and adolescents. In: Payne H (ed) Dance movement therapy: theory and practice. Tavistock/Routledge, London, p 39–80
- Payne H (ed) 1993 Handbook of inquiry in the arts therapies: one river, many currents. Jessica Kingsley, London
- Payne H L 1994a Dance movement therapy. In: Jones D (ed) Innovative therapy. Open University, Milton Keynes
- Payne H 1994b Eating distress, women and integrative movement psychotherapy. In: Dokter D (ed) Arts therapies and clients with eating disorders: fragile board. Jessica Kingsley, London, p 208–225
- Payne H 1995 The DMT group as personal development in training in higher education. Unpublished PhD thesis. University of London, Institute of Education
- Payne H 2001 Authentic movement and supervision. E-motion ADMT UK Quarterly XIII(4):4–7
- Pearson J (ed) 1996 Discovering the self through drama and movement: the Sesame approach. Jessica Kingsley, London

- Penfield K 1992 Individual movement psychotherapy: dance movement therapy in private practice. In: Payne H (ed) Dance movement therapy: theory and practice. Tavistock/Routledge, London, p 163–182
- Penfield K 2001 Movement as a way to the unconscious. In: Seale Y, Strong I (eds) Where analysis meets the arts. Karnac Books, London
- Preston-Dunlop V 1963 Handbook for modern educational dance. MacDonald and Evans, London
- Priebe S, Röhricht F 2001 Specific body image pathology in acute schizophrenia. Psychiatry Research 101:289–301
- Reich W 1960 An introduction to orgonomy: selected writings. Noonday, New York
- Ritter M, Low K G 1996 Effects of dance/movement therapy: a meta-analysis, The Arts in Psychotherapy 23:249–260
- Rolf I 1975 Structural integration. Viking, New York
- Sandel S, Johnson D 1983 Structure and process of the nascent group: dance movement therapy with chronic patients. The Arts in Psychotherapy 10:131–140
- Sanderson P 1984 Modern educational dance revisited. Physical Education Review 7(1):80–82
- Sanderson P 1986 Current issues in dance education. Momentum 10(3):2–10
- Sanderson P 1996 Dance within the national physical education curriculum of England and Wales. The European Physical Education Review 2(1):54–63
- Sanderson P 2001 Age and gender issues in adolescent attitudes to dance. European Physical Education Review 7(2):137–155
- Sanderson P 2002 An appreciation of the life of Irene Dilks, dancer and educator. Research in Dance Education 2(1):103–105
- Sanderson P, Meakin D C 1983 Dance in English secondary schools today. The Journal of Aesthetic Education 17(1): 69–83
- Schmais C 1985 Healing processes in group dance/movement therapy. American Journal of Dance Therapy 8:17–36
- Sherborne V 1990 Developmental movement for children. Cambridge University Press, Cambridge
- Siegel E V 1984 Dance movement therapy: mirrors of ourselves. The psychoanalytic approach. Human Sciences Press, New York
- Spitz R 1965 The first year of life. International Universities Press, New York
- Stanton-Jones K 1992 An introduction to dance movement therapy in psychiatry. Tavistock/Routledge, London
- Sullivan H S 1955 The interpersonal theory of psychiatry. W W Norton, New York
- Whitehouse M 1979 C G Jung and dance-therapy: two major principles. In: Bernstein P L (ed) Eight theoretical approaches in dance/movement therapy, vol I. Kendall/Hunt, Iowa
- Whiting H T A 1973 Review: personality assessment through movement. Laban Art of Movement Guild Magazine
- Yalom I D 1970 The theory and practice of group psychotherapy. Basic Books, New York

Conclusions

In this book we have offered an introduction to arts therapies in a way that clarifies what arts therapies practices are and what they are not, how they are practised and why. We have also outlined and discussed what is common and what is different amongst different approaches. For example, as an introduction to the professional development of the field, we have seen that over the centuries, there have been dynamic changes in the philosophy and rationale of the 'why' and 'how' of using the arts as healing (Ch. 1). Within the 20th century, artists, art teachers, psychotherapists/psychiatrists, other health professionals and hospital artists have moved such ideas forward and contributed to the emergence of separate arts therapies disciplines, that is music therapy (MT), art therapy (AT), dramatherapy (DT) and dance movement therapy (DMT). With the emergence of the arts therapies professional bodies in the last 50 years, there has been a strong shift towards organised action that has translated into: the development of training courses, articulation of clear professional requirements, and acumination of professional experience and research studies within a number of settings and with a number of client groups. The current expansion in the above areas suggests strong professional development and a gradual recognition from the wider community of the contribution of arts therapies to well-being. The registration of arts therapists with the Health Professions Council (HPC) offers additional guarantees of good practice; arts therapies are regulated and monitored by an independent body in a way that protects the public from possible abuse or malpractice.

We have also seen (Ch. 2) that professionalisation of the arts therapies field has created practices that are substantially different from the work undertaken by community artists or hospital artists, arts teachers, other therapists and/or other health professionals. The most important difference from these fields is the fact that arts therapists have specific training and experiences that enable them to make safe and potentially beneficial use of the arts with vulnerable clients. Such a specific knowledge base and experience of using the arts in therapy is not present in the work of any other professional groupings. Furthermore, while redefining the field as a whole we have identified key characteristics of most arts therapies practices such as the use of the arts, creativity, imagery, imagination, symbolism and metaphors, non-verbal communication, the client–therapist relationship and therapeutic aims. Although most of these aspects can be also detected in neighbouring fields such as the arts and psychotherapy, they have been combined and further developed within arts therapies in a unique way (Ch. 3).

Nevertheless, we have argued that the therapeutic nature of arts therapies lies in the presence of therapeutic underpinnings and consistent methodological principles that guide practices, safeguard the process and the client, and give meaning to the content of the sessions (Ch. 4). As Kossolapow et al (2001) (reviewed by Karkou, 2002) has claimed, there is a need to identify and describe therapy practices in order to improve conceptual understanding of a rapidly evolving field, and create solid foundations. Given the dynamic nature of the field, pinpointing the overall foundations of arts therapies can be elusive. Furthermore, describing therapeutic principles and conceptual frameworks that go beyond one discipline to the arts therapies field as a whole is even more challenging. Nevertheless, the results from our study suggest that there are a number of common therapeutic frameworks that are relevant to all arts therapies disciplines. We have called these frameworks 'therapeutic trends' and we have identified six as the most important ones (Ch. 4): humanistic, eclectic/integrative, psychoanalytic/psychodynamic, developmental, artistic/creative, active/directive. Other important therapeutic frameworks that can be found within arts therapies literature, such as models stemming from family/systemic therapy, transpersonal psychology, personal construct theory, narrative therapy, anthropology, social psychology and neuroscience have not been covered in this book due to lack of sufficient empirical data. We believe, however, that some of these conceptual frames are becoming increasingly relevant to arts therapies, and that they will have a significant impact upon future developments within arts therapies practice.

The therapeutic trends we have already conceptualised during our research survey can be seen as a first mapping of the current arts therapies practice. Research results suggest that there is indeed a tendency to work in different ways with different client groups and in different settings. We have also seen how the age of the practitioners and their backgrounds play an important role on the type of arts therapies preferred. Finally, we have seen that the degree to which these trends are preferred in each discipline also varies. Comparative results amongst different arts therapies disciplines in relation to these trends are shown in Figure 9.1. These results can be treated as a comprehensive summary of similarities and differences amongst disciplines. For example, although all arts therapies disciplines share common beliefs regarding the main therapeutic trends we have identified, there is a varying degree of agreement with these ideas depending on the arts therapies discipline under discussion. Some reasons for these differences have been identified in the chapters dealing with separate arts therapies disciplines in Section 2, such as separate historical developments and preferences of work of the pioneers in each field, varying degrees of support received from neighbouring fields and psychotherapy in particular, different choices and alliances made by separate arts therapies professional associations, separate theoretical advancements achieved in each field, and specific areas of work stressed by each arts therapies discipline.

We find that these differences can offer unique approaches to treatment and a wide range of options for clients. However, we also perceive them as potentially offering useful examples of practice for the arts therapists themselves. For example:

■ The relatively strong emphasis upon models of health, body-based work and creativity within DT and DMT, can remind other arts therapists that humanistic and at times multi-modal approaches can be more appropriate ways of working with certain client groups (e.g. children or adults with no apparent difficulties) and in certain working environments (e.g. mainstream schools or in private practice). According to a recent document produced by the Department of Health (DoH 2004), where psychological therapies are concerned, empathy and flexibility on the part of the therapist are highly regarded amongst the majority of service users. Such principles have been fundamental to the emergence of all arts therapies and it will

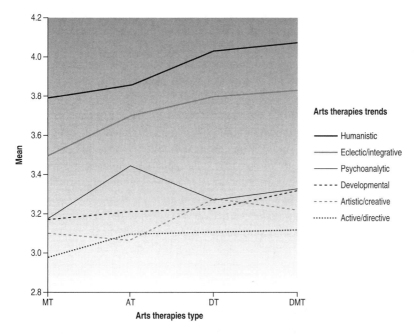

Figure. 9.1: *Main therapeutic trends according to each of the arts therapies disciplines.*
The higher the score, the stronger the agreement with this group of statements (a five-point scale was used ranging from strongly agree = 5 to strongly disagree = 1).
It is apparent that, although overall, each trend holds significance for all arts therapies disciplines, there are also a number of differences. ANOVAs performed for the arts therapies trends suggest the following statistically significant differences:
The humanistic trend has greater relevance to DT and DMT in comparison with MT (p = 0.002 and 0.012 respectively). Furthermore, DT places greater emphasis upon such principles than AT (p = 0.016).
There is a relative preoccupation of AT with psychoanalytic/psychodynamic theory, compared to MT (p = 0.000) and DT (p = 0.003).
DT emphasises artistic/creative practices more than other arts therapies types and AT in particular (p = 0.017).
Finally, the eclectic/integrative approach is relevant for all arts therapies but not as important for MT (in comparison with AT p = 0.018, with DT p = 0.003 and with DMT p = 0.024).

be important not to neglect them within the current climate of rapid professionalisation of the field.

▦ The fact that art therapists have a strong alliance with psychoanalytic/psychodynamic thinking can highlight the need for all arts therapists to hold a clear psychotherapeutic rationale for their work and develop practices that are coherent and psychologically sound. We have already discussed the relevance of psychoanalytic/psychodynamic thinking for working with clients with mental health problems and in hospital-based environments. Art therapists have been on the frontline of this type of work and their experience cannot be ignored. Furthermore, BAAT (the British Association of Art Therapists), as the largest arts therapies association with substantial experience of battles for professional recognition, can offer experience of how to recruit and organise practitioners and pursue professional rights.

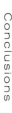

- The emphasis of dramatherapists upon utilising artistic/creative frameworks for informing their practice can remind other arts therapists not to neglect the artistic components of their work. The arts are the very first thing that attracts many practitioners to the field and at times they are the very first thing that is responsible for therapeutic change in the client. Flexible ways of working in the community, consultancy work and work with institutions is an additional lesson that can be learnt from the DT field.
- Finally, MT can offer knowledge and experiences of undertaking extensive research work in MT practice and creating a public profile that can be useful for all arts therapists. In terms of clinical practice, the relative aversion of music therapists to eclectic/integrative principles can remind arts therapists that within a postmodern era that values diversity, it is important to retain a clear sense of professional identity that is not in danger of fragmentation or diffusion and at the same time does not lose essential flexibility.

After borrowing useful ideas, theoretical frames and existing knowledge from neighbouring fields, it is important for arts therapies to strengthen theoretical and practical development that stems from within the arts therapies field itself. Calls for defining arts therapies with language that originates from arts therapies can be found in the relevant literature beyond the MT field. For example, Jones (1996) and Meekums (2002) suggest that discipline-specific developments offer sufficient theoretical justifications of DT and DMT practice respectively without the need to borrow ideas from other fields. We suggest that discipline-specific professional identity can be further strengthened if commonalities and distinctive practices amongst different arts therapies are clearly outlined. We also find that when weaknesses in existing discipline-specific practice are found or new areas of work are being developed, the first place where arts therapists can look for further understanding and development can be the arts therapies field as a whole. The concept of discourse (i.e. ways of thinking or talking about things) introduced by Foucault (1967) and valued by current postmodern thinking within the arts therapies field, can extend beyond the boundaries of the session and the client–therapist relationship to unfolding ways of thinking and/or talking about different arts therapies disciplines and approaches. It is expected that the outcome from an extensive and in-depth dialogue will enable clearer articulation of theory and contribute to further advancements in practice that relies less upon other fields and more upon arts therapies practice. Such discussions are not always easy; they can create tensions between the supporters of one approach/discipline over another. However, as Landy (1995) puts it, this tension can be seen as a 'creative tension' that is useful for further development and change. We expect that ideas raised and discussed in this book will make a small contribution in this direction and that this will become useful for arts therapies practitioners, educationalists, other health professionals and ultimately, arts therapies clients.

References

- Department of Health (DoH) 2004 Organising and delivering psychological therapies. Department of Health, London
- Foucault M 1967 Madness and civilisation: a history of insanity in the age of reason. Tavistock, London
- Jones P 1996 Drama as therapy: theatre as living. Routledge, London
- Karkou V 2002 Review: arts – therapies – communication: on the way to a communicative European arts therapy. Inscape 7(1):43–45
- Kossolapow L, Scoble S, Waller D (eds) 2001 Arts – therapies – communication: on the way to a communicative European arts therapy, vol. 1. Lit Verlag, Munster
- Landy R J 1995 Isolation and collaboration in the creative arts therapies – the implications of crossing borders. The Arts in Psychotherapy 22(2):83–86
- Meekums B 2002 Dance movement therapy. Sage, London

Conclusions

Appendix 1

Research Methodology

Introduction

This book arose from extensive research work in the field of arts therapies over a number of years. A large part of this study was completed at the University of Manchester, School of Education and was funded by the Economic and Social Research Council (ESRC). It was part of the PhD work of one of the authors of this book and was completed under the supervision of the other author. A more recent part of the research work was undertaken during the writing of this book and was financially supported by the Department of Art and Arts Therapies at the University of Hertfordshire.

Philosophical underpinnings

The philosophical perspective of the study has been strongly influenced by 'New Paradigm' research and 'Grounded Theory' in particular (Glaser & Strauss 1967). Grounded theory encourages researchers to avoid concepts, theories and preconceived ideas at an early stage, allowing the practitioners' own voices to be heard. The research design of the study was therefore 'grounded' in the field in that the perspectives of as many practising arts therapists as possible were taken on board from the early stages of the work as well as throughout the progress of the study. Initial aims and research questions were refined and hypotheses were stated in an emergent way (i.e. they were formulated as the process of the study was unfolding). Consequently, the research design remained flexible and creativity, a key notion for arts therapies practice and research in arts therapies (Meekums 1993), became also a key notion for this study.

For example, despite influences from grounded theory, methodological loyalties were avoided. Instead, the study valued 'methodological plurality' that was expressed through a combination of strategies: semi-structured interviews and survey and case studies were used, which were guided by the overall aims and emerging research questions. Both qualitative and quantitative methods were used depending on the best possible way of collecting data each time. This is regarded as sound practice amongst researchers in education, social sciences, and psychotherapy and is increasingly acknowledged within arts therapies research (see Ansdell & Pavlicevic 2001).

Research design

Broadly speaking, the research design had three stages that developed as the study progressed and research questions were refined. The first stage involved collecting and analysing information from leading practitioners in the field regarding their practice (semi-structured interviews); the second involved trying out the results from stage one against the perceptions of the wider community of practising arts therapists in the UK in order to recognise major patterns of practice for the field as a whole (survey through questionnaires, N = 580); a final stage involved moving back to the field and collecting examples of practice that reflected these patterns (case studies through interviews and observations). Stages one and two were funded by ESRC and completed at the University of Manchester during the period 1994–1998. The final part of the research was prepared with financial support from the Department of Art and Arts Therapies, at the University of Hertfordshire (2001–2002). In both cases, a nation-wide scope was retained aiming to describe British arts therapies practice as fully as possible.

Stage 1: Interviews

Semi-structured interviews were completed with leading arts therapists in the UK, who acted as key-informants (N = 12). They were chosen on the basis of their contribution to the arts therapies field as evidenced in their published work and their involvement in arts therapies training courses (purposive sampling). The main areas dealt with during the interviews were: theory, methodology and assessment procedures followed by the interviewees.

All of the interviews were transcribed and analysed using a subjective content analysis (Bliss et al 1983). The analysis was initially based on predefined domains closely related to the interview questions. However, these main areas were used only as a working frame allowing other categories and subcategories to emerge through scanning the data. No quantification was made. Several refinements of the categories followed by continuously moving forwards and backwards in relation to the collected material. This procedure was similar to what Strauss & Corbin (1990) call 'a comparison method'.

Statements were extracted from the transcripts, regrouped based on their conceptual relevance to the rest of the statements, and double-checked between the primary researcher and the supervisor and against relevant literature. Lists of statements were finally devised that dealt with: (a) theory (main influences, theoretical principles and aims), (b) methodology (c) initial assessment and evaluation of the therapeutic process.

Stage 2: Survey

A questionnaire was devised, piloted and eventually distributed to all practising arts therapists in the UK (initial N = 1448). The questionnaire included the lists of statements revealed from stage 1 and refined through the pilot study. Against each statement participants were asked to state their degree of agreement/disagreement on a scale from 5 to 1. The questionnaire also included additional questions about arts therapists' practice (e.g. type of arts therapies, client group, age of clients, settings) and their background (sex and age, level of arts therapies training, other qualifications and other formal training). Finally it included open-ended questions regarding the main topics covered. Quantitative data collected from the returned questionnaires (final N = 580) were coded and analysed using the Statistical Package for the Social Sciences (SPSS). Descriptive statistics, factor analysis, two-way Multivariate Analyses of Variants (MANOVAs) and Canonical Correlations were performed on this data. Subjective content analysis was used for the qualitative data collected.

Results from the above analyses can be regarded as fairly conclusive due to what was perceived as an unexpectedly high, for the arts therapies field, response rate (39%). Moreover, the response rate was acceptable because: (i) the sample consisted of four different groups of participants, i.e. art therapists, music therapists, dramatherapists, dance movement therapists, all of whom were organised in separate professional associations; (ii) the survey was national; and (iii) practitioners were contacted once only.

Stage 3: Case studies

A number of case studies were completed (N = 20) aiming to identify the way in which results from stage 2 were expressed in practice in terms of case vignettes, therapeutic tools and clients' artwork. Explanations about practice were also sought. Key informants from stage 1 were contacted again and additional participants were identified using the same criteria as before (i.e. their contribution to the arts therapies field through published work and their involvement in arts therapies training). An additional criterion was included which was diversity of practice (purposive sampling). The inclusion of additional participants was due to the fact that results from stage 2 suggested a wide range of available practices. It was also expected that in the interim period since the completion of stage 2, further changes and growth in the field had taken place. We attempted to accommodate these changes through additional data collection from a fairly large sample for a case study methodology.

With the above criteria in mind, all training courses in the UK were contacted and asked for participation, most of which responded positively. The case studies completed included interviews and, where appropriate, observations. Case vignettes were collected and organised on the basis of results from the survey and relevant literature. A selection of these vignettes was eventually included in this book alongside participants' explanations of their practice (Section 2). Permission for the use of client's artwork proved too difficult to pursue and attempts to get this were eventually dropped. A number of therapeutic tools were collected, most of which were about assessment and evaluation, a topic that has been only marginally covered in the book.

Summary

There are two major reports that are available regarding the above research work. For stages 1 and 2, interested readers can consult the PhD thesis held with the University of Manchester (Karkou 1998). For stage 3, there is an unpublished report submitted to the University of Hertfordshire (Karkou 2002).

References

* Ansdell G, Pavlicevic M 2001 Beginning research in the arts therapies: a practical guide. Jessica Kingsley, London
* Bliss J, Monk M, Ogborn J 1983 Qualitative data analysis for educational research. Croom Helm, Beckenham
* Glaser B G, Strauss A L 1967 The discovery of grounded theory: strategies for qualitative research. Aldine, Chicago
* Karkou V 1998 A descriptive evaluation of the practice of arts therapies. Unpublished PhD thesis, University of Manchester, School of Education
* Karkou V 2002 Report: from theory to practice. Unpublished report submitted to the University of Hertfordshire
* Meekums B 1993 Research as an act of creation. In: Payne H (ed) Handbook of inquiry in the arts therapies: one river, many currents. Jessica Kingsley, London, p 130–137
* Strauss A, Corbin J 1990 Basics of qualitative research: grounded theory procedures and techniques. Sage, Newbury Park

Appendices

Appendix 2

Training Courses

The training courses available in the UK that offer professional qualifications to arts therapists and licence to practice are the following. Notes are made for courses for which full accreditation and/or validation was not completed at the time of publication. Many more courses can be found in other parts of the world. The most established ones can be found in the USA, Europe, Middle East (i.e. Israel), Japan and Australia.

University	AT (Source: British Association of Art Therapists – BAAT 2004)			DMT[1] (Source: Association for Dance Movement Therapy – ADMT UK 2004)		
	Department/faculty	Degree	Length of course	Department/faculty	Degree	Length of course
Queen Margaret University College, Edinburgh http://www.qmuc.ac.uk	Department of Occupational Therapy and Art Therapy, Faculty of Social Sciences and Health Care	Master (MSc) in AT MPhil/PhD options	2 years full-time or 3 years part-time	–	–	–
Queen's University, Belfast http://www.qub.ac.uk	Graduate School of Education	Master (MSc) in AT	3 years part-time	–	–	–
Northern Programme for Art Psychotherapy (validated by the Leeds Metropolitan University) http://www.sct.nhs.uk/arttherapy.html	Faculty of Health, Centre for Psychological Therapies in partnership with Sheffield Care Trust	Master (MA) in Art Psychotherapy Practice	2 years full-time or 3 years part-time	–	–	–
University of Hertfordshire http://www.herts.ac.uk	Department of Art and Art Therapy, Faculty of Art and Design	Master (MA) in AT MPhil/PhD options	2 years full-time or 3 years part-time	–	–	–

Institution	Department/Unit	Qualification	Duration	Department/Unit	Qualification	Duration
Goldsmith's College (validated by the University of London) http://www.goldsmiths.ac.uk	Unit of Psychotherapeutic Studies, Professional and Community Education (PACE)	Diploma/Master (MA) in Art Psychotherapy MRes MPhil/PhD options	2 years full-time (Diploma) 2 terms full-time (MA) Part-time options	Unit of Psychotherapeutic Studies, Professional and Community Education (PACE)	Diploma/Master (MA)	2 years full-time (Diploma) 2 terms full-time (MA) (also: part-time options)
University of Derby http://www.derby.ac.uk	School of Education, Health and Sciences	Diploma/Master (MA) MPhil/PhD options	2 years full-time (Diploma) 2 trimesters for Master Part-time options	School of Education, Health and Sciences	Diploma/Master (MA)[2], MPhil/PhD options	2 years full-time (Diploma) 2 trimesters (Master) Part-time options
Roehampton University http://www.roehampton.ac.uk	School of Psychology and Therapeutic Studies	Master(MA) in AT[2] MPhil/PhD options	3–4 years part-time	School of Psychology and Therapeutic Studies	Diploma/Master (MA) MPhil/PhD options	1–2 years part-time

[1] Dance Voice in Bristol is currently developing a postgraduate training course in DMT which has received validation from the University of Derby and is awaiting accreditation from ADMT UK (see http://www.dancevoice.org.uk).

[2] Subject to accreditation from either the Health Professions Council (HPC) or, in the case of DMT, from the professional association, i.e. ADMT UK.

University	MT (Source: British Society for Music Therapy – BSMT 2004)			DT (Source: British Association of Dramatherapists – BADth 2004)		
	Department/ faculty	Degree	Length of course	Department/ faculty	Degree	Length of course
Guildhall School of Music and Drama (validated by City University) http://www.gsmd.ac.uk	Department of Music Therapy	Diploma (DipMTh)	1 year full-time or 2 years part-time	–	–	–
The Nordoff–Robbins Music Therapy Centre, London (validated by City University) http://www.nordoff-robbins.org.uk	–	Master (MMT) MPhil/PhD options	2 years full-time	–	–	–
Queen Margaret University College http://www.qmuc.ac.uk	School of Health Sciences in partnership with the Nordoff–Robbins Music Therapy Trust	Master (MSc) in MT MPhil/PhD Options	2 years full-time 3 years part-time			
University of Bristol http://www.bristol.ac.uk	Department of Music Faculty of Arts	Diploma	2 years part-time	–	–	–

Institution	Department	Qualification	Duration	Department	Qualification	Duration
Anglia Polytechnic University http://www.anglia.ac.uk	Music Department, School of Arts and Letters	Diploma/ Master (MA) MPhil/PhD options	1 year full-time (Diploma) Extra time for Master	—	—	—
Royal Welsh College of Music and Drama http://www.rwcmd.ac.uk	School of Music	Diploma/ Master (MA) options	1 year full-time or 2 years part-time (Diploma) Extra time for Master	—	—	—
Roehampton University http://www.roehampton.ac.uk	School of Psychology and Therapeutic Studies	Diploma Master (MA) MPhil/PhD options	18 months full-time or 2.5 years part-time (Diploma) Extra time for Master	School of Psychology and Therapeutic Studies	Diploma/ Master (MA) MPhil/ PhD options	3 years part-time (Diploma) 18 months (Master)
University of Derby http://www.derby.ac.uk	School of Education, Health and Sciences	Diploma[1] Master (MA) MPhil/PhD options	2 years full-time (Diploma) 2 trimesters for Master Part-time options	School of Education, Health and Sciences	Diploma/ Master (MA) MPhil/ PhD options	2 years full-time (Diploma) 2 trimesters for Master Part-time options

Continued

University	MT (Source: British Society for Music Therapy – BSMT 2004)			DT (Source: British Association of Dramatherapists – BADth 2004)		
	Department/ faculty	Degree	Length of course	Department/ faculty	Degree	Length of course
Sesame Institute (validated by the Open University) http://www.cssd.ac.uk	–	–	–	Central School of Speech and Drama	Master (MA) in Drama and Movement Therapy	3 semesters full-time
Millbrook House (University of Plymouth) http://www2.plymouth.ac.uk/millbrook	–	–	–	School of Health Professions, Faculty of Health and Social Work	Master (MA)	2–3 years part-time
The Northern Trust for Dramatherapy (validated by The University of Manchester) email: ntd@supanet.com	–	–	–	–	Diploma	3 years part-time

[1]Subject to accreditation from the Health Professions Council (HPC).

Appendix 3

Useful Addresses

Art therapy (AT)

Professional associations

In the UK

British Association of Art Therapists (BAAT)
Contact address: BAAT, 24–27 White Lion Street, London, UK N1 9PD
Tel: 00 44 (0)20 7686 4216
Fax: 00 44 (0)20 7837 7945
e-mail: info@baat.org
website: http://www.baat.org

International
The following are some examples of professional associations that can be found on the internet (many more AT associations are available around the world):
American Art Therapy Association: http://www.arttherapy.org
Australian National Art Therapy Association: http://www.anata.org.au
Canadian Art Therapy Association: http://www.catainfo.ca/
Canada: Association of Art Therapy of Quebec: http://iquebec.ifrance.com
Denmark: Institute of Art Therapy: http://www.kunstterapi.dk
France: Association Romande Arts Expression et Therapies:
http://www.araet.ch/
France: Federation of Art Therapy: http://ffat.free.fr/
German Association of Art Therapy: http://www.dgkt.de/frameset.htm
Italy: Art Therapy Italiana: http://www.rcvr.org/assoc/artherapy/
Latvian Art Therapy Association: http://www.arttherapy.lv/
Switzerland: International Association for Art, Creativity and Therapy:
http://www.igkgt-iaact.com/
A longer list of professional associations can be found at:
http://www.arttherapy.co.za/associations.htm
Information about approved training courses in each country can be found through contacting directly the respective professional association.

Professional AT journals

Inscape, The British Association of Art Therapy Journal:
http://www.baat.org/inscape.html
Art Therapy: Journal of the American Art Therapy Association:
http://www.arttherapy.org/aboutaata/journal.htm
The Canadian Art Therapy Association Journal:
http://www.catainfo.ca/journal.php

Other relevant journals
Raw Vision: http://www.rawvision.com/
Journal of Art Education: http://www.naea-reston.org/publications-artedu.html

Other relevant addresses
International Networking Group of Art Therapists:
http://www.emporia.edu/ingat/information.htm
Art Therapists Practice Research Network:
http://www.baat.org/atprn.html
Northern Ireland Group for Art as Therapy:
http://www.geocities.com/nigat_uk
Adamson Collection:
http://www.slamart.org.uk/p2_artsprojects/adamson_collection.htm
Artworks in Mental Health: http://www.artworksinmentalhealth.co.uk
The Cunningham-Dax Collection: http://www.mhri.edu.au/dax/
The Champernowne Trust: http://champerowne@aol.com
See also addresses listed for other arts therapies.

Dance movement therapy (DMT)

Professional associations

In the UK

Association for Dance Movement Therapy UK (ADMT UK)
Contact address: ADMT UK, c/o Quaker Meeting House, Wedmore Vale,
  Bristol, UK BS3 5HX
e-mail: queries@admt.org.uk
website: http://www.admt.org.uk

International
The following are some examples of professional associations that can be
found on the internet (many more DMT associations are available around
the world):

American Dance Therapy Association (ADTA): http://www.adta.org
Argentine Association of Dance Therapy:
http://www.brecha.com.ar/asoc_arg.htm
Australia: Dance Therapy Association of Australia: http://www.dtaa.org
Finnish Dance Therapy Association: http://www.tanssiterapia.net/
Germany: Dance Therapy Professional Association:
http://www.dancetherapy.de/
Italy: Art Therapy Italiana: http://www.rcvr.org/assoc/artherapy/
Japan Dance Therapy Association:
http://www.jadta.net/dance/index.html
Netherlands: Hogeschool voor muziek en dans: http://www.hmd.nl/
Spanish Association of Dance Movement Therapy (ADMTE):
http://www.danzamovimientoterapia.com
Swedish Dance Therapy Association: http://www.dansterapi.info/

Information about approved training courses in different countries can be found through contacting directly the respective professional association.

Professional DMT journals and newsletters

Body, Movement, Dance in Psychotherapy:
http://www.tandf.co.uk/journals/titles/17432979.asp
American Journal of Dance Therapy:
http://www.wkap.nl/journalhome.htm/0146-3721
Moving On: Quarterly Journal of the Dance Movement Therapy
Association of Australia, http://www.dtaa.org
A Moving Journal: Ongoing Expressions of Authentic Movement:
http://www.movingjournal.org/
e-motion: ADMT UK newsletter: http://www.admt.org.uk

Other relevant journals

Body and Society: http://tcs.ntu.ac.uk/body/
Dance Theatre Journal: http://www.laban.org/dance_theatre_journal.phtml
Journal of Bodywork and Movement Therapies:
http://intl.elsevierhealth.com/journals/jbmt
Research in Dance Education:
http://www.tandf.co.uk/journals/titles/14647893.asp

Other relevant addresses

International Institute for Dance Therapy: http://www.dancetherapy.com/
Voice of Dance: http://www.voiceofdance.com
DanceUK: http://www.danceuk.org/links/links.asp
Jabadao: community dance: http://www.jabadao.org/code.html
Foundation for Community Dance: http://www.communitydance.org.uk
Marian Chace Foundation: http://www.adta.org/chace.html
Authentic Movement Institute: http://www.authenticmovement-usa.com/
Laban Collection:
http://www.laban.org/laban/library_and_archive/archive.phtml
See also addresses listed for other arts therapies.

Dramatherapy (DT)

Professional associations

In the UK

The British Association of Dramatherapists (BADth)
Contact address: 41 Broomhouse Lane, London SW6 3DP
Tel/Fax: 00 44 (0)20 7731 0160
e-mail: info@badth.org.uk
website: http://www.badth.org.uk

International

National Association for Drama Therapy: http://www.nadt.org
Greece: Dramatherapy in Greece and Cyprus: http://www.dramatherapy.gr

Korea: Dramatherapy in Korea: http://www.dramatherapy.co.kr/

Information about approved training courses in each country can be found through contacting directly the respective professional association. Also at: http://freespace.virgin.net/david.pratt3/pages/Dramatherapy/Dramatherapy_training_courses.htm

Professional DT journal and newsletter

Dramatherapy: the journal of the Association for Dramatherapists: http://www.badth.org.uk
Dramascope: The National Association for Drama Therapy Newsletter: http://www.nadt.org

Other relevant journals

New Theatre Quarterly: http://titles.cambridge.org/journals/journal_catalogue.asp?historylinks=ALPHA&mnemonic=NTQ
The Drama Review (TDR): http://www.jstor.org/journals/00125962.html
Research in Drama Education: http://www.tandf.co.uk/journals/titles/13569783.asp

Other relevant addresses

The Dramatherapy Network: http://www.dramatherapy.net
The International Playback Theatre Network: http://www.playbacknet.org/iptn/index.htm
The International Theatre of the Oppressed Organisation (Augusto Boal), based in the Netherlands: http://www.theatreoftheoppressed.org
The puppetry home page: http://sagecraft.com/puppetry
The Healing Story Alliance: http://www.healingstory.org/
The roundabout – drama and movement therapy: http://www.roundabout.nildram.co.uk/links.htm
The WWW Virtual Library: Theatre and Drama: http://vl-theatre.com
Applied and Interactive Theatre Guide: http://www.tonisant.com/aitg/
British Psychodrama Association: http://www.psychodrama.org.uk/
The United Kingdom Society for Play and Creative Arts Therapies: http://www.playtherapy.org.uk

See also addresses listed for other arts therapies.

Music Therapy (MT)

Professional associations and societies

In the UK

Association of Professional Music Therapists (APMT)
Contact address: APMT, 61 Church Hill Road, East Barnet, Herts EN4 8SY, UK
Tel/Fax: 00 44 (0)20 8440 4153
e-mail: APMToffice@aol.com
website: www.apmt.org

British Society for Music Therapy (BSMT)
Contact address: BSMT, 61 Church Hill Road, East Barnet, Hertfordshire,
EN4 8SY, UK
Tel/Fax: 00 44 (0)20 8441 6226
e-mail: info@bsmt.org
website: http://www.bsmt.org

International
The following are some examples of professional associations that can be found
on the internet (many more MT associations are available around the world):
American Music Therapy Association: http://www.musictherapy.org
Argentina: Association for Training and Research in Music Therapy:
http://www.geocities.com/Paris/Metro/8395/
Argentinean Association of Music Therapy:
http://www.musicoterapia.org.ar
Australian Music Therapy Association Inc: http://www.austmta.org.au
Austrian Association of Music Therapists:
http://free.pages.at/oebm/frameset.htm
Belgian Association of Music Therapy: http://www.muziektherapie.net/
Brazilian Union of Associations of Music Therapy: http://www.go.to/ubam
Canadian Association for Music Therapy (CAMT):
http://www.musictherapy.ca
Danish Association of Music Therapists: http://www.musikterapi.org
Danish Society for Music Therapy:
http://www.dansk-forbund-for-musikterapi.dk
Finland: Association of Professional Music Therapists:
http://www.musiikkiterapia.net
Finnish Society for Music Therapy:
http://personal.inet.fi/yhdistys/risto.jukkola/
French Association of Music Therapy:
http://psydoc-fr.broca.inserm.fr/formatio/musico/cim.html
German Association on Physiology of Music and Performing Arts Medicine:
http://www.dgfmm.org/
German Society for Music Therapy: http://www.musiktherapie.de
Germany: Professional Association of the Musiktherapeutinnen and
Musiktherapeuten: http://www.musiktherapie-bvm.de
Greece: Hellenic Music Therapy and Creative Expression Society:
http://www.geocities.com/artmusictherapy/index.htm
Italian Confederation of Music Therapy Associations:
http://www.musicaterapia.it
Japanese Music Therapy Association: http://www.jmta.jp/
Korean Music Therapy Association: http://www.musictherapy.or.kr/
Korean Association for Music Therapy:
http://www.kamt.com/mainpg.htm
Netherlands: Music Therapy organisations: http://www.musictherapy.nl and
http://www.stichtingmuziektherapie.nl/
New Zealand Society for Music Therapy: http://www.musictherapy.org.nz
Norwegian Association for Music Therapy: http://www.musikkterapi.no

Spain: Catalonian Association of Music Therapy:
http://www.bcn.es/tjussana/acmt/
Sweden: Association for Professional Music Therapists:
http://www.fmt-metoden.se/
Swiss Professional Association of Music therapy:
http://www.berbu.ch/subdomains/musiktherapie/

A longer list of professional associations can be found at:
http://www.musictherapyworld.de

Information about approved training courses in each country can be found through contacting directly the respective professional association.

Professional MT journals and newsletters

The British Journal of Music Therapy: http://www.bsmt.org/journal.htm
The Nordic Journal of Music Therapy: http://www.hisf.no/njmt/index.ssi
The Australian Journal of Music Therapy:
http://www.austmta.org.au/publications
Spanish Journal of Music Therapy: http://www.xarxabcn.net/acmt/rc.htm
Music Therapy Matters (AMTA newsletter):
http://www.musictherapy.org/products/pubs.html
Voices – A World Forum for Music Therapy (electronic journal):
http://www.voices.no
International Latin-American Journal of Music Therapy:
http://www.geocities.com/Paris/Metro/8395/ ilajmt-g.html
Music Therapy Today (e-magazine): http://www.musictherapyworld.de
British Society for Music Therapy Bulletin:
http://library.berklee.edu:8080/ipac20/periodicals/Brit_Soc_for_Music_The
r_Bul.php

Other relevant journals

Music Education Research:
http://www.tandf.co.uk/journals/titles/14613808.asp
European Music Journal: http://www.music-journal.com
Music Perception: An Interdisciplinary Journal:
http://www.ucpress.edu/journals/mp
MuSICA Research Notes: http://www.musica.uci.edu/mrn/issues.html
Psychology of Music: http://pom.sagepub.com/
Electronic Music Journals and Newspapers:
http://www.music.indiana.edu/collections/e-journals.html

Other relevant addresses

World Federation of Music Therapy: http://www.musictherapyworld.de
European Music Therapy Confederation:
http://www.musictherapyworld.de
The Bonny Foundation: http://www.bonnyfoundation.org
http://www.euphonica.com/
Archive on Analytical Music Therapy (Mary Priestley):
http://www.temple.edu/musictherapy/dbs/amt_priestley.htm

International Trust for Nordoff–Robbins:
http://www.nordoff-robbins.org.uk/html/body_worldwide.html
See also addresses listed for other arts therapies.

Arts therapies

Professional associations

Australian Creative Arts Therapies Association (ACATA):
http://mc2.vicnet.net.au/home/acata/index.html
Dutch Association for Creative Therapy:
http://www.creativetherapiedans.nl
Irish Association of Creative Arts Therapists:
http://www.iacat.ie/about.html
New Zealand: Creative Therapies Association of Aotearoa:
http://www.creativetherapies.org.nz/index.html
Peru: EQUIPO de Terapias de Arte:
http://terapiasdearte.perucultural.org.pe/
The Israeli Association of Creative and Expressive Therapies (YAHAT):
http://www.yahat.org
USA: National Coalition of Creative Arts Therapies Associations:
http://www.nccata.org
USA: The National Expressive Therapy Association:
http://www.expressivetherapy.com/index_other.html

Other associations, groups and networks

European Consortium for Arts Therapies Education (ECArTE):
http://www.uni-muenster.de/Ecarte/
Professional Association for Arts, Music and Dance Therapy (Berufsverband
f?r Kunst-, Musik-und Tanztherapie), based in Germany:
http://www.muenster.de/~bkmt/
European Association for Arts Therapies (Associazone Europea per le Arti
Terapie), based in Italy: http://www.artiterapie.org/index.htm
International Expressive Arts Therapy Association: http://www.ieata.org/
KenVac: the Netherlands research centre: http://kenvak.hszuyd.nl/index.jsp
Scottish Arts Therapies Forum: http://www.satf.org.uk
Arts in Therapy International Alliance: http://arts-in-therapy.blogspot.com
Arts in therapy network: http://artsintherapy.com/default.asp
International Society for the Psychopathology of Expression and Art
Therapy: http://www.online-art-therapy.com
The International Arts-Medicine Association:
http://members.aol.com/iamaorg
The National Association for Poetry Therapy: http://www.poetrytherapy.org
Phototherapy: http://www.phototherapy-centre.com
National Network for the Arts in Health: http://www.nnah.org.uk/
Arts in Health and Wellbeing: http://www.dryw.freeserve.co.uk/
United Kingdom Council for Psychotherapists (UKCP):
http://www.psychotherapy.org.uk
British Association of Counselling and Psychotherapy (BACP):
http://www.bacp.co.uk/research/conference2005/index.html

Professional and academic journals

Arts in Psychotherapy Journal: http://www.elsevier.nl/locate/issn/01974556
The virtual arts therapies network:
http://www.derby.ac.uk/research/vart/journal/index.html
Music, Dance and Art Therapy: Magazine for artistic therapies in education, social and health service (in German: Musik-,Tanz-und Kunsttherapie): http://www.hogrefe.de/mtk/
Italian Journal of Arts Therapies, produced by the European Association for Arts Therapies (in Italian: Arti Terapie):
http://www.artiterapie.org/ita/pubblicazioni/ info_pub.htm
Pratt Institute Creative Arts Therapy Review:
http://www.pratt.edu/ad/ather/general/right.html
International Journal of Arts Medicine:
http://www.mmbmusic.com/MMB/ijam_home.html

Counselling and psychotherapy journals

The following web pages provide long lists of relevant journals:
http://www.psychwatch.com/therapy_journals.htm
http://www.psychwatch.com/counsel_journals.htm

Governmental addresses

Health Professions Council (HPC): http://www.hpc-uk.org/
List of HPC registered members: http://www.hpc-uk.org/register/
NHS Careers Information: http://www.nhscareers.nhs.uk/nhs-knowledge_base/data/4914.html
Subject Benchmark statement: health care programmes: Arts Therapies:
http://www.qaa.ac.uk/crntwork/benchmark/nhsbenchmark/artsTherapy.htm
Standards of proficiency: http://www.hpc-uk.org/publications/standards/
Standards_of_Proficiency_Arts_Therapists.pdf
National Institute of Clinical Effectiveness (NICE): http://www.nice.org.uk

Other relevant addresses

Practical Resources for therapy and education: speechmark:
http://www.speechmark.net/
International Arts resources from Artslynx: http://www.artslynx.org/

Subject Index

All entries refer to arts therapies in general unless otherwise stated.
Page numbers followed by 'b,' 'f' and 't' indicate boxes, figures and tables respectively.

Index

Index